ATLAS OF
NEURO-OPHTHALMOLOGY

Thomas C Spoor MD FACS

Professor Emeritus Ophthalmology and Neurosurgery
Wayne State University School of Medicine
Oculoplastic, Orbital and Neuro-ophthalmic Surgery
St John Macomb Hospital
Warren
USA

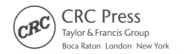

CRC Press
Taylor & Francis Group
Boca Raton London New York

CRC Press is an imprint of the
Taylor & Francis Group, an **informa** business

CRC Press
Taylor & Francis Group
6000 Broken Sound Parkway NW, Suite 300
Boca Raton, FL 33487-2742

First issued in paperback 2019

© 2004 by Taylor & Francis Group, LLC
CRC Press is an imprint of Taylor & Francis Group, an Informa business

No claim to original U.S. Government works

ISBN-13: 978-1-85317-773-6 (hbk)
ISBN-13: 978-0-367-39434-9 (pbk)

A CIP record for this book is available from the British Library.

Library of Congress Cataloging-in-Publication Data

Data available on application

Composition by J&L Compsition, Filey, North Yorkshire

Visit the Taylor & Francis Web site at
http://www.taylorandfrancis.com

and the CRC Press Web site at
http://www.crcpress.com

Contents

Dedication

To my female dominant society: wife Deanne, daughter Kristen and mother Edna, thank you for your love, help and support.

Thanks also to Mary Tluczek, my secretary for more years and more books than either of us care to remember and Trina Fennel medical illustrator par excellence whose illustrations have enhanced five books and countless lectures, courses and presentations.

Preface

There have been several generations of great neuro-ophthalmology texts ranging from major treatises like the multiple Walsh and Hoyt's (later Miller/Newman's/Walsh and Hoyt's). Lesser texts, no offense, that are not as detailed or compulsive have been equally excellent but not as encyclopedic. Some texts have been unreadable and totally impractical, while others have been excellent office references. Beauty is in the eye of the beholder.

Neuro-ophthalmology is like extraocular motility, you get it or you do not. If you do not get it and do not understand the big picture, you should not be practicing this subspecialty. If you are trying to be a good generalist and practice some neuro-op that's great, but get the picture. In the world of great neuro-imaging it is hard to miss a brain tumor, but it is easy to be a bit obtuse beating around the bush looking for an appropriate diagnosis. I will show you examples of visual loss caused by pituitary tumors and attributed to macular degeneration, and visual loss secondary to huge tumors attributed to psychosis, diagnosed by well-respected university professors. Stop learning and the best imaging in the world is no substitute for clinical acumen and judgement. The best teacher in neuro-ophthalmology is time, which unfortunately does not help the undiagnosed and untreated patient.

This book is the result and completion of my career in neuro-ophthalmology. It has been a lot of fun, I have helped many people and have hurt a few, but it has been a great ride. Over the years I have taken thousands of clinical photographs for use in teaching residents and fellows. Here I hope to pass these photos to posterity so that others may benefit from my triumphs and mistakes. It has been tremendous, I have no regrets and I hope the next generation enjoys practicing neuro-ophthalmology as much as I have.

Thanks to my mentor and former preceptor, Dr Jack Kennerdell. I am still using some of his slides salvaged from my fellowship year at the University of Pittsburgh, some of which appear in this book, sometimes annotated and sometimes not, but remembered and appreciated just the same. Thanks also to my entourage of fellows and international fellows from 1984 to 2003. Their hard work, and excellent, compulsive patient care was responsible for much of my success and for a few of my failures. It was however great fun, and made the practice of both academic and clinical neuro-ophthalmology much more rewarding.

There are many compulsively referenced neuro-ophthalmology texts but I have referenced few in this atlas. However, I have made a point to reference topics that might be controversial, to direct the reader to primary sources so that they can make their own decisions. In today's world of computerized information retrieval it is very easy to research a subject, so I feel no need or obligation to reference every statement I make. If you disagree, research the issue and draw your own conclusions. All I wish to do is expose you to a great subspecialty and lure you into a deeper thought process.

Thomas C Spoor

Abbreviations

AAION	arteritic anterior ischemic optic neuropathy	IOP	intraocular pressure
ACE	angiotensin-converting enzyme	IR	inferior rectus (muscle)
AIBSE	acute idiopathic blind-spot enlargement	LHON	Leber's hereditary optic neuropathy
AIDS	acquired immune deficiency syndrome	LTG	low-tension glaucoma
AION	arteritic ischemic optic neuropathy	MAR	melanoma-associated retinopathy
AMPE	acquired monocular elevator palsy	MEWDS	multiple evanescent white-dot syndrome
APMPPE	acute posterior multifocal placoid pigment epitheliopathy	MG	myasthenia gravis
		MLF	median longitudinal fasciculus
AR	Argyll Robertson (pupils)	MR	medial rectus (muscle)
AZOOR	acute zonal occult outer retinopathy	MRI	magnetic resonance imaging
CACD	cancer-associated cone dysfunction	MS	multiple sclerosis
CAR	cancer-associated retinopathy	NAION	non-arteritic anterior ischemic optic neuropathy
CME	cystoid macular edema		
CMV	cytomegalic inclusion virus	NLP	no light perception
CPEO	chronic progressive external ophthalmoplegia	OD	right eye
		ONSD	optic nerve sheath decompression
CRAO	central retinal artery occlusions	ONTT	Optic Neuritis Treatment Trial
CRVO	central retinal vein occlusions	OS	left eye
CSF	cerebrospinal fluid	OU	both eyes
CT	computerized tomography	PCA	posterior communicating artery
DON	dysthyroid optic neuropathy	PION	posterior ischemic optic neuropathy
ERG	electroretinogram	PPRF	parapontine reticular formation
ERM	epiretinal membranes	PR	paraeoplastic retinopathies
ESR	erythrocyte sedimentation rate	PTC	pseudotumor cerebri
FTA-ABS	fluorescent treponemal antibody absorption	RAPD	relative afferent pupillary defect
		riMLF	rostral interstitial nucleus of the medial longitudinal fasciculus (muscle)
GCA	giant cell arteritis		
HIV	human immunodeficiency virus	RPE	retinal pigment epithelium
HMO	health maintenance organization	SLE	systemic lupus erythmatosus
ICA	internal carotid artery	SR	superior rectus (muscle)
ICP	intracranial pressure	STA	superficial temporal artery
INH	isoniazid	TAO	thyroid-associated orbitopathy
INO	internuclear ophthalmoplegia	VDRL	venereal disease research lab
IO	inferior oblique (muscle)	WBC	white blood count
IOI	idiopathic orbital inflammation	WEBINO	wall-eyed bilateral internuclear ophthalmoplegia
IONDT	Ischemic Optic Neuropathy Decompression Trial		

Chapter 1   Pupils

INTRODUCTION

The appearance of a patient with a dilated pupil in the ophthalmologist's or neurologist's office raises the possibility of an acute neurologic emergency (Fig. 1.1); however, this is very rarely the case. An isolated pupillary abnormality is more often than not a benign event, with much more ophthalmologic than neurologic significance. On the other hand, pupillary involvement accompanied by other neurologic findings (Figs 1.2 and 1.3), obvious or subtle, may portend a very serious neurologic problem. A practical, intelligent approach to evaluating pupillary abnormalities will save the patient unnecessary procedures and anxiety. Examination of the pupil also helps to differentiate the various causes of visual dysfunction. A relative afferent pupillary defect (RAPD) is the sine qua non of optic nerve dysfunction and its presence or absence helps differentiate visual loss due to optic neuropathies from maculopathies and occipital lobe pathology.

Examination of the pupil with magnification, preferably with a slit lamp, may avoid unnecessary testing, anxiety and expense. Obvious synechiae (Fig. 1.4a), vermilliform motions, sphincter rupture or dysfunction

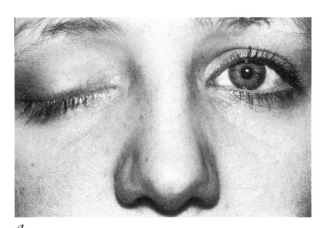

a

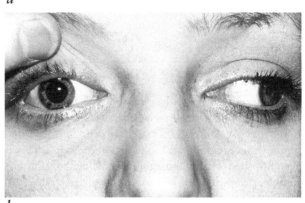

b

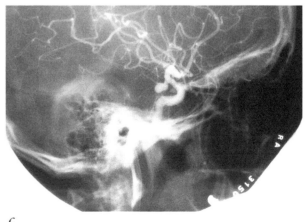

c

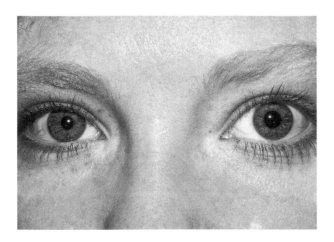

Figure 1.1 *An isolated, dilated pupil is rarely a neurologic emergency (a).*

Figure 1.2 *A patient with an obvious pupil involving third-nerve palsy (a and b) due to a posterior-communicating internal carotid artery aneurysm evidenced on cerebral angiogram (c).*

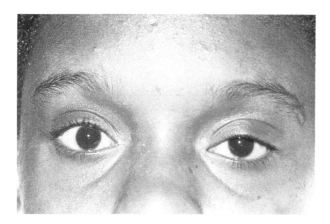

Figure 1.3 *Intracranial aneurysms may also present as a much more subtle third-nerve palsy. Note the pupil is involved to the same degree as the extraocular motility.*

from trauma or intraocular surgery are obvious ophthalmologic causes of abnormal pupils and require no further neurologic evaluation.

FUNCTION

The pupil functions like the f-number of a camera. It regulates the amount of light reaching the retina (analogous to the film in a camera), increases the depth of focus, and diminishes chromatic and spherical aberrations. This is accomplished by the antagonistic actions of the iris sphincter and dilator. The iris sphincter is attached to the iris border in a circumferential pattern and is innervated by the parasympathetic nervous system. The iris dilator muscles are weaker, radially arranged and innervated by the sympathetic nervous system. The pupil is constantly moving, responding to changes in ambient lighting and innervation. This constant movement (hippus) is normal and needs to be differentiated from the early release of a RAPD.

ANATOMY

PUPILLARY REACTION TO LIGHT[1]

Afferent pupillary function depends on the integrity of the retinal receptors, the retinal ganglion cells and their axons in the optic nerve, chiasm and tract (Fig. 1.5). Like the visual fibers, approximately one half of the fibers

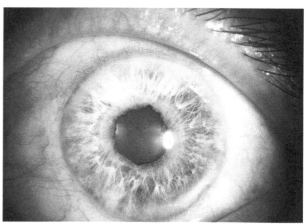

a

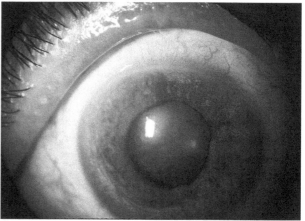

b

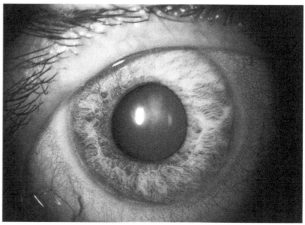

c

Figure 1.4 *Slit-lamp examination may reveal an obvious ophthalmologic cause of the abnormal pupil–iris sphincter atrophy (a), iritis with posterior synechiae (b) or rubeosis iridis (c).*

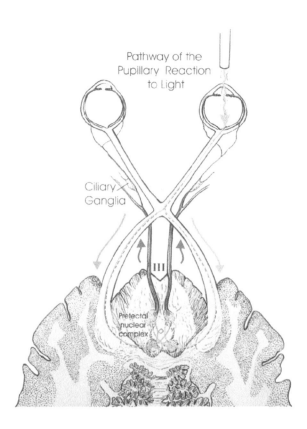

Figure 1.5 *Pupillary reaction to light: pupillary fibers synapse in the pretectal nuclei, then pass crossed and uncrossed to the intercalated neurons, which in turn synapse with the Edinger-Westphal nuclei.*

cross in the optic chiasm. Unlike the visual fibers, the pupillary fibers do not synapse at the lateral geniculate body but leave the optic tracts before it and pass through the brachium of the superior colliculus to the pretectal nuclei in the rostral midbrain. Intercalated neurons connect to the Edinger-Westphal nucleus dorsally, above the aqueduct of Sylvius, through the posterior commissure and ventrally through the peri-aqueductal gray matter (Fig. 1.5).

The Edinger-Westphal nucleus originates parasympathetic, visceral efferent fibers to the iris sphincter (pupillary constriction) and ciliary muscles (accommodation). These fibers join the fibers from other oculomotor subnuclei, forming the fascicle of the third nerve, exit the midbrain, and pass to and through the cavernous sinus. The pupillary fibers lie superficially in the intrapeduncular oculomotor nerve, hence are susceptible to compression along the interpeduncular course of the oculomotor nerve (Fig. 1.6). As the oculomotor nerve divides into a superior and inferior branch as it enters the orbit, the inferior branch carries the parasympathetic

fibers to the ciliary ganglion via the branch to the inferior oblique muscle. The preganglionic parasympathetic fibers synapse in the ciliary ganglion. Postganglionic parasympathetic fibers then pass to the iris sphincter and ciliary muscles via the short ciliary nerves (Fig. 1.6).

The Edinger-Westphal nucleus, the oculomotor nerve, ciliary ganglion and short ciliary nerves are also the final common pathway for the near synkinesis. When viewing a close object the eyes must converge, the lenses accommodate and the pupils constrict. Many more ciliary ganglion cells innervate accommodation than innervate pupillary constriction (30:1). Damage to the near synkinesis occurs commonly after head trauma and results in accommodative convergence insufficiency (Fig. 1.7) (see Chapter 7).

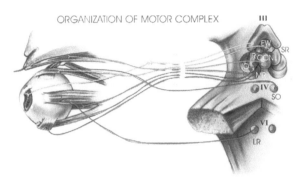

Figure 1.6 *Pupillary fibers from the Edinger-Westphal nucleus travel from the midbrain to the orbit as part of the interpeduncular third nerve.*

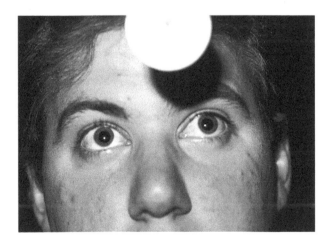

Figure 1.7 *Severe convergence insufficiency with loss of convergence, accommodation and pupillary miosis at near.*

NORMAL LIGHT AND NEAR REACTION (FIG. 1.5)

When light is directed into one eye then both pupils constrict equally. The midbrain cannot determine where the light is coming from and equal parasympathetic innervation is directed at both pupils. Likewise, as the eyes converge, both pupils constrict equally. The degree of constriction to light should equal the degree of constriction to near. Pupils never constrict more to light than they do to near. If pupils constrict more during the near response than in response to light, light-near dissociation is present.

LIGHT-NEAR DISSOCIATION

Light-near dissociation of the pupils may occur in patients with normal vision or decreased visual function. This dissociation of the pupillary reactions—greater constriction to the near response than to the light response—occurs most commonly with bilateral optic neuropathies or compression of the optic chiasm. Both optic nerves are dysfunctional and visual function is compromised (Fig. 1.8).

Light-near dissociation may also occur in patients with normal vision due to midbrain dysfunction. The classic etiology is tabes dorsalis due to tertiary syphilis,

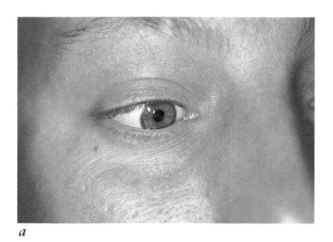
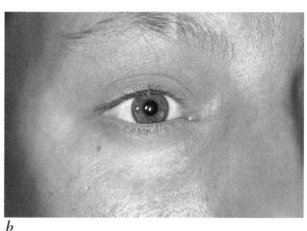

Figure 1.8 *Light-near dissociation of the pupils due to a bilateral optic neuropathy. The pupils constrict more to near stimulus (a) than they do to light stimuli (b).*

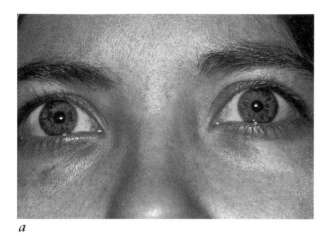
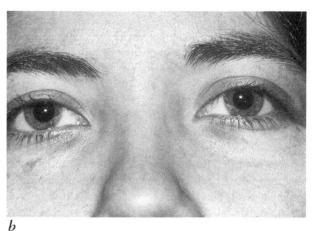

Figure 1.9 *RAPD: when light is directed into the normal eye, both pupils constrict (a). As the light is directed into the eye with the optic neuropathy, the normal pupil paradoxically dilates (b).*

but similar lesions may also occur in diabetics due to a presumed defect in the midbrain light-reflex pathway. The classic findings are miotic pupils with little to no reaction to light and definite constriction at near.

RAPD

RAPD is the sine qua non of an optic neuropathy. Optic nerve dysfunction in one eye results in a decreased amount of light transmitted to the midbrain when light is directed into the involved eye. This results in a paradoxical dilatation of the involved pupil. Light is directed into the normal eye but both pupils constrict equally (Fig. 1.9a). The light is then directed into the eye with optic nerve dysfunction and the pupil in the involved eye paradoxically dilates (Fig. 1.9b). Less light is transmitted to the midbrain, so pupillary dilatation occurs. A subtle RAPD may be detected by utilizing the swinging flashlight test while observing the pupil in question with slit-lamp magnification and an external light source (transillumination).[2] Neutral density filters may also be useful in quantitating or detecting subtle RAPD.[1]

If the involved eye also has efferent pupillary dysfunction and the involved pupil is dilated, an inverse RAPD may be detected. Light is shone into the dilated pupil with presumed optic nerve dysfunction (Fig. 1.10a): if optic nerve function is compromised, less light is detected by the midbrain and the normal pupil paradoxically dilates (Fig. 1.10a). When light is directed into the normal eye, its pupil briskly constricts; the pupil in the involved eye remains dilated (Fig. 1.10b). The presence of anisocoria may obscure the recognition of an RAPD.[3]

Remember that you are eliciting an RAPD comparing a normal optic nerve with a dysfunctional optic nerve. If neither optic nerve is compromised then an afferent pupillary defect will not be evident. If both optic nerves are compromised, an RAPD may not be evident, but light-near dissociation of the pupils will be (Fig. 1.8).

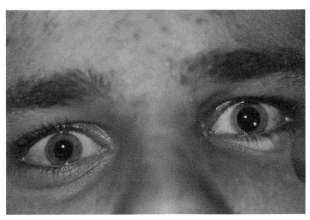

a

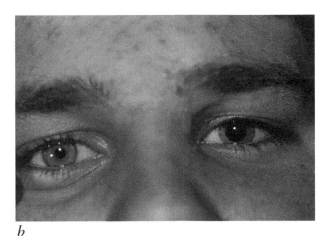

b

Figure 1.10 *Inverse RAPD. Light is directed into the eye with the dilated pupil and optic neuropathy. The normal contralateral pupil paradoxically dilates (a). As light is directed into the normal pupil it briskly constricts while the abnormal pupil remains dilated (b).*

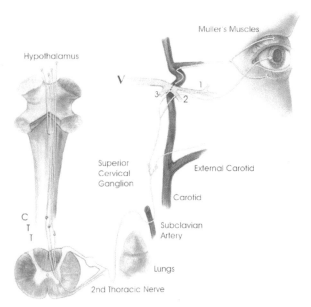

Figure 1.11 *Sympathetic pathway for pupillary dilatation (see text).*

SYMPATHETIC PATHWAY (FIG. 1.11)

Sympathetic pupillary innervation arises in the hypothalamus. These first-order hypothalamic neurons descend through the brainstem and the cervical spinal cord to synapse in the intermedio-lateral gray column. Axons exit the spinal cord (C-8 through T-2) via the ipsilateral ventral rami as preganglionic sympathetic fibers. These enter the brain via the sympathetic chain, passing through the superior mediastinum and stellate ganglion to synapse in the superior cervical ganglion. Postganglionic sympathetic axons arise in the superior cervical ganglion and ascend in the carotid plexus along the internal carotid artery to the cavernous sinus. In the cavernous sinus the sympathetic axons join the third, sixth and fifth nerves to innervate structures in the eye and orbit. Fibers destined for pupillary dilatation accompany the sixth nerve, then join branches of the ophthalmic (V1)

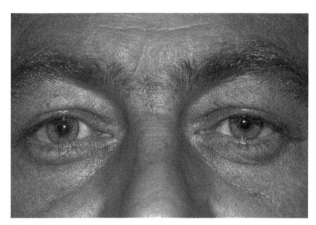

a

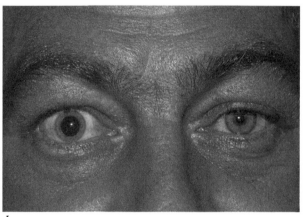

b

Figure 1.12 *Patient with mild ptosis and miosis due to sympathetic denervation (left Horner's syndrome) (a). After instillation of 4% cocaine to both eyes, the normal pupil dilates; the Horner's pupil remains miotic (b).*

and long ciliary nerve to reach the iris dilator muscles. Sympathetic fibers to the upper and lower eyelids (Muller's muscles) join branches of the third nerve to reach the eyelids. Some sympathetic axons, those controlling sweating of the lower face, accompany the external carotid and then the facial arteries.

Dysfunction of the sympathetic pathways causes a Horner's syndrome consisting predominately of mild ptosis (Muller's muscle) and miosis (iris dilator), accompanied by facial anhidrosis and lower eyelid ptosis (elevation). The latter two are rarely of clinical importance and are usually overlooked. Mild ptosis of the upper eyelid and a miotic pupil are the hallmarks of Horner's syndrome (Fig. 1.12a).

Various pharmacologic tests have been described to differentiate a Horner's pupil from physiologic miosis (cocaine test), and attempts have been made to differentiate pre- and postganglionic Horner's pupils based on reactions to hydroxyamfetamine drops.

Physiologic anisocoria and upper eyelid ptosis are common, especially in older individuals. The cocaine test is useful for differentiating physiologic miosis from miosis due to sympathetic denervation. Cocaine blocks the uptake of norepinephrine (noradrenaline) at the iris dilator, but dilates a normal pupil. Dysfunction anywhere along the sympathetic chain decreases the norepinephrine (noradrenaline) release by the third-order neuron and cocaine will not dilate the pupil. The cocaine drop test confirms the presence of miosis due to sympathetic denervation (Fig. 1.12b) but does not help localize where the dysfunction is occurring.

The hydroxyamfetamine test was an attempt to differentiate a preganglionic Horner's pupil, which is indicative of chest or neck pathology, from a postganglionic Horner's pupil with a more benign prognosis. If the third-order neuron is dysfunctional, the pupil will not dilate for there is no presynaptic norepinephrine (noradrenaline) to release. If the pupil dilates after instillation of hydroxyamfetamine drops, the third-order neuron is intact; therefore, Horner's syndrome results from dysfunction of the first- or second-order (preganglionic) neuron. The sequential drop test was standard for evaluating a patient with Horner's syndrome until Maloney et al[4] demonstrated that the diagnostic specificity for postganglionic Horner's pupils was only 84%. Sixteen percent of patients whose pupils failed to dilate had a preganglionic lesion. This datum and the fact that hydroxyamfetamine drops are no longer commercially available have rendered this test all but obsolete, except for the most diehard neuro-ophthalmologists.

Usually, the clinical diagnosis of Horner's syndrome is obvious—the ptosis is minimal and the pupillary miosis is obvious, and the degree of anisocoria increases as the

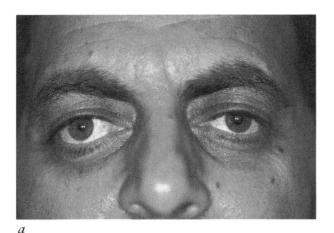

a

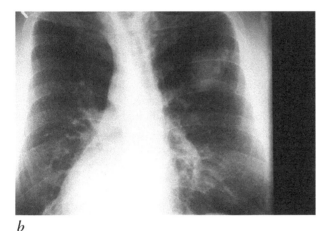

b

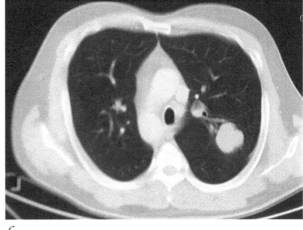

c

Figure 1.13 *A patient with a history of heavy cigarette smoking presented with mild ptosis and miosis (a). A chest x-ray (b) and a CT scan (c) demonstrated carcinoma of the lung.*

illumination decreases. The anisocoria increases in darkness as the sympathetic nerves are stimulated to dilate the pupil. The cause and severity of a Horner's syndrome can usually be determined by history and associated neurologic signs.

A patient with a history of smoking and a Horner's syndrome needs a chest x-ray and a chest computerized tomography (CT) scan (Fig. 1.13). An apical lung tumor may cause sympathetic dysfunction. A patient with a painful Horner's syndrome needs a magnetic resonance (MR) angiography of the neck to rule out a dissecting carotid artery aneurysm or carotid thrombosis (Fig. 1.14).[5,6] Patients with spontaneous or traumatic dissection of the cervical cerebral arteries may present with headache and neck pain (65%), ischemic cerebral symptoms (84%) and local neurologic signs including Horner's syndrome (31%).[5]

A 30-year-old receptionist in a neurologist's office was referred for a second opinion relative to a painful Horner's syndrome (Fig. 1.14a). An MR angiogram of the neck demonstrated a dissection of the internal carotid artery (Fig. 1.14b).[6] Patients with a Horner's syn-

drome accompanied by dysfunction of the third, fourth, fifth or sixth cranial nerves need an MR angiogram with contrast directed at the cavernous sinus (Fig. 1.14).

ANISOCORIA[7]

When a patient is referred for evaluation of unequally sized pupils (anisocoria), first determine whether the larger or the smaller pupil is abnormal. If the dilated pupil is abnormal the anisocoria will increase in brighter light, since the brighter light stimulates the parasympathetic system to constrict the pupil, the normal pupil will constrict further and the degree of anisocoria will increase. If the small pupil is abnormal, dimming the lights will stimulate the sympathetic dilatation of the pupil and the pupil in the normal eye will dilate more, increasing the degree of anisocoria.

After determining that the larger pupil is abnormal and reacts sluggishly to light, determine whether there is

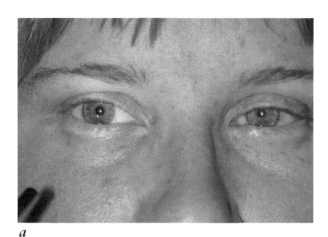
a

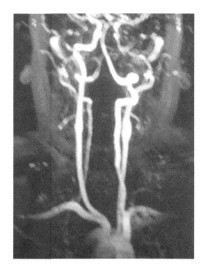
b

Figure 1.14 *A patient presented with a painful Horner's syndrome—a carotid artery dissection until proven otherwise (a). An MR angiogram demonstrates dissection of the internal carotid artery (b).*

any evidence for oculomotor nerve dysfunction. Is there any ptosis evident? Is extraocular motility normal? It is extremely uncommon for a third-nerve palsy to present as an isolated, dilated pupil without other evidence for third-nerve dysfunction (ptosis, diplopia). Although the classic patient with third-nerve compression has total ptosis and an abducted eye that cannot elevate, depress or adduct (Fig. 1.2), the associated third-nerve findings may be much more subtle (Fig. 1.3).

Examine the pupil at the slit lamp or with another source of magnification. Is the iris sphincter adherent to the anterior lens capsule by posterior synechiae or iris sphincter atrophy (Fig. 1.4)? Has there been previous intraocular surgery disrupting the appearance of the pupils? Is the pupillary sphincter intact, does it constrict as a unit or is there evidence for segmental denervation

(vermilliform movements). If so, a tonic pupil is present and the diagnosis can be confirmed by evidence for denervation supersensitivity. The dilated pupil will constrict dramatically after instillation of a dilute (1/10–1/15%) pilocarpine solution. The normal pupil will not constrict (Fig. 1.15).

TONIC PUPILS

Patients with tonic pupils often complain about sensitivity to light, difficulty focusing at near (accommodation fibers) and reading. Tonic pupils are always painless. Anisocoria is often noted by the patient or noticed by

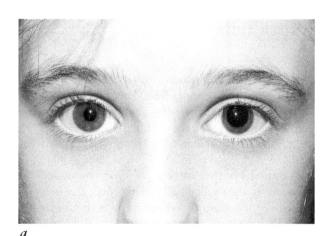
a

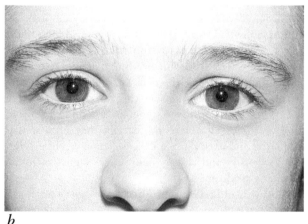
b

Figure 1.15 *A patient presenting with a dilated pupil and loss of accommodation (a). Miosis after instillation of dilute pilocarpine drops confirms the diagnosis of tonic pupil (b). The normal pupil does not constrict.*

another individual (Fig. 1.15). Segmental iris paralysis and vermilliform motion of the iris is diagnostic on slit-lamp examination. Response to dilute pilocarpine is confirmatory.

If the iris sphincter appears normal, there is no associated extraocular motility dysfunction and the pupil does not constrict after instillation of dilute pilocarpine solution, instill 1% pilocarpine into the eye. If the pupil does not constrict then pharmacologic blockade is present (Fig. 1.16). The patient either intentionally or inadvertently has placed mydriatic drops in their eye. If the pupil constricts to 1% pilocarpine it is either normal or dilated due to an acute tonic pupil (no time for denervation supersensitivity to occur) or an oculomotor nerve paresis.

If the anisocoria is greater in the dark and the pupils react normally to light the defect is due to sympathetic denervation or physiologic anisocoria. Check for exacerbation of the anisocoria in dim illumination. Patients with physiologic anisocoria will have an equal degree of anisocoria regardless of whether the illumination is ambient, dim or bright. Patients with sympathetic denervation will have a significant increase in anisocoria in the dark. If there is still a question of sympathetic denervation, a cocaine test is confirmatory (Fig. 1.12).

UPPER MIDBRAIN LESIONS (PARINAUD'S SYNDROME)

Lesions affecting the dorsal midbrain disrupt axons entering into the pretectal region and cause light-near

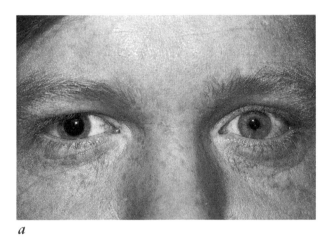

a

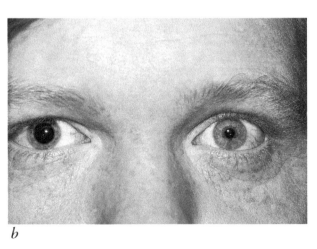

b

Figure 1.16 *A patient referred for iatrogenic anisocoria (a). The pupil fails to constrict after instillation of 1% pilocarpine (b); also note that the normal left pupil is more miotic.*

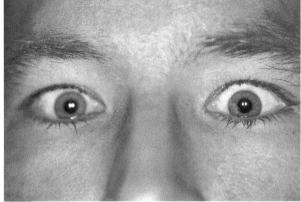

a

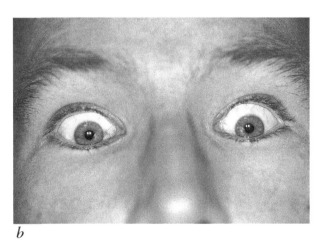

b

Figure 1.17 *Dorsal midbrain syndrome. Upper eyelids are retracted with attempted upgaze, and pupils are mid-dilated and poorly reactive to light (a). The near pupillary reaction is greater than the pupillary reaction to light (b).*

dissociation of the pupils. Pupils are often mid-dilated, have a diminished light response and an intact near response (Fig. 1.17). The whole or part of the near response may be abnormal with defective convergence, accommodation and miosis (Fig. 1.17). The diagnosis is usually obvious by associated features of dorsal midbrain dysfunction: upgaze paresis, convergence retraction nystagmus and upper eyelid retraction (Fig. 1.18). Neuroimaging is mandatory since dorsal midbrain syndrome is most commonly caused by pineal area tumors or hydrocephalus (Fig. 1.18). Hydrocephalus in infants may present as an upgaze palsy due to compression of the midbrain: this is known as sunset sign.

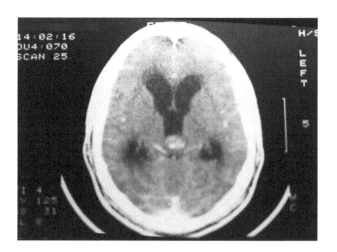

Figure 1.18 *CT scan demonstrating a pinealoma.*

SUMMARY

Evaluation of the patient with abnormal pupils requires common sense. A dilated pupil with no associated motility findings is rarely of neuro-ophthalmologic importance. There is usually a local cause for this pupillary dysfunction and an extensive neuroradiologic evaluation is rarely necessary. An intelligent pupillary examination is much more valuable than a plethora of neuroimaging studies. The etiology of the abnormal pupil may often be easily revealed by an intelligent office examination.

A painless Horner's syndrome in a nonsmoker is almost always benign unless accompanied by pain or oculomotor dysfunction. A painful Horner's syndrome or a Horner's syndrome occurring in a smoker requires appropriate neuroimaging studies.

For an encyclopedic reference containing more information than you will ever need to know about the pupil see Lowenfeld.[8]

REFERENCES

1. Girkin CA. Evaluation of the pupillary light response as an objective measure of visual function. *Ophthalmol Clin North Am* 2003; **16**:143–53.
2. Glazer-Hockstein C, Brucker AJ. The detection of a relative afferent pupillary defect. *Am J Ophthalmol* 2002; **134**:142–3.
3. Lam BL, Thompson HS. An anisocoria produces a small relative afferent pupillary defect in the eye with the smaller pupil. *J Neuro-ophthalmol* 1999; **19**:153–9.
4. Maloney WF, Younge BR, Moyer NJ. Evaluation of the causes and accuracy of pharmacologic localization in Horner's syndrome. *Am J Ophthalmol* 1980; **90**:394–402.
5. Bassi P, Lattuudu P, Gomitoni A. Cervical cerebral artery dissection: a multicenter prospective study. *Neurol Sci* 2003; **24** (Suppl 1): S4–S7.
6. Kline LB. The neuro-ophthalmologic manifestations of spontaneous dissection of the internal carotid artery. *Semin Ophthalmol* 1992; **7**:30–7.
7. Thompson HS, Pilley SF. Unequal pupils: a flow chart for sorting out anisocorias. *Surv Ophthalmol* 1976; **21**:45–8.
8. Lowenfeld IE. The Pupil: Anatomy, Physiology and Clinical Applications. (Wayne State University Press: Detroit, 1993.)

Chapter 2 **Visual loss**

Many neuro-ophthalmologists insist on a lengthy, detailed examination of the patient. The present author prefers a concise, problem-solving oriented approach, attempting to elicit the patient's major concerns and problems. Why are you here today? What questions can I answer for you that will make your wait worthwhile? What bothers you most? Questions like these allow determination of exactly what concerns the patient and why he/she has been referred to your office. A patient's answers might include, 'My vision is not as sharp as it used to be', 'I see double', or 'I have headaches'. These leads allow the patient's major concerns to be focused on instead of wasting time searching elsewhere. There is a place for the extensive neuro-ophthalmologic examination but in the present author's opinion the majority of neuro-ophthalmic consultations can be handled quickly in an efficient, problem-solving manner. The long drawn-out examination may be saved for obscure, difficult cases. If you know what you are doing and what you are looking for, a brief, problem-oriented history and examination is usually effective.

VISUAL LOSS

Progressive visual loss still demands an explanation. The explanation may be quite simple, e.g. corneal endothelial dystrophy or cataract that had been missed by a cursory, undilated slit-lamp examination (Fig. 2.1). Remember the whole eye and think from external to internal.

REFRACTION

Refracting remains the bane of many ophthalmologists' existence but it is still an important part of any ophthalmologic or neuro-ophthalmologic examination. Streak retinoscopy, keratometry and an automated refractor may uncover some really simple ocular causes of decreased vision. Examples include high astigmatism, keratoconus, irregular astigmatism, subtle nuclear sclerotic and posterior subcapsular cataracts. Corneal changes such as irregular astigmatism, punctate epithelial keratopathy, tear film abnormalities, stromal infiltration and endothelial dystrophies, may cause significant,

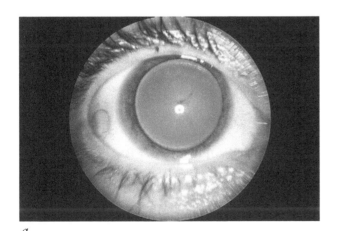
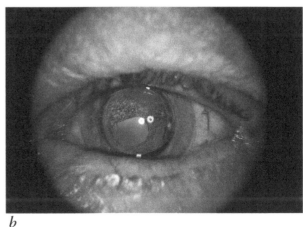

a   *b*

Figure 2.1 *Patients referred for progressive visual loss. Dilated fundus examination with retroillumination revealed this not too subtle cararact (a), another with an eccentric capsulotomy and a partially occluded pupillary axis (b).*

and often undiagnosed, visual loss. A careful slit-lamp examination is usually diagnostic.

PUPILS

A relative afferent pupillary defect (RAPD) is the sine qua non of optic nerve dysfunction. Detecting a RAPD differentiates optic nerve dysfunction from macular dysfunction. Shine a light into the normal eye and both pupils constrict (Fig. 2.2a), redirect the light into the involved eye and the pupil paradoxically dilates (Fig. 2.2b). The presence of a RAPD confirms that the visual dysfunction results from an optic neuropathy. A subtle RAPD may be detected using slit-lamp magnification or neutral density filters. Patients with bilateral optic nerve or chiasmal dysfunction may not demonstrate a RAPD or may have a very subtle RAPD, since both optic nerves are involved to a similar extent. These patients will have light-near dissociation of their pupils. Bilateral optic neuropathies and chiasmal compression are much more common causes of light-near dissociation than midbrain lesions from tertiary syphilis [Argyll Robertson (AR) pupils]. Remember that you can not diagnose AR pupils unless visual function is equal and there is no optic nerve dysfunction. Have a patient fixate on a distant target (Fig. 2.3a), shine a light into one eye and grade the pupillary reaction 1–4 (Fig. 2.3b). Shine the light on the other eye and similarly grade the pupillary reaction. Swing the light from eye to eye and look for a RAPD (Fig. 2.2). If none is evident and the pupils appear to have a sluggish light reflex, ask the patient to fixate at near. Have the patient hold their thumb in front of their nose and look at it (Fig. 2.3c). Remember that a totally blind individual can do this based on proprioception. If the patient states that they cannot do this, suspect malingering. Compare the pupillary response to light with the near reaction. If the near reaction is brisker than the light reaction, this represents light-near dissociation and indicates bilateral optic nerve or chiasmal dysfunction.

CATARACTS

It is amazing how often patients are referred for evaluation of progressive visual loss and the cause is a subtle nuclear sclerotic or posterior subcapsular cataract (Fig. 2.1a). These can usually be detected with a dilated slit-lamp examination or streak retinoscopy. Subtle nuclear

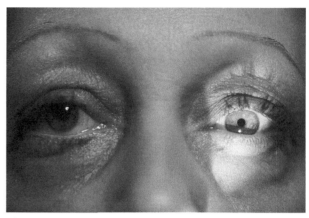

a

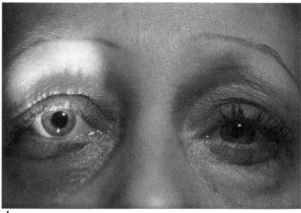

b

Figure 2.2 *An RAPD (a). The normal right eye is illuminated and both pupils constrict. The light is switched to the left eye with the optic neuropathy; both pupils paradoxically dilate (b).*

sclerosis may be harder to detect, but a myopic refractive shift should increase your suspicion. These changes can often be detected by looking through the patient's dilated pupil with a dimmed, indirect ophthalmoscope without a condensing lens. A clump of nuclear sclerosis will be evident.

OPTIC NEUROPATHY VERSUS MACULOPATHY

Patients with unexplained (non-cataractous or corneal) visual loss are either referred to a retinal specialist or a neuro-ophthalmologist. The retinal specialist looks for a maculopathy and does the requisite fluorescein angiogram. When this is negative, the patient is referred to

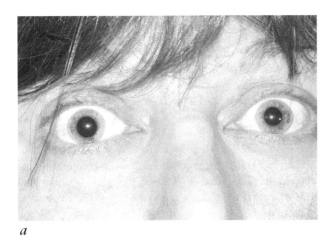

a

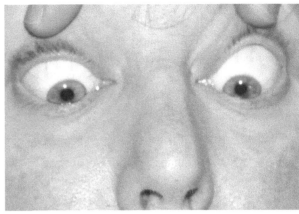

c

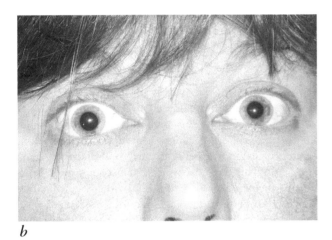

b

Figure 2.3 *Light-near dissociation due to bilateral optic nerve dysfunction. The patient has sluggish, mid-dilated pupils and when either eye is illuminated, both pupils constrict (a). The degree of constriction is noted (b) and compared with the degree of constriction at near (c). Greater constriction at near indicates bilateral optic nerve or chiasmal dysfunction.*

the neuro-ophthalmologist. The neuro-ophthalmologist, on the other hand, performs the requisite visual field and orders the neuroimaging study, if these are negative the patient is referred to the retinal specialist. This is not cost-effective medical care.

Initially differentiating between macular and optic nerve disease can avoid this situation. Patients with maculopathies often complain of metamorphopsia (distortion of images). There is often central visual loss or a relative central scotoma on visual field testing. Photopsias are a prominent symptom, i.e. light bothers the eye, and there is no RAPD. This, of course, must be sought prior to dilating the patient's pupils.

Maculopathies are diagnosed by a careful examination of the macula. Fluorescein angiography may be diagnostic or confirmatory. Careful examination of the macula and fluorescein angiogram may be normal in patients with subtle maculopathies. The diagnostic key is that these patients do not have a RAPD compatible with their degree of visual loss.

Regardless of your subspecialty, it is important to have a logical method for evaluating the patient with visual dysfunction. The retinal specialist may neglect to look at the pupils prior to ordering the fluorescein angiogram, while the neuro-ophthalmologist may miss the central serous choroidopathy prior to ordering the gadolinium-enhanced magnetic resonance imaging (MRI) scan with attention to the optic nerve and chiasm. The patient in Fig. 2.1 had actually been referred from a comprehensive ophthalmologist for progressive visual loss. The cause (many dollars later) was a nuclear sclerotic cataract evident on careful dilated slit-lamp examination. When all else fails, examine the patient. Do not put on your subspecialty blinders and fail to examine the entire eye. A recent patient was referred for evaluation of a superior visual field defect. A quick look with the indirect ophthalmoscope revealed a retinal detachment that was obvious even to the examining neuro-ophthalmologist.

CASE STUDY 1

A 42-year-old nurse complained of distorted vision. She complained that 'Things just do not look right'. Visual acuity was decreased to 20/25. There was no RAPD. Dilated examination with a 78-diopter lens revealed a perifoveal retinal pigment epithelial defect that appeared inflammatory (Fig. 2.4a). Fluorescein angiography revealed no neovascularization (Fig. 2.4b).

Comment: Metamorphopsia is almost always due to macula disease and not optic nerve dysfunction.

CASE STUDY 2

A 38-year-old lady presented with decreased vision to 20/100. There was no evidence for a RAPD. Visual field demonstrated a relative central scotoma. Dilated fundus examination appeared normal. Fluorescein angiography demonstrated classic appearance of central serous choroidopathy (Fig. 2.5). Symptoms resolved spontaneously. Central serous chorioretinopathy is more common in males than females. Males are commonly type A personalities (like those reading and the one writing this book). Other risk factors include psychotropic medications, corticosteroid use and systemic hypertension. Patients present with decreased vision and metamorphopsia. Careful dilated fundus examination reveals a serous detachment of the macula (Fig. 2.5a). This may be very subtle and certainly missed upon cursory fundus examination through undilated pupils. Fluorescein angiography is diagnostic (Fig. 2.5b–d), demonstrating detachment of the neurosensory retina. This entity may be confused with optic neuritis. The patients may have that same intense personality, but there is no pain upon eye movement or RAPD evident in patients with central serous chorioretinopathy. Examine the pupils before dilating the patient's eyes.

Fluorescein angiography can be very helpful in diagnosing visual loss from central serous choroidopathy and cystoid macula edema (Fig. 2.6). These patients may have a nearly normal fundus examination, but the fluorescein angiogram is again diagnostic.

CYSTOID MACULAR EDEMA (CME)

Patients with CME are usually obvious, often seen with decreased vision after cataract surgery or an episode of ocular inflammation. They present with decreased vision and metamorphopsia. Fluorescein angiography demonstrates the diagnostic petaloid pattern of macular edema (Fig. 2.6). This diagnosis is easy. It becomes more difficult when the edema is either old or the result of nicotinic acid ingestion. Leakage may not be evident on a fluorescein angiogram. Examination of the macula may appear normal except for some subtle, mild pigment epithelial changes (Fig. 2.7).

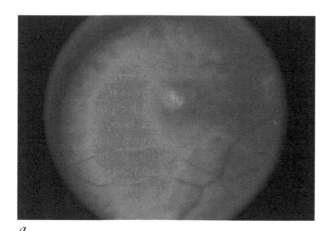

a

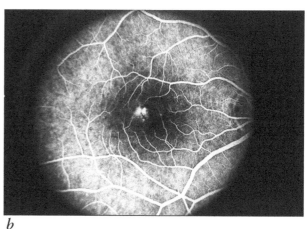

b

Figure 2.4   *The fundus, demonstrating an inflammatory lesion in the right macula (a). Fluorescein angiogram demonstrating a retinal pigment epithelial defect but no subretinal neovascularization (b).*

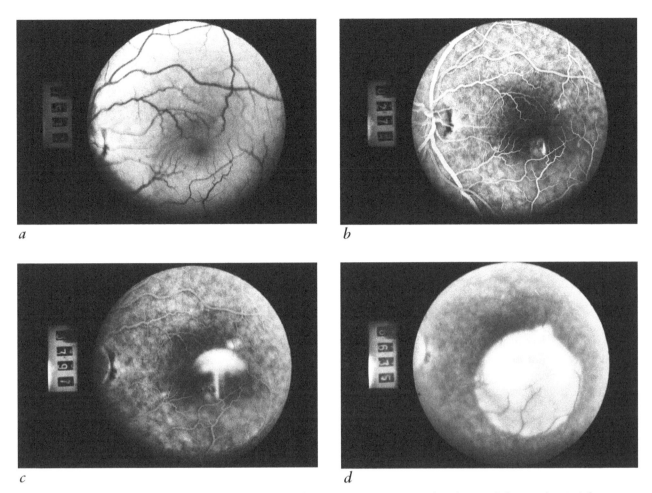

Figure 2.5 *Central serous choroidopathy. Red-free image demonstrating an apparent detachment of the macula (a). A fluorescein angiogram demonstrating an early retinal pigment epithelial defect (b), then the classic smokestack retinal pigment epithelial defect (c) and subsequent filling of the exudative macular detachment (d).*

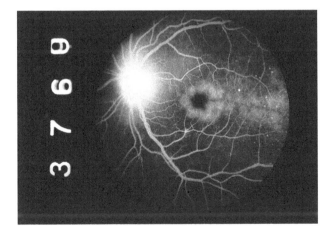

Figure 2.6 *Cystoid macular edema; classic petaloid appearance shown on this late-phase fluorescein angiogram.*

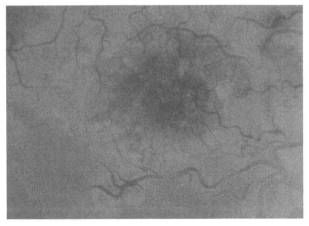

Figure 2.7 *Subtle retinal pigmentary changes in a patient with longstanding cystoid macular edema treated with laser photocoagulation.*

DIABETIC MACULOPATHY

Diabetic patients with visual loss usually have very evident exudates in their macula (Fig. 2.8) compatible with their degree of visual dysfunction. Some patients with pre-proliferative retinopathy may have macular ischemia secondary to capillary non-perfusion and a normal fundus examination. Fluorescein angiography will demonstrate capillary non-perfusion and establish the diagnosis.

ACUTE POSTERIOR MULTIFOCAL PLACOID PIGMENT EPITHELIOPATHY (APMPPE)

A neurologist referred a 21-year-old lady with normal neuro-imaging for evaluation of papilledema (Fig. 2.9a). Visual fields demonstrated bilateral central scotomas, thought to be atypical for papilledema and pseudotumor cerebri (Fig. 2.9b). There were more multiple gray pigmentary changes in the macula than would be expected from papilledema (Fig. 2.9c). The visual field demonstrated bilateral central scotomas—most atypical for papilledema.

Fluorescein angiography demonstrated multiple retinal pigment epithelial defects thought to be typical for APMPPE (Fig. 2.9d). Treatment with systemic corticosteroids hastened restoration of her visual function and normalization of fundus appearance 1 month later (Fig. 2.9e).

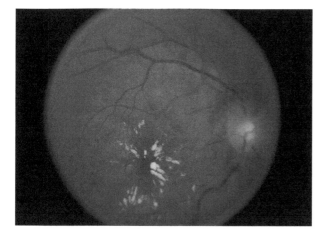

Figure 2.8 *Obvious diabetic exudative maculopathy.*

These multiple gray-white lesions at the level of the retinal pigment epithelium result from dysfunction of the choroidal vasculature. Choroidal vascular insufficiency would also account for the optic disc swelling evident in this patient. Associated systemic symptoms include headache, transient ischemic attacks, dysacousis, tinnitus, cerebral vasculitis, stroke and aseptic meningitis.[1]

COMMENTS

Neuro-ophthalmologic disorders and macular disorders are not mutually exclusive. There is a certain amount of crossover between the two and the patient is better served if each practitioner is aware of the other's subspecialty. Key diagnostic survival points are that patients with macular disease usually complain of metamorphopsia, painless visual loss and photopsia. There is almost never a RAPD, unless there is so much macular pathology that the diagnosis is obvious (Fig. 2.10) and there is no pain with eye movements. When fundus examination appears normal, fluorescein angiography may be very helpful.

MACULOPATHIES

MACULAR DYSTROPHIES

Cone dystrophies usually commence in middle age, may be sporadic or familial and are often perplexing to the neuro-ophthalmologist unless the diagnosis is actually considered and an electroretinogram (ERG) obtained. These patients may have decreased vision, loss of visual field, dyschromatopsia, and complain of difficulty seeing in the daylight, photopsias and photophobia. Fundus examination may be normal or there may be some temporal optic disc pallor and depigmentation of the retinal pigment epithelium, often accompanied by profound loss of visual acuity and field (Fig. 2.11a). An afferent pupillary defect, if present, is less than would be expected for the degree of visual loss. Visual loss may be progressive, which is especially perplexing for the neuro-ophthalmologist. This may be very difficult to distinguish from an optic neuropathy presenting as progressive loss of central vision with an often normal fundus examination. Visual loss may be stationary or progressive. It may also be very asymmetrical, first affecting one eye and then the other, as in the following case.

A 47-year-old lady was referred complaining of decreased vision in the left eye. Visual acuity progressively deteriorated to 20/400 and the visual field was markedly impaired. An afferent pupillary defect was present but less than would be expected for the degree of visual loss. MRI was normal, with scattered areas of demyelination. Optic neuritis was diagnosed and she was treated with a course of high-dose intravenous methylprednisolone with no improvement in her visual acuity or visual field.

She returned 3 years later with vague visual complaints in her only sighted right eye. Visual acuity and field progressively deteriorated, and neuroimaging was again negative. She was referred for a second opinion and an ERG was obtained, the flicker response was markedly depressed and cone dystrophy was diagnosed. Follow-up examination revealed a hint of temporal optic disc pallor and altered macular pigment epithelium. This is a diagnosis that most neuro-ophthalmologists miss only once, as they then become more attuned to the history of photophobia—a key to subjective diagnosis, photopsia and complaints of decreased vision in daylight. Vision may decrease to 20/30–20/200, dyschromatopsia and a central scotoma on visual fields may be evident. Fundus changes are often very subtle and often manifest as subtle fine granularity of the macular pigment accompanied by peripapillary pigment atrophy. An ERG is diagnostic and demonstrates reduction of the flicker response (cone function) and reduction of the B-wave. Unfortunately, in the early stages of the disease, the ERG may be normal.

FUNDUS FLAVIMACULATUS

Fundus flavimaculatus, or Stargardt's disease, usually presents in early adulthood and is autosomal recessive. Patients have marked loss of central vision and a distinctive fundus and fluorescein angiography appearance (Fig. 2.12a–c).

X-LINKED JUVENILE RETINOSCHISIS

This is a congenital disorder presenting in childhood with visual loss and a distinctive foveal stellate pattern of superficial cysts with radial stria. The fluorescein angiogram may demonstrate mottling of the retinal pigment epithelium or appear normal. The B-wave is diminished on ERG.

INFLAMMATORY MACULOPATHIES

Acute Macular Neuroretinopathy

Whilst reviewing material for this chapter, a young lady was referred to the present author's practice looking for a reason for her metamorphopsia in her right eye. The vision was not quite right and she had difficulty reading with the right eye. Neuro-ophthalmic examination, including visual field, was normal. A small, discrete central field defect was present on an Amsler grid. Careful dilated fundus exam with a 78-diopter lens demonstrated a discrete petalloid defect in her fovea compatible with acute macular neuroretinopathy (Fig. 2.13).

Big Blind-Spot Syndrome

These patients have the acute onset of photopsias and an accompanying enlarged blind spot on visual field testing. Visual acuity is normal. Females are more often affected than males. Blind-spot enlargement is caused by displacement of the peripapillary retina by a swollen or normal optic nerve.

Acute Idiopathic Blind-Spot Enlargement (AIBSE)

Patients present with complaints of photopsias. The blind spot is enlarged and there is no evidence for optic disc swelling. The steep borders of the blind-spot enlargement may mimic a bitemporal defect and elicit the erroneous diagnosis of chiasmal syndrome. The photopsias resolves but the visual field defects may persist.

Multiple Evanescent White-Dot Syndrome (MEWDS)

Female patients present with acute, unilateral visual loss, scotomas and multiple evanescent white lesions at the level of the retinal pigment epithelium. The optic disc may be inflamed and stain on fluorescein angiography. There is significant overlap between these syndromes to prompt Gass[2] to clump them all under the moniker of acute zonal occult outer retinopathy (AZOOR). This includes AIBSE, MEWDS, acute macular neuroretinopathy and multifocal choroiditis. These acute causes of focal loss of outer retinal function result in non-neurologic causes of abnormal visual fields that may or may not be accompanied by an abnormal-appearing fundus. They should be considered in young females complaining of photopsias accompanied by visual field defects with minimal or no fundus changes or localizing pupillary signs (RAPD).

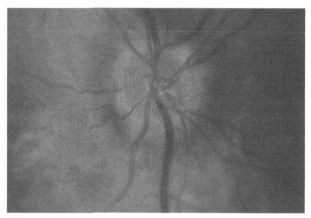
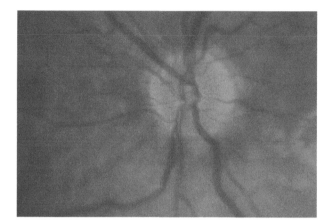

a

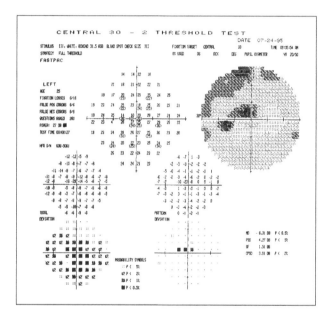

b

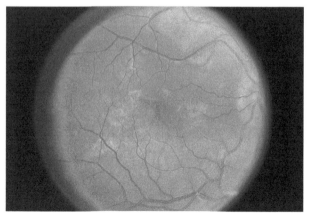
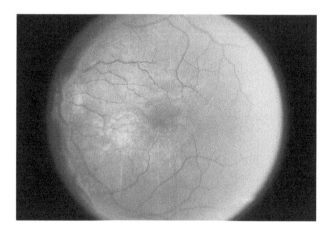

c

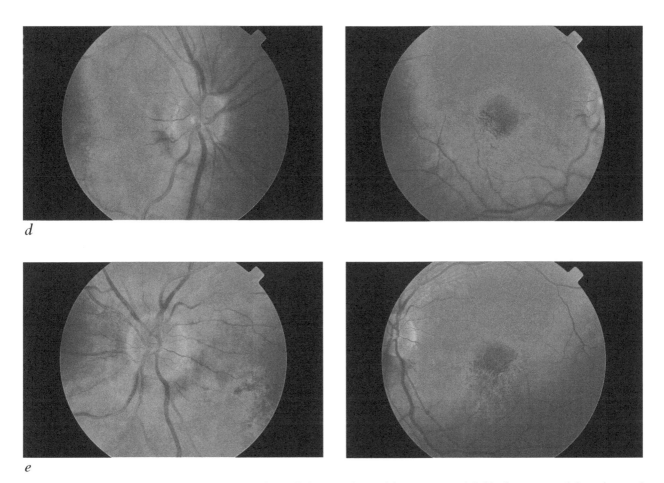

d

e

Figure 2.9 *A patient referred for evaluation of papilledema and visual loss (a). Visual fields demonstrate bilateral central scotomas in addition to enlarged blind spots (b). The fundus demonstrates multiple pigmented lesions (c). Fluorescein angiogram demonstrates multiple retinal pigment epithelial defects (d), compatible with AMPPE. Resolution of optic disc swelling and normalization of fundus appearance 1 month later (e).*

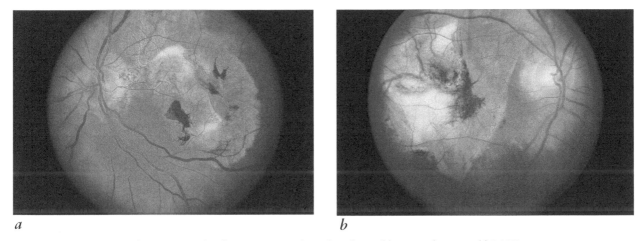

a   *b*

Figure 2.10 *Patients with severe macular degeneration with profound visual loss may have a mild RAPD.*

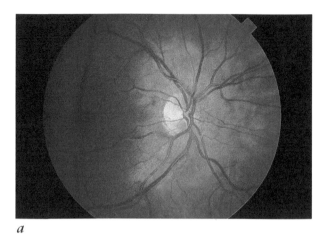

a

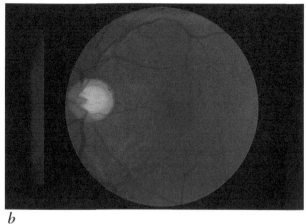

b

Figure 2.11 *Cone dystrophy may present as bilateral loss of visual acuity and visual field in a patient with minimal fundus changes including temporal pallor and macular pigment changes.*

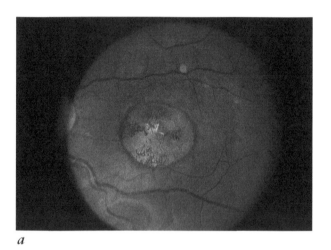

a

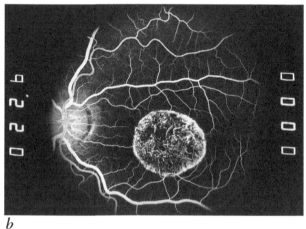

b

Figure 2.12 *Fundus flavimaculatus. Distinctive fundus appearance (a) and fluorescein angiogram (b) in a patient with decreased vision (20/400) and central scotomas on visual field.*

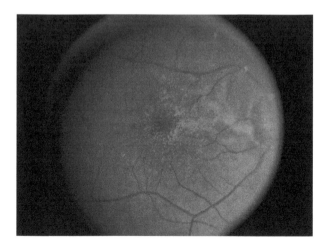

Figure 2.13 *Subtle, petaloid defect in the fovea in a patient with acute macular neuroretinopathy.*

PARANEOPLASTIC RETINOPATHIES (PR)

PR occur as a remote effect of a systemic malignancy. An immune phenomenon causes photoreceptor dysfunction that may mimic an optic neuropathy. These syndromes are rarely diagnosed upon initial presentation for they commonly occur prior to the diagnosis of the underlying malignancy.

Patients complain of photopsias, but visual acuity may be normal or markedly reduced, and color vision is reduced. A photo-stress test may be abnormal. Central visual fields are often normal, and visual field loss is manifest as mid-peripheral scotomas that may eventually coalesce into a classic ring scotoma. Goldmann visual field or a 30–60°

automated visual field should be obtained. These arcuate-type defects are retinal in origin, so they do not respect the horizontal or vertical midline. Initial ophthalmologic examination is often normal. Ocular findings may include a mild vitritis, attenuated retinal vessels, mild optic disc pallor, granular appearance of the retinal pigment epithelium, and peripheral retinal pigmentation. ERG, when obtained, demonstrates diffuse retinal dysfunction. An ERG demonstrating diffuse retinal dysfunction in a patient with acute visual loss indicates a paraneoplastic syndrome. Patients with retinitis pigmentosa, the classic cause of diffuse retinal dysfunction on ERG, have slowly progressive visual field loss and good central vision. There are several distinct types of paraneoplastic retinopathy each having distinguishing signs and symptoms.[3]

CANCER-ASSOCIATED RETINOPATHY (CAR)

CAR is primarily rod dysfunction. Patients present with visual loss and nyctalopia. The scotopic ERG is markedly abnormal (rod function). Visual loss is relentless.

CANCER-ASSOCIATED CONE DYSFUNCTION (CACD)

These patients present with decreased vision, dyschromatopsia, and complaints of glare and photosensitivity. Vision is primarily reduced in bright light (cones). Visual fields demonstrate central scotomas (loss of macular cones) and the ERG has a reduced flicker response (cone function).

MELANOMA-ASSOCIATED RETINOPATHY (MAR)

Patients with known cutaneous melanoma present with photopsias, night blindness and floaters. Visual acuity is usually 20/40 or better. Visual fields may demonstrate central or arcuate scotomas or peripheral constriction. ERG demonstrates bipolar cell dysfunction. The dark-adapted ERG reveals absent B-waves and normal cone amplitudes. There is no relentless loss of vision.

RETINITIS PIGMENTOSA

Although retinitis pigmentosa is basically a retinal disorder, these patients may present to the comprehensive ophthalmologist or neuro-ophthalmologist complaining of nyctalopia or be referred with constricted visual fields.

A 34-year-old physician was referred by his ophthalmologist for evaluation of visual field constriction. He was essentially asymptomatic, continuing to drive and practice family medicine. Visual fields were markedly constricted and there was concern that this may be caused by elevated intracranial pressure, in spite of the normal-appearing optic discs. Examination revealed markedly constricted visual fields and a very abnormal fundus with only the macular anatomy appearing normal (Fig. 2.14). Bone spicule pigmentation was subtle and quite peripheral. ERG was extinguished and retinitis pigmentosa diagnosed. Usually, the diagnosis and fundus appearance is more typical (Fig. 2.15).

A 45-year-old lady was referred with constricted visual fields, abnormal optic discs and headache. Visual acuity

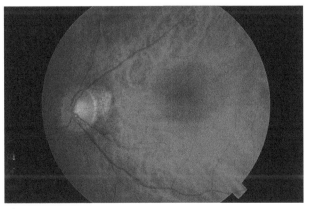

a

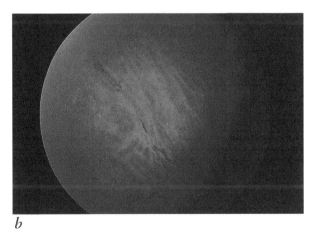

b

Figure 2.14 *Subtle retinitis pigmentosa: this patient presented with an asymptomatic, severely constricted visual field. Only the macula appeared normal on fundus examination (a), but scattered bone spicule pigmentation was present in the periphery (b).*

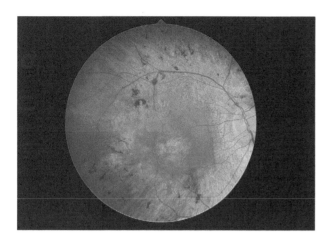

Figure 2.15 *Typical and obvious retinitis pigmentosa.*

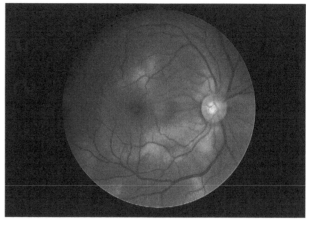

Figure 2.16 *Commotio retinae.*

was 20/20 in both eyes (OU). Visual fields were constricted and a bilateral vitritis was present, as were pigmentary changes in the near peripheral fundus. After an extensive and non-productive evaluation, an ERG was obtained and found to be extinguished, establishing the diagnosis of retinitis pigmentosa.

TRAUMATIC MACULOPATHY

These patients have acute visual loss and obvious commotio retinae (Fig. 2.16). Visual function may remain abnormal, with a normal-appearing fundus and possible evidence for subtle retinal pigment epithelium (RPE) mottling.

SOLAR MACULOPATHY

This is characterized by bilateral central scotomas and decreased central vision caused by staring directly at the sun. There is often a history of psychiatric imbalance or hallucinogenic drug use.

INTRAOPERATIVE PHOTIC RETINOPATHY

These patients present with a paracentral scotoma following intraocular surgery. Examination reveals an oval, yellow-to-white deep retinal lesion that stains intensely with fluorescein. RPE mottling ensues and the scotoma remains. Fortunately, central vision is often spared since the eye is usually partially depressed during intraocular

surgery. The etiology is intense light from the operating microscope focused on the retina. This most commonly occurs during prolonged intraocular procedures by less experienced surgeons.

TOXIC RETINOPATHIES

Toxic retinopathies may present with visual loss and an initially normal-appearing fundus. Common etiologies include digoxin, chloroquine/hydroxychloroquine, thioridazine, quinine and desferrioxamine. If undetected retinal changes ensue, the visual loss may be permanent. Patients with digoxin toxicity complain of yellow vision (xanthopsia) and scintillating scotomas. They may have dyschromatopsia and paracentral scotomas. Chloroquine and hydroxychloroquine may cause a dose-related pigmentary retinopathy. This is initially reversible, but may progress to pigment mottling in the macula (bullseye maculopathy; Fig. 2.17) with loss of central vision and central scotomas. Poliosis and corneal whorls are associated findings. Thioridazine causes pigmentary deposits in the cornea and anterior lens capsule, and a pigmentary retinopathy. Isotretinoin may cause nyctalopia, blurred vision, dyschromatopsia and a compendium of other ophthalmologic dysfunctions including dry eye and optic neuritis.[4] High doses of nicotinic acid (1.5–5 g/day) may cause visual loss due to cystoid macula edema that does not leak fluorescein. Symptoms and signs resolve after stopping the medication. History of drug ingestion facilitates a timely diagnosis.

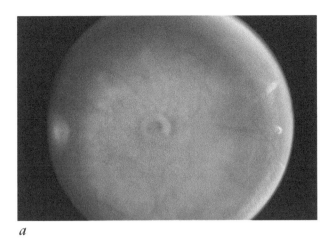

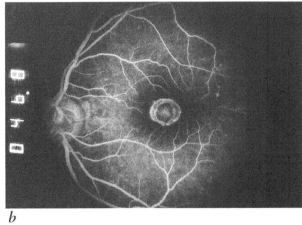

a   *b*

Figure 2.17   *Bullseye maculopathy (a). Fluorescein angiogram highlighting the bullseye defect (b).*

MACULAR HOLES

Vitreoretinal traction on the fovea may cause macular cysts and holes (Fig. 2.18). Progressive decrease in vision and a central scotoma are the hallmarks of this disorder that predominately affects elderly females. Idiopathic macular holes may be subtle (Fig. 2.19) or obvious (Fig. 2.18) and may be detected by careful funduscopic examination. Patients complain of blurred vision and metamorphopsia. Careful examination of the macula usually demonstrates the suspicious lesion. Treatment when necessary is surgical and beyond the scope of this text.

MACULAR EPIRETINAL MEMBRANES

Epiretinal membranes (ERM) develop at the vitreo-retinal interface by proliferating retinal glial cells that have reached the retinal surface through a break in the internal limiting membrane. They may be idiopathic or secondary to retinal surgery, ocular inflammation and trauma. Idiopathic ERM is found in otherwise healthy elderly patients and are bilateral in 10% of cases.

ERM may be divided into cellophane maculopathy and macular pucker depending upon the density of the membrane and the degree of retinal distortion. Cellophane maculopathy (Fig. 2.20) consists of a thin

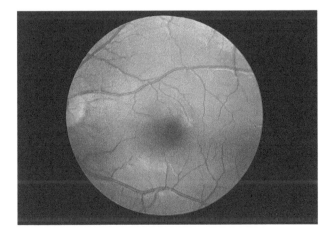

Figure 2.18   *Macular hole.*

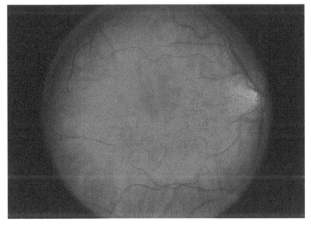

Figure 2.19   *Subtle macular hole.*

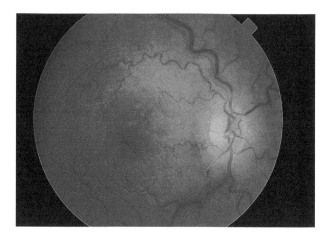

Figure 2.20   *Cellophane maculopathy.*

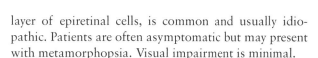

Figure 2.21   *Epiretinal membrane.*

layer of epiretinal cells, is common and usually idiopathic. Patients are often asymptomatic but may present with metamorphopsia. Visual impairment is minimal.

Thickening and contraction of the epiretinal membrane causes macular pucker. It may be idiopathic or secondary. Patients present with decreased central vision and metamorphopsia. There is evidence for distortion of the retinal blood vessels and wrinkling of the retina (Fig. 2.21). If symptoms are progressive and severe, surgical removal of the membrane usually improves the metamorphopsia and may improve visual acuity.[5]

RETINAL VASCULAR DISORDERS

Retinal vascular occlusions may be obvious (Fig. 2.22) or subtle (Fig. 2.23). A central retinal artery occlusion may not have a typical appearance if seen early before the cherry-red spot has had time to develop (Fig. 2.23). Branch retinal artery occlusions may be asymptomatic or very symptomatic depending which branches are occluded (Fig. 2.24). A lady was referred with complaints of visual loss occurring during cerebral angiography. Visual acuity was normal and visual fields demonstrated a central scotoma respecting the horizontal midline (Fig. 2.25a); talc emboli were evident in the perifoveal arterioles (Fig. 2.25b). One month later, her examination was totally normal except for the residual visual field defect.[6]

Occlusion of a cilioretinal artery may decimate central vision but with a relatively normal fundus; whereas central retinal artery occlusion with sparing of the cilioretinal artery may spare central visual acuity accom-

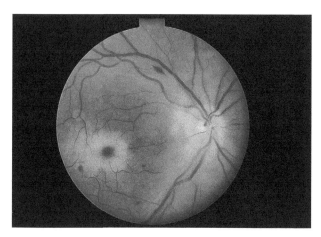

Figure 2.22   *Obvious CRAO with retinal edema and a cherry-red spot.*

panied by a markedly abnormal fundus examination (Fig. 2.26).

The ophthalmic artery is the first intracranial branch of the carotid artery (Fig. 2.27). After it enters the orbit it divides into the central retinal artery, long ciliary arteries, lacrimal artery and numerous short ciliary arteries. The short ciliary arteries supply blood to the prelaminar optic nerve and the choroid; the central retinal artery enters the eye, dividing and providing blood supply to the retina. The long ciliary arteries supply the anterior segment of the eye (Fig. 2.27). Occlusion of the ophthalmic artery or its branches results in a distinct clinical picture.

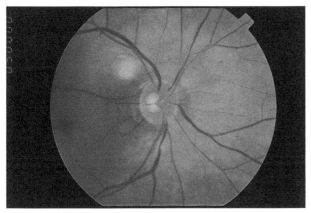

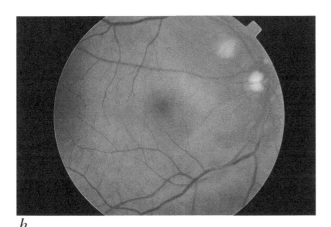

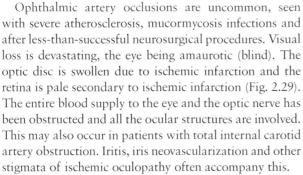

Figure 2.23 *Early, more subtle, CRAO with cotton-wool spots and minimal macular edema (a); 26 hours later, the cherry-red spot begins to appear (b).*

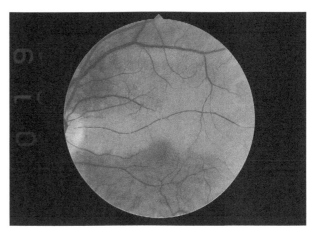

Figure 2.24 *A very symptomatic occlusion of a branch retinal artery due to its location in the macula.*

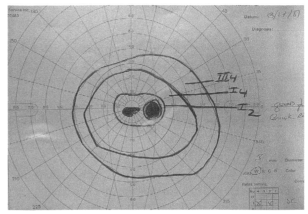

a

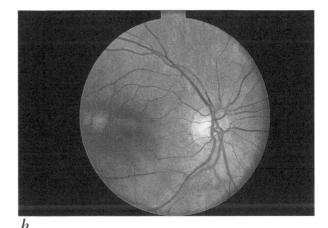

b

Figure 2.25 *Visual field demonstrates a central scotoma respecting the horizontal midline (a); talc emboli present in the superior perifoveal arterioles (b).*

Ophthalmic artery occlusions are uncommon, seen with severe atherosclerosis, mucormycosis infections and after less-than-successful neurosurgical procedures. Visual loss is devastating, the eye being amaurotic (blind). The optic disc is swollen due to ischemic infarction and the retina is pale secondary to ischemic infarction (Fig. 2.29). The entire blood supply to the eye and the optic nerve has been obstructed and all the ocular structures are involved. This may also occur in patients with total internal carotid artery obstruction. Iritis, iris neovascularization and other stigmata of ischemic oculopathy often accompany this.

Isolated central retinal artery occlusions (CRAO) are much more familiar to the ophthalmologist. The central retinal artery supplies the retina. Occlusion infarcts the retina; partial occlusion infarcts parts of the retina. The clinical picture is predictable. Patients with a total CRAO have devastating, but not total, visual loss. The

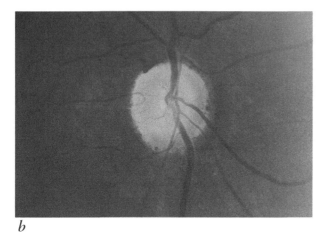

a

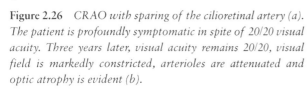

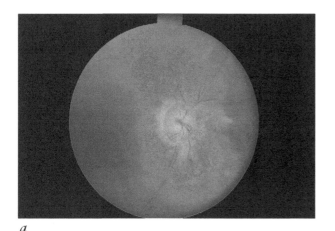

b

Figure 2.26 *CRAO with sparing of the cilioretinal artery (a). The patient is profoundly symptomatic in spite of 20/20 visual acuity. Three years later, visual acuity remains 20/20, visual field is markedly constricted, arterioles are attenuated and optic atrophy is evident (b).*

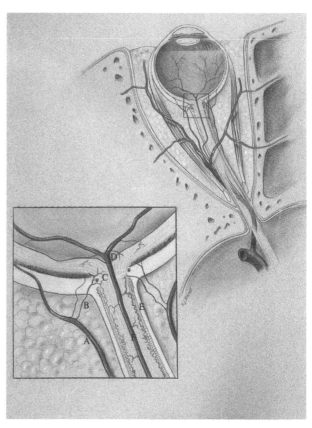

Figure 2.27 *Ophthalmic artery branches in the orbit and eye.*

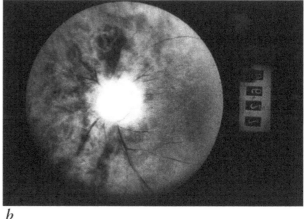

a   *b*

Figure 2.28 *Total obstruction of the ophthalmic artery (a). No blood flow is evident on fluorescein angiogram (b).*

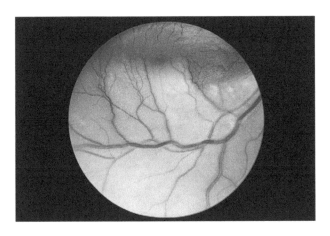

Figure 2.29 *Inferior retinal artery occlusion presenting as a superior visual field defect.*

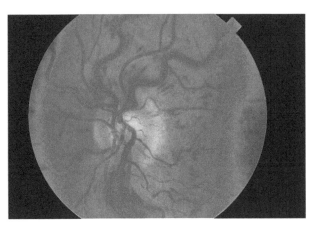

Figure 2.30 *Obvious CRVO.*

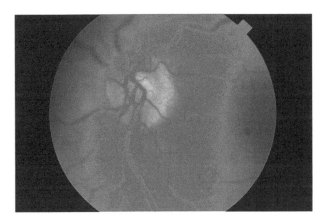

Figure 2.31 *Same patient as in Fig. 2.30 (1 month earlier) manifests dilated retinal veins and a perimacular hemorrhage.*

retina appears white and edematous. The macula, with its choroidal blood supply, maintains its normal color (cherry-red spot; Fig. 2.22). The optic nerve appears normal, since its blood supply is from the short ciliary (choroidal) circulation (Figs 2.22 and 2.23). CRAO is usually a very apparent diagnosis in the setting of dramatic visual loss. It may not be very typical with visual loss and a less-than-obvious initial retinal examination (Fig. 2.23a); however, with time, the clinical picture is usually quite typical (Fig. 2.23b).

Branch retinal artery occlusions often present more subtly. The author saw the patient in Fig. 2.29 while a junior resident. He was a postman complaining of difficulty reading the numbers on mail boxes above eye level. Fundus examination confirmed infarction of the inferior retina due to an inferior retinal artery occlusion (Fig. 2.31). Angiography demonstrated significant occlusion of the extracranial internal carotid artery as the source of the offending embolus.

Variations upon the theme of branch retinal artery occlusions provide for an interesting array of visual complaints and ophthalmoscopic findings. Cilioretinal arteries may be obstructed causing loss of central vision and a relatively normal-appearing fundus, except for the small area of infarction. They may also be obstructed by excessive optic disc edema, causing central visual loss in excess of the degree of optic nerve swelling.

Central retinal vein occlusions (CRVO) are usually obvious (Fig. 2.30), but may be more subtle when partial or when seen early (Fig. 2.31).

CAROTID INSUFFICIENCY

Severe, total carotid artery insufficiency is fortunately rarer now than it was 20 years ago. Ocular ischemic syndrome, consisting of iritis, iris neovascularization, cataract, and an ischemic retina and optic nerve, is uncommon. These patients have a very typical fundus appearance (Fig. 2.32) with large blot retinal hemorrhages just peripheral to the superior and inferior retinal vascular arcades. This may progress to venous stasis retinopathy secondary to carotid insufficiency. Patients with very severe ischemia may actually develop cystoid macular edema (Fig. 2.33) and iris neovascularization (Fig. 2.34). Retinal and ocular

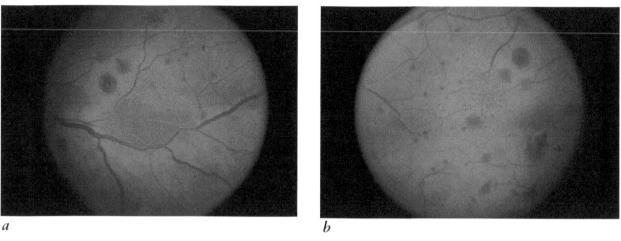

a   *b*

Figure 2.32 *Typical fundus appearance of venous stasis secondary to carotid insufficiency.*

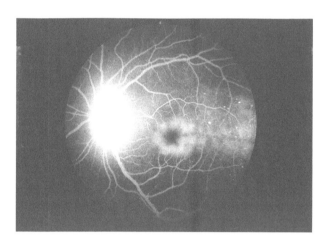

Figure 2.33 *Cystoid macular edema secondary to carotid insufficiency.*

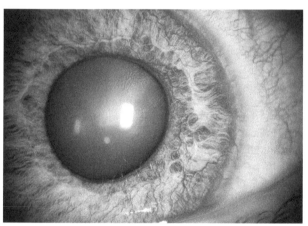

Figure 2.34 *Iris neovascularization secondary to carotid insufficiency.*

ischemia is almost always diagnosed after a dilated fundus examination and ancillary, often non-invasive, testing.

Treatment is revascularization of the carotid artery either by carotid endarterectomy or an extracranial–intracranial bypass procedure. The best treatment is prevention of this extreme form of atherosclerotic disease.

Giant cell arteritis (GCA) is dealt with in detail in Chapter 6. Patients with GCA may have marked ocular hypoperfusion prior to any manifestations of ischemic oculopathy. Fluorescein angiography may demonstrate marked delay in choroidal filling due to occlusion of the short ciliary vessels. This fluorescein angiographic feature is almost diagnostic of GCA.

OPTIC NEUROPATHIES

Each optic nerve consists of axons originating from retinal ganglion cells. These axons pass from the eye into the orbit and extend intracranially to combine with axons from the opposite eye, forming the optic chiasm and tracts, and finally synapse at the lateral geniculate bodies (Fig. 2.35). Each optic nerve consists of approximately one million axons. Axons from each eye combine to form the optic chiasm. Nasal fibers cross to the contralateral side to join the temporal fibers that pass uncrossed through the optic chiasm joining with the

The Visual Sensory System

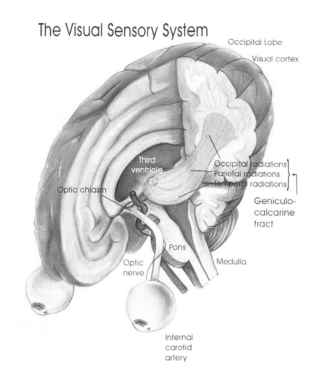

Figure 2.35 *Visual pathways from the eye to the occipital lobe of the brain.*

VISUAL PATHWAYS

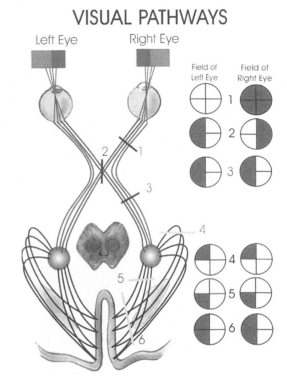

Figure 2.36 *Visual pathways and visual field defects.*

crossed nasal fibers to form the optic tracts and synapse at the lateral geniculate body (Figs 2.35 and 2.36). Damage or injury to these very long axons anterior to their crossing in the chiasm results in unilateral visual dysfunction, i.e. an optic neuropathy. Optic neuropathies are the mainstay of neuro-ophthalmology and will be covered in detail in several chapters.

Damage to the optic chiasm or tracts results in bilateral visual field defects (Fig. 2.36). Distinctive visual field defects result from the location of the injury in the optic tracts or optic chiasm (Fig. 2.36). Patients with optic nerve, chiasm or tract damage will have a RAPD or light-near dissociation of their pupils accompanying the visual defects (Figs 2.2, 2.3 and 2.36). Injury to the posterior visual pathways—optic radiations to occipital lobes—likewise result in bilateral homonymous hemianopic visual field defects (Fig. 2.36), but pupillary reactions are normal. There is no evident RAPD or light-near dissociation of the pupils.

Patients with optic neuropathies have visual dysfunction accompanied by a RAPD. If there is no evidence for a RAPD or light-near dissociation, there is no optic nerve dysfunction, i.e. look elsewhere. Be very careful,

however, if the patient has had previously documented normal vision and you cannot correct the vision to normal. The following case is illustrative (Fig. 2.37).

A 36-year-old lady was referred by her ophthalmologist for evaluation of decreased vision. He could not correct her visual acuity to any better than 20/25 and had corrected her to 20/20 several years previously. Ocular examination was totally normal. Two observers were unable to detect any pupillary abnormalities. Visual fields were normal on two occasions. After several months of repeated examinations, an exacerbated examiner detected a subtle RAPD and obtained another computerized tomography (CT) scan, which demonstrated a subtle, enhancing intrasellar mass (Fig. 2.37c and d) proving to be an intrasellar meningioma at surgery (Fig. 2.37e).

Comment: Follow-up examinations are very important when evaluating patients with subtle visual complaints. Sooner or later, the pathology will become apparent. It is better to detect it yourself rather than have your competitor make the elusive diagnosis.

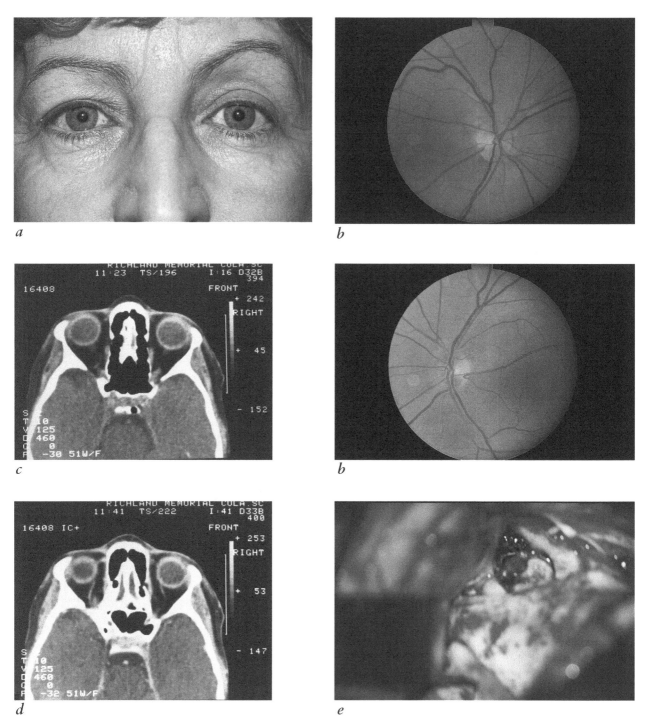

Figure 2.37 *Patient presenting with vague visual complaints and a hysterical personality (a), a normal fundus examination (b) and visual fields (c). CT scans demonstrate subtle intrasellar enhancement [without (c) and with (d) contrast enhancement]. Intraoperative photograph demonstrates effacement of the optic chiasm by an intrasellar meningioma (e).*

JUNCTIONAL SCOTOMAS AND BITEMPORAL HEMIANOPIAS

The most important visual field that is performed on a patient with an optic neuropathy is performed upon the uninvolved eye. This concept originally purported by J Lawton Smith is as valid today as it was many years ago. Only by testing the uninvolved eye will one diagnose the junctional scotoma (anterior chiasmal compression) or bitemporal hemianopia indicative of chiasmal compression.

OPTIC CHIASM

Nasal fibers from one eye combine with temporal fibers from the opposite eye to form the optic chiasm (Figs 2.36 and 2.38). The optic chiasm is situated above the sella turcica and the enclosed pituitary gland in 80% of individuals, located over the tuberculum sella (prefixed) in 15% of individuals and located over the dorsum sellae in 5% of individuals. Fig. 2.39 demonstrates the relationship of the chiasm to the cavernous sinus, carotid arteries and pituitary gland. It is evident that pituitary masses, meningiomas on the anterior or posterior clinoids, and carotid artery aneurysms can cause not only chiasmal dysfunction but also extraocular motility dysfunction. Fig. 2.35 also demonstrates the relationship between the optic nerves, chiasm and optic tracts, the third ventricle and the surrounding intracranial structures.

Chiasmal syndromes range from subtle junctional scotomas due to compression or inflammation of the optic nerve anterior chiasmal junction, to classic bitemporal hemianopias, to central (macular) bitemporal hemianopias due to compression of the posterior chiasmal notch by an enlarged third ventricle. The following cases—examples of a variety of chiasmal visual field defects—are illustrative.

A patient was recently referred with a mildly elevated sedimentation rate for evaluation of an atrophic optic disc and a biopsy of her superficial temporal artery to rule out GCA. Visual acuity was bare light perception in the left eye. The left optic disc was atrophic and the right one appeared normal (Fig. 2.40a). Visual fields were all but obliterated in the left eye, but an obvious superior temporal quadrant defect was evident in the right visual field (Fig. 2.40b). Neuroimaging demonstrated an enlarged, enhancing intraorbital and intracranial optic nerve (Fig. 2.40c) involving the anterior optic chiasm,

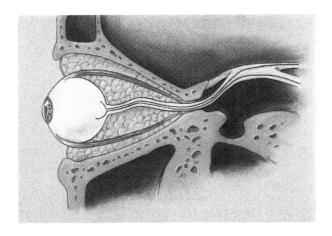

Figure 2.38 *Diagram illustrating the relationship of the optic chiasm to the sella turcica.*

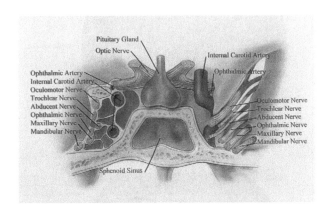

Figure 2.39 *Coronal section demonstrates the relationship between the optic chiasm to the pituitary gland and the sphenoid sinus beneath it and the cavernous sinus structures laterally.*

resulting in the junctional visual field defect (Fig. 2.40b). Biopsy confirmed the diagnosis of sarcoidosis (Fig. 2.40d).

A 40-year-old man complained of decreased vision in his left eye. There was an obvious RAPD and optic atrophy on the left side (Fig. 2.41a). He was referred with a diagnosis of glaucoma. Visual field examination demonstrated a temporal scotoma respecting the vertical midline. Visual field on the right eye demonstrated a very subtle temporal scotoma, subjectively solicited (Fig. 2.41b). The first CT scan was negative, 1 month later the bitemporal visual field defects were obvious (Fig. 2.41c), and the third CT scan demonstrated an enhancing suprasellar mass (Fig. 2.41d), which proved to be a meningioma.

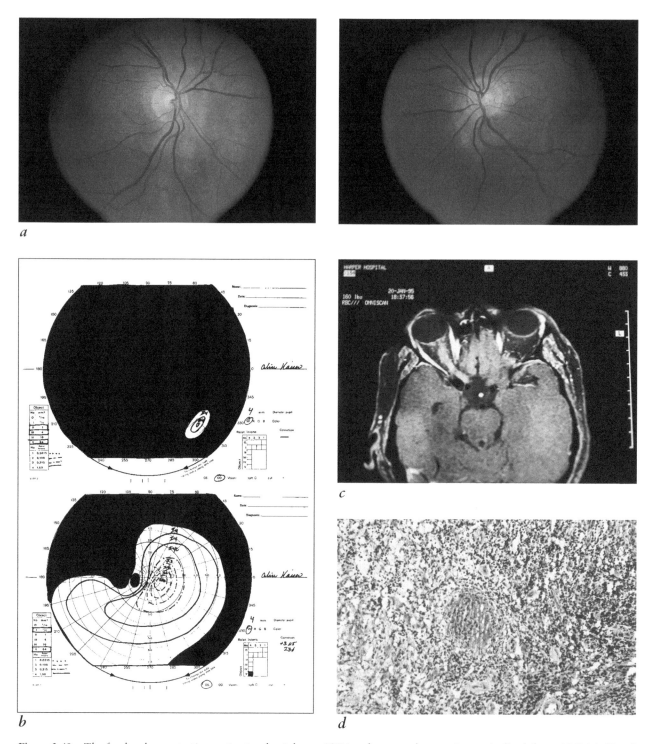

Figure 2.40   *The fundus demonstrating optic atrophy right eye (OD) and a normal-appearing optic disc left eye (OS) (a). Visual fields demonstrate almost complete loss of vision OD; a junctional scotoma is evident OS (b). Enhancement of the intraorbital and intracranial optic nerve is evident on a gadolinium-enhanced MRI (c). Biopsy specimen demonstrates non-caseating granulomas compatible with sarcoidosis (d).*

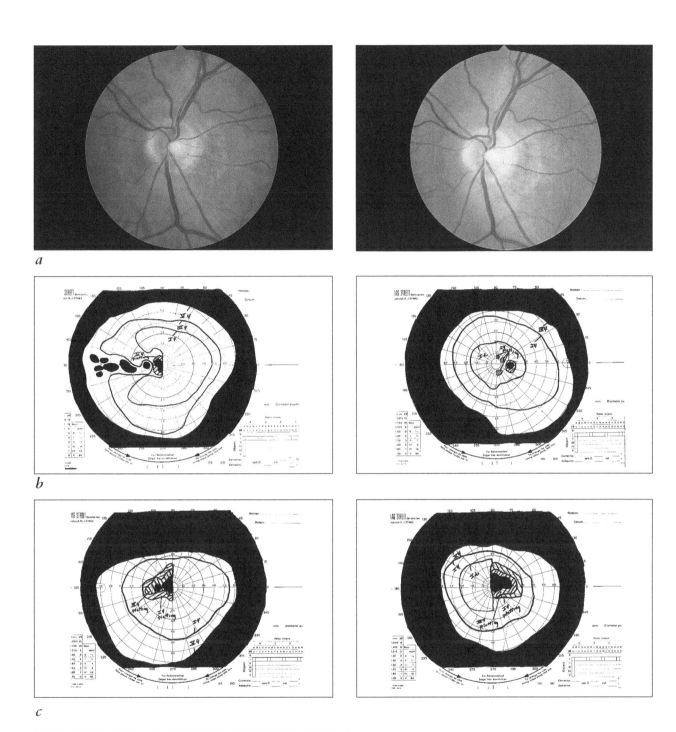

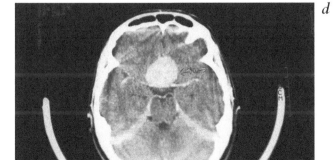

Figure 2.41 *The fundus demonstrating optic atrophy OS and a normal-appearing right optic nerve (a). Visual fields demonstrate a subtle bitemporal defect (b), progressing to an obvious bitemporal hemianopia (c). A CT scan demonstrates a large enhancing suprasellar mass (d).*

A 65-year-old man was referred with a central retinal vein occlusion with an atypical appearance (Fig. 2.45a). The rather extensive visual loss (bare light perception) prompted a CT scan, demonstrating a markedly enlarged optic nerve compatible with an optic nerve sheath meningioma (Fig. 2.42b). Visual field on the sighted left eye demonstrated a superior temporal defect (junctional scotoma; Fig. 2.42c), indicating intracranial and chiasmal involvement not yet evident on the imaging studies. Rapid progression of the junctional scotoma prompted a biopsy, confirming the diagnosis of malignant glioblastoma of the optic pathways (Fig. 2.42d).

Comment: Chiasmal syndrome–bitemporal hemianopia due to chiasmal compression by tumor should be an obvious diagnosis but is often missed even by skilled examiners.

A 63-year-old man was followed for several years for complaints of decreased vision in his left eye. The obvious cause was age-related macular degeneration (Fig. 2.43a). Referral for a second opinion prompted a visual field examination in the contralateral normal eye, and a bitemporal defect was very evident (Fig. 2.43b). Neuroimaging confirmed the diagnosis of a compressive chiasmal lesion (Fig. 2.43c). The obvious diagnosis may not be so obvious in neuro-ophthalmology. Check the visual field in the 'normal' eye and save yourself potential embarrassment. Before ascribing visual loss to age-related macular degeneration, make sure that there is sufficient macular damage to justify the decrease in visual acuity (although patients with apparently very severe macular degeneration are sometimes able to read the Snellen chart surprisingly well). The corollary is seldom true. If you do not see significant macular disruption on examination and fluorescein angiogram, look for another reason for the visual dysfunction.

A 43-year-old psychiatric nurse saw her ophthalmologist with complaints of 'funny vision' in both eyes. Nothing was evident on initial examination. She kept complaining and was referred to a local university. The visual field examination was not repeated ('important to contain costs') and there were no obvious localizing signs (Fig. 2.44a). She was told that she was crazy and should consider taking some of the medications that she was dispensing to her psychiatric patients. She was angered and sought a second opinion at another university. A screening visual field demonstrated an obvious bitemporal hemianopia (Fig. 2.44b) and subsequent neuroimaging revealed an obvious compressive mass lesion (Fig. 2.44c). Avoiding the second visual field in the spirit of cost containment is not a good idea and may prove very embarrassing. It is also important to remember, especially in neuro-ophthalmology, two basic axioms of medicine: first, crocks get sick; and second, a patient is innocent until proven guilty (i.e. there is real disease or visual dysfunction present until proven otherwise).

FUNCTIONAL VISUAL LOSS [7–10]

This leads to the subject of malingering, dysfunctional patients and hysterical visual loss. Let's deal with hysteria first. This is very uncommon. The classic tubular fields, failing to enlarge with increased distance or spot size, must be very uncommon. I am not sure that I have seen a bona fide case of hysterical visual loss in more than 20 years of neuro-ophthalmic practice.

Adolescents claiming decreased vision or visual field as a response to environmental stress is very common, easily detected and treated by giving the patient a reasonable way out (the magic drops to alleviate the spasm and make the vision better).[7] These patients are eager for treatment. By the time they have seen the subspecialist they have been through the diagnostic mill and are eager to resolve their problems; they have had all the attention that they can stand. A careful examination, power of suggestion, documentation that they can see, and a placebo medication to cure their 'spasm' usually suffices. Let me stress that diagnosis of functional visual dysfunction is predicated upon a careful, unbiased examination.

A 12-year-old girl complained of headaches and decreased vision. Her parents were divorcing at the time, and anxiety and stress reactions were the logical explanation. Her family doctor sent her to the psychiatrist, the social worker and her parish priest. All failed to diagnose her craniopharyngioma, which effectively blinded her.

Children complaining of headaches and visual dysfunction must be taken seriously. The author has seen a number of children who have passed through managed care systems with headaches and progressive loss of vision (actually documented), and never diagnosed as having a compressive intracranial mass. By the time the craniopharyngioma was diagnosed vision had been lost in one or both eyes.

A 10-year-old boy complained of headaches for several months. Decreased vision in the left eye was thought to be due to amblyopia. Visual complaints in the good eye prompted a second opinion. Examination revealed a temporal visual field defect in the right eye, an obvious RAPD in the nearly blind left eye and obvious optic atrophy (Fig. 2.45a). Neuroimaging demonstrated a large, cystic compressive lesion (Fig. 2.45b). Early diagnosis of

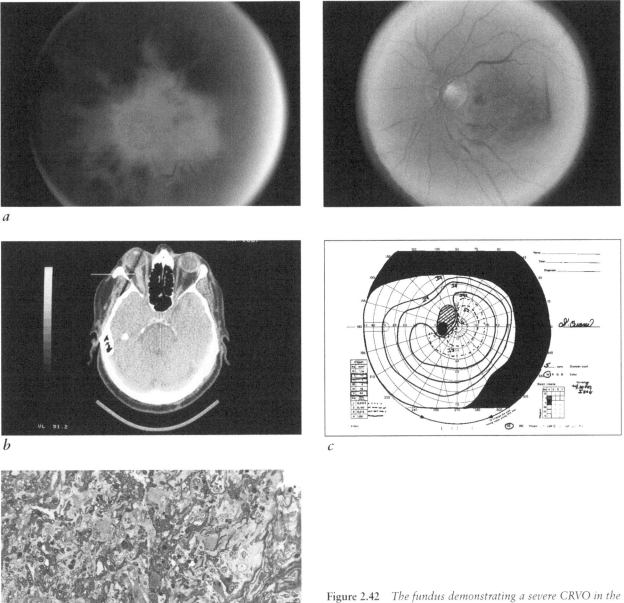

Figure 2.42 *The fundus demonstrating a severe CRVO in the right eye and a normal-appearing left eye (a). A CT scan demonstrates an enlarged right optic nerve (b). Visual field demonstrates a junctional scotoma in the left eye (c). Biopsy specimen demonstrates a malignant glioblastoma (d).*

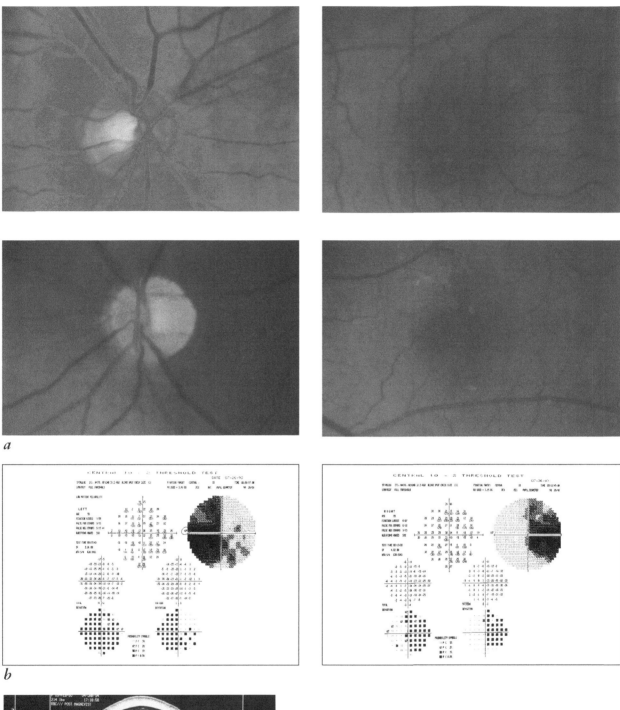

a

b

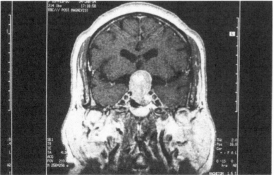

c

Figure 2.43 *Optic discs and macula appear normal OD; mild macular degeneration is evident OS (a). Obvious bitemporal visual field defects (b). A CT scan demonstrates a large pituitary mass with suprasellar extension (c).*

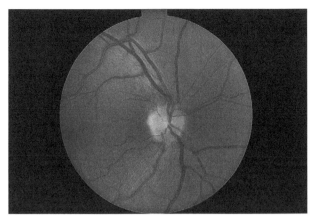

a

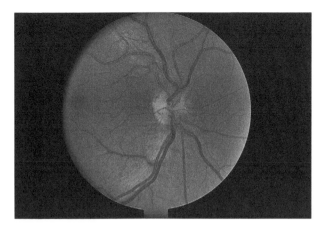

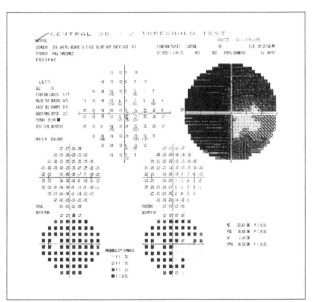

b

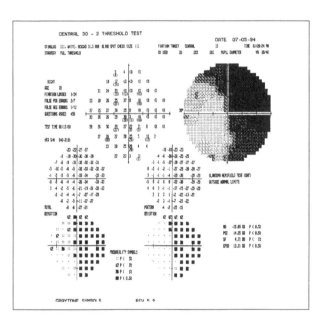

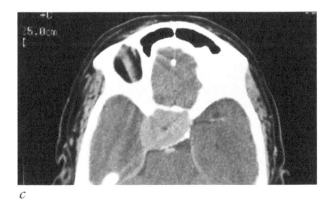

c

Figure 2.44 *Normal-appearing optic discs and fundus (a). Visual fields demonstrate an obvious bitemporal hemianopia (b). A CT scan reveals a large, enhancing suprasellar mass (c).*

these lesions is key to preserving visual function. The atrophic optic disc rarely recovers significantly.

Malingerers, on the other hand, are the bane of the neuro-ophthalmologist's existence. These patients may be very difficult to effectively evaluate and treat. By definition, they are feigning visual dysfunction for secondary gain—financial or otherwise—usually trying to bilk the system for workman's compensation or settle a personal injury lawsuit. Unilateral claimed visual dysfunction is usually easy to detect. Bilateral, feigned visual dysfunction may be very difficult and expensive to detect and prove. These patients are usually obvious. It is important to be sure that there is no true/true and unrelated cause contributing to visual dysfunction (a patient claims bare hand motion visual acuity and has a 20/25 intracanalicular meningioma). Malingerers may also have real and unrelated disease to the bane of the examiner. The most difficult to deal with are those with known real disease who embellish their symptoms and refuse to read below the 20/200 line (legal blindness). You know from your examination that the objective find-ings do not correlate with the degree of claimed visual dysfunction but proving this may be nearly impossible.

Once neuroimaging and a careful examination have ruled out real disease, what do you do with the obvious malingerer? Defer your opinion until after the next examination! Neuro-ophthalmology can be very humbling and it is less so if you are less dogmatic in your pontifications.

As a senior fellow, I was called by the junior resident one evening inquiring about a patient seen in the Emergency Room that evening. She was an older lady (65 years of age), diabetic, living alone and missing her family. She complained that she could not see well, claimed hand motion visual acuity, and the resident could detect no localizing signs. Examining her the following morning, I could get her to read 20/400 and 20/800 at near (for those in the know, that's the equivalent of finger counting). Her visual fields were definitely not localizing (Fig. 2.46a) but were quite abnormal. She could, however, recognize the resident who had examined her the previous night from the other side of the clinic. Her examination was otherwise totally unremarkable. While awaiting the return of

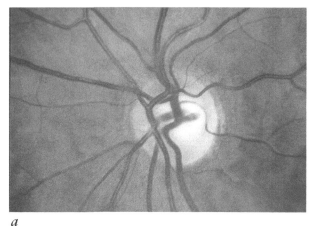

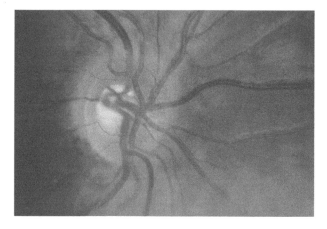

a

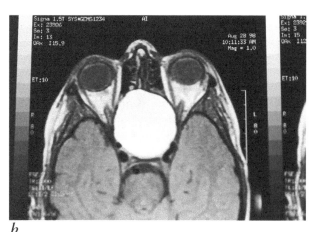

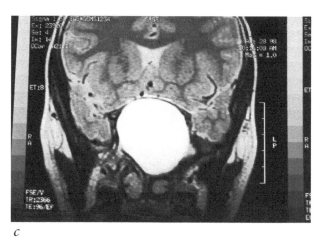

b   *c*

Figure 2.45 *The fundus demonstrating optic atrophy OD and a normal-appearing left optic disc (a). An MRI scan—axial (b) and coronal (c)—demonstrating a large cystic mass compressing the optic chiasm.*

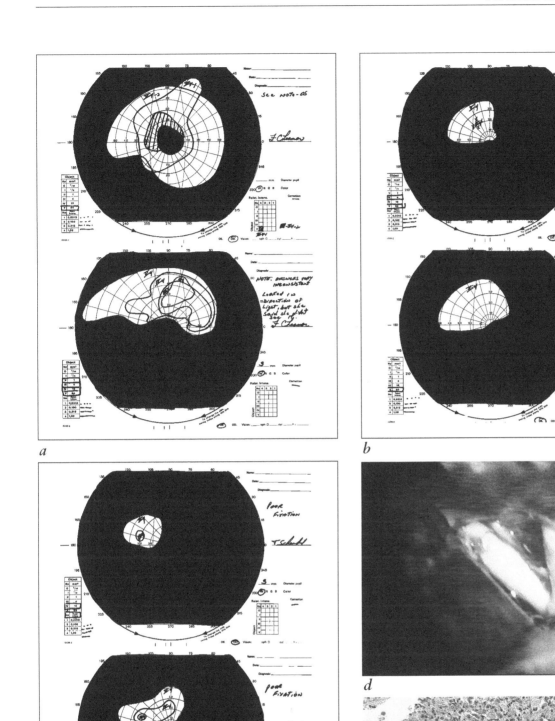

a

b

c

d

e

Figure 2.46 *Abnormal non-localizing visual fields (a), progressively deteriorating (b and c). Surgical photograph demonstrating an enlarged, atrophic intracranial optic nerve (d). A biopsy specimen demonstrating glioblastoma of the optic nerve (e).*

my preceptor, she underwent a complete and negative neuroradiologic evaluation. Upon his return she underwent further evaluation, including a negative temporal artery biopsy. The neuro-ophthalmologist thought that her visual fields demonstrated an obvious occipital flavor (Fig. 2.46b), but this did not explain her marked loss of central vision. Her vision continued to deteriorate (Fig. 2.46c) and her headaches increased. A neurosurgical consultant offered to explore her anterior visual pathways. The present author was convinced that they were doing a craniotomy on a malingerer and crowed when no compressive lesion was evident. However, the intracranial optic nerve did appear enlarged and atrophic (Fig. 2.46d), and was biopsied despite my objections.

A primary glioblastoma of the optic pathways was evident on histopathologic examination (Fig. 2.46e). Always certain; often wrong. Progressive loss of visual acuity or field still demands an explanation.

POSTERIOR VISUAL PATHWAY DYSFUNCTION

Posterior visual pathways—the optic radiations—extend from the lateral geniculate bodies to the occipital lobes of the brain, passing through the temporal and parietal lobes in the process (Fig. 2.47). Lesions affecting the visual pathways will cause distinctive, bilateral visual field defects (Fig. 2.48). Injury to the optic radiations in the temporal lobe result in a distinctive superior quadrantanopia (Fig. 2.49), since the inferior fibers pass through the temporal lobe as Meyer's loop (Fig. 2.47). Injury to the radiations in the parietal lobe results in an inferior quadrantanopia due to injury to the superior fibers of the optic radiations (Fig. 2.50). Occipital lobe injury results in very congruous homonymous hemianopias, either involving just central vision (occipital tip lesion) or the entire hemifield (Fig. 2.51). The occipital etiology of these defects is usually evident on neuro-imaging studies (Figs 2.52 and 2.53). Bilateral occipital infarction or injury results in bilateral visual field defects (Fig. 2.54). Hypotensive infarction of the occipital tip—

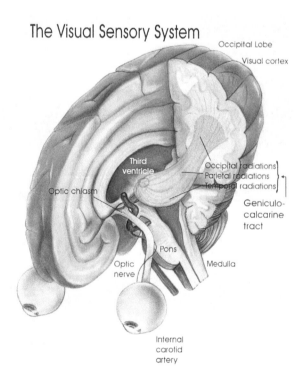

Figure 2.47 *Posterior visual pathways from the lateral geniculate body to the occipital lobe.*

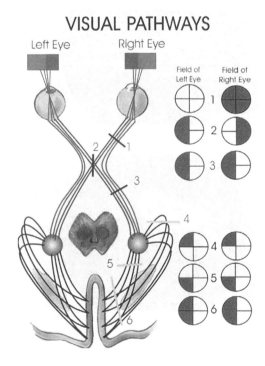

Figure 2.48 *Lesions of the posterior visual pathways result in bilateral, homonymous visual field defects.*

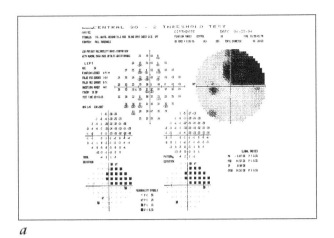 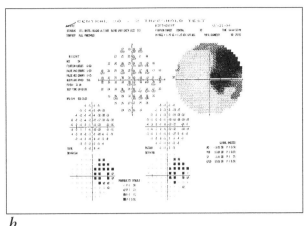

Figure 2.49 *Superior temporal quadrantanopias may be caused by temporal lobe lesions, but much more commonly by occipital lobe infarctions.*

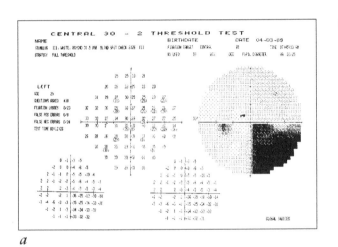 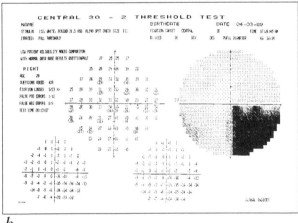

Figure 2.50 *Parietal lobe lesions may cause inferior quadrantanopias, but an occipital etiology is more common.*

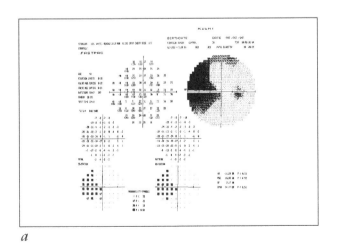 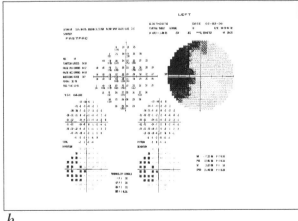

Figure 2.51 *Visual fields demonstrate a left homonymous hemianopia cuased by the vascular malformation present in the right occipital lobe.*

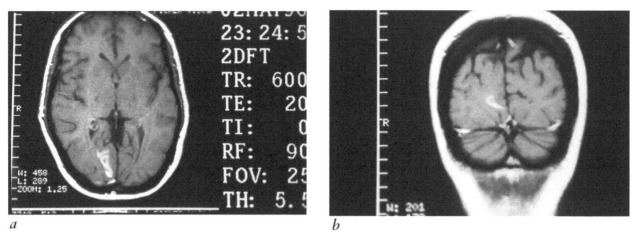

Figure 2.52 *Vascular malformation in the right occipital lobe: axial (a) and coronal (b).*

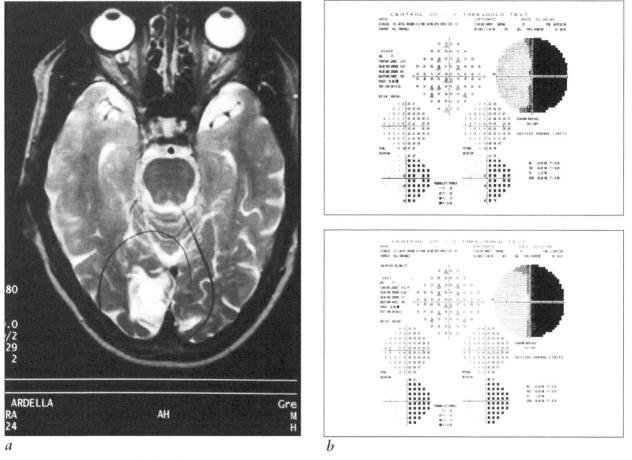

Figure 2.53 *Large occipital lobe infarction (a) causing a complete homonymous hemianopic visual field defect (b).*

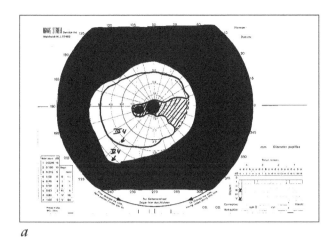

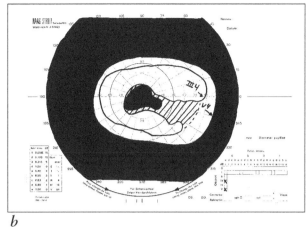

a   *b*

Figure 2.54   *Bilateral homonymous visual field defects caused by a hypotensive infarction of the tip of the occipital lobe.*

a watershed between posterior cerebral and middle cerebral circulation (Fig. 2.55)—causes a bilateral central scotoma, often involving fixation (Figs 2.54 and 2.55).

In the present author's experience, posterior visual pathway dysfunction, especially occipital lobe visual dysfunction, is often overdiagnosed by the neurologist and underdiagnosed by the ophthalmologist. Posterior visual pathway dysfunction is always bilateral, the pupils have normal reactions (there is no RAPD or light-near dissociation) and the optic discs are normal. There may be associated obvious or subtle neurologic signs.

Patients with minor occipital lobe strokes may have asymptomatic superior or inferior quadrantanopias (Figs 2.49 and 2.50), often subjectively localized to only one eye. Again, the visual field in the 'normal' eye may be diagnostic. A visual field is a valuable screening test in any patient complaining of visual dysfunction without an obvious reason.

An 81-year-old lady was referred with vague visual complaints and a putative diagnosis of GCA. Visual fields had a distinct homonymous hemianopic flavor (Fig. 2.56). An MRI demonstrated a rather massive and relatively asymptomatic occipital lobe meningioma causing her visual symptoms (Fig. 2.57). The homonymous nature of her visual field defects became more obvious with practice. The clinician has to take a bit of poetic license when interpreting visual fields, especially initial automated fields in elderly individuals. Look for respect of the vertical midline (posterior visual pathways) or the horizontal midline (retina and optic nerve). Repeat visual field tests are often much more localizing or much more normal. Do not overreact to an initial visual field unless the pathology is obvious. Many initial abnormal visual fields caused by an inattentive or

Circulation to Occipital Tip

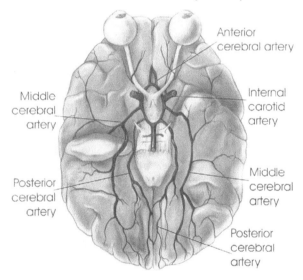

Figure 2.55   *Diagram illustrating that the occipital tip (macular vision) is a watershed between the posterior and middle cerebral circulations, making it susceptible to hypotensive infarctions with resultant bilateral loss of central vision (see Fig. 2.57).*

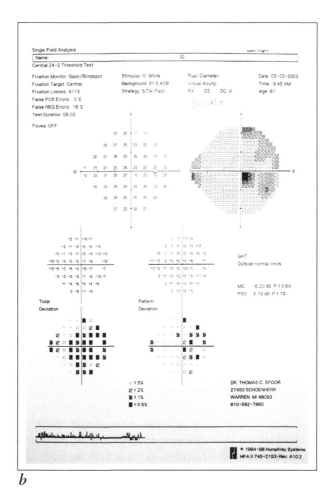

Figure 2.56   *Visual fields demonstrate a subtle, incongruous right homonymous hemianopia.*

ill-informed patient are normal when tested again. Remember that a visual field requires a cooperative, informed and responsive patient to be of diagnostic value.

Patients with multiple strokes may have multiple visual field defects. The key to diagnosing posterior visual pathway dysfunction is thinking of the diagnosis, ordering a visual field and obtaining neuroimaging studies of the appropriate area (Figs 2.52 and 2.57). With today's emphasis on stroke prevention, such efforts may be lifesaving.

Always examine the patient's fundus prior to interpreting a visual field. The present author will not interpret a visual field without a fundus examination. A dilated fundus examination often elucidates a perplexing visual field (Figs 2.58 and 2.59). You really cannot properly interpret a visual field without examining the patient, and attempts to do so are fraught with error. Those referring physicians who ask you to do so should be asked to refer their patients elsewhere. There is nothing cost-effective about making unnecessary diagnostic and management errors.

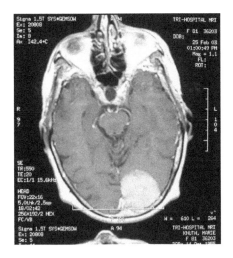

a

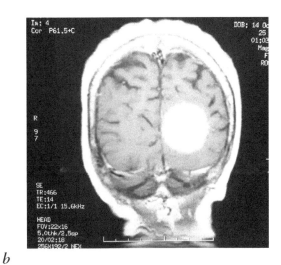

b

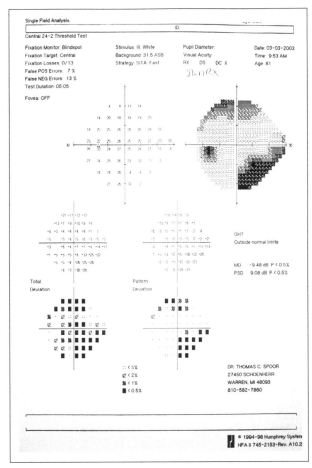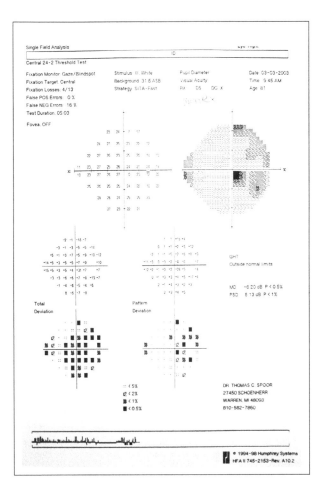

c

Figure 2.57 *MRI scans—axial (a) and coronal (b)—demonstrating a not-so-subtle occipital lobe meningioma as the cause of the subtle visual field defects (c).*

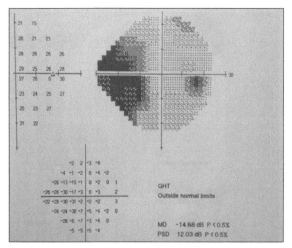

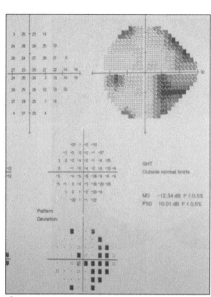

a

b

Figure 2.58   *A patient referred with abnormal, non-localizing visual fields caused by choroidal osteomas.*

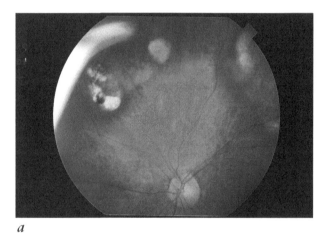

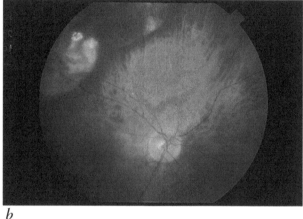

a

b

Figure 2.59   *The fundus demonstrating obvious etiology for the visual field defects shown in Fig. 2.61.*

REFERENCES

1. Comu S, Verstraeten T, Rinkoff JS. Neurologic manifestations of acute posterior multifocal placoid epitheliopathy. *Stroke* 1996; 27:996–1001.

2. Gass JD. Acute zonal occult outer retinopathy. *J Clin Neuro-Ophthal* 1993; 13:79–97.

3. Chung SM, Selhorst JB. Cancer associated retinopathy. *Ophthalmol Clinics N Am* 1992; 5:587–96.

4. Fraunfelder FT, Fraunfelder FW, Edwards R. Ocular side effects possibly associated with isotretinoin use. *Am J Ophthalmol* 2001; 132:299–305.

5. Kanski JJ, Stanislaw AM. Diseases of the macula. (Mosby: Philadelphia, 2002.)

6. Spoor TC, Hammer ME. Retinal embolism following percutaneous femoral angiography. *J Clin Neuro-Ophthalmol* 1982; 2:49–54.

7. Clarke NW, Noel LP, Barriciak M. Functional visual loss in children: a common problem with an easy solution. *Can J Ophthalmol* 1996; 31:311–13.

8. Moster ML, Galetta SL, Schatz NJ. Physiologic 'functional' visual loss. *Surv Ophthalmol* 1996; 40:395–9.

9. Thompson HS. Functional visual loss. *Am J Ophthalmol* 1985; 100:209–13.

10. Keltner JL. The California syndrome: a threat to all. *Arch Ophthalmol* 1988; 106:1053–4.

Chapter 3 The optic nerve

ANATOMY

Each optic nerve is composed of approximately one million axons from retinal ganglion cells. These axons exit the eye through the lamina cribrosa—where they are most susceptible to damage from either elevated intraocular or intracranial pressure—intermingle with axons from the opposite eye to form the optic chiasm and optic tracts, and finally synapse at the lateral geniculate bodies. Optic atrophy results from damage to the ganglion cell (ascending) or to the axon anywhere along its course from the eye to the lateral geniculate body (descending).

The optic nerve fibers arise from the retinal ganglion cells, are unmyelinated in the eye and extend along the retina as the nerve fiber layer to exit the eye as the optic nerve (Fig. 3.1a–c). The axons forming the optic nerve retain their retinal relationships. Superior temporal and nasal fibers form the superior optic nerve, inferior retinal fibers form the inferior optic nerve and the papillomacular fibers form the temporal optic nerve (Fig. 3.1b). Temporal retinal fibers arch around the papillomacular bundle to form the superior and inferior optic nerves. The increased density of fibers at the superior and inferior poles of the optic nerve is clinically significant, and swelling is an early sign of optic disc edema (Fig. 3.2) in

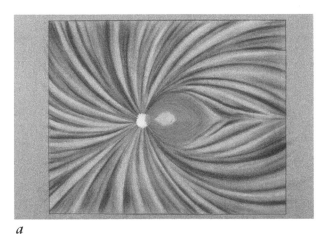

a

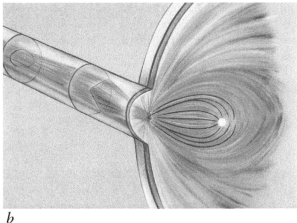

b

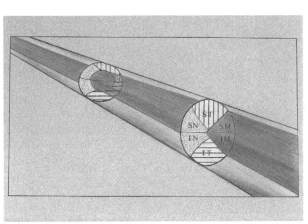

c

Figure 3.1 *Optic nerve fibers in the retina (a); optic nerve fibers (b) turning posteriorly to form the optic nerve; medial rotation of optic nerve fibers (c).*

papilledema. The nasal retinal fibers enter the optic nerve in a less dense radial pattern. As the optic nerve crosses the orbit to approach the optic chiasm, the nerve fibers gradually rotate, positioning the papillomacular fibers in the center of the optic nerve and the temporal fibers in the temporal optic nerve (Fig. 3.1c). By the time the optic nerve fibers reach the optic chiasm, the temporal fibers are positioned to pass through the chiasm uncrossed, while the nasal fibers are positioned to facilitate crossing in the chiasm.

The optic nerve is approximately 50–60 mm long from the back of the eye to the optic chiasm. It can be divided into four distinct segments: intraocular, intraorbital, intracanalicular and intracranial (Fig. 3.3).

INTRAOCULAR OPTIC NERVE

The intraocular optic nerve measures 1.5 by 1.0 mm in diameter and 1 mm in length. This surface layer, consisting of unmyelinated axons of retinal ganglion cells, is the portion of the nerve visible with the ophthalmoscope. These axons turn posteriorly to exit the globe perpendicular to the surface layer. These unmyelinated axons, divided into fascicles by astrocytes, form the prelaminar portion of the optic nerve surrounded by retina and choroid (Fig. 3.4). The nerve fibers, divided into fascicles, pass through the multiple fenestrations in the sieve-like lamina cribrosa, formed by connective tissue from the surrounding sclera and distal dura mater of the optic nerve sheath. The lamina cribrosa is the site of optic nerve injury caused by both elevated intraocular pressure (glaucoma) and elevated intracranial pressure.

INTRAORBITAL OPTIC NERVE

Posterior to the lamina cribrosa, oligodendrocytes ensheath the optic nerve in concentric wrappings of myelin, increasing its diameter to 3–4 mm. Myelination marks the beginning of the intraorbital optic nerve (Fig. 3.5a and b).

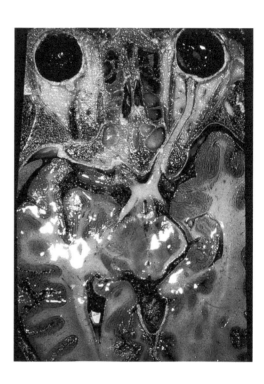

Figure 3.3 *Axial fresh cadaver section demonstrating the four segments of the optic nerve: intraocular, intraorbital, intracanalicular and intracranial.*

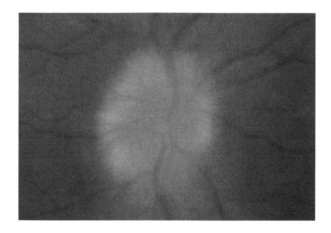

Figure 3.2 *Early papilledema demonstrating swelling at the superior and inferior poles of the optic nerve where the nerve fibers are densest.*

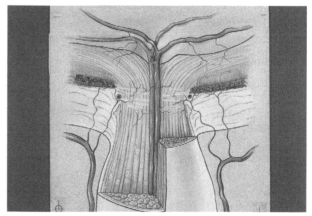

Figure 3.4 *Retinal ganglion cell axons exiting the eye to form the optic nerve.*

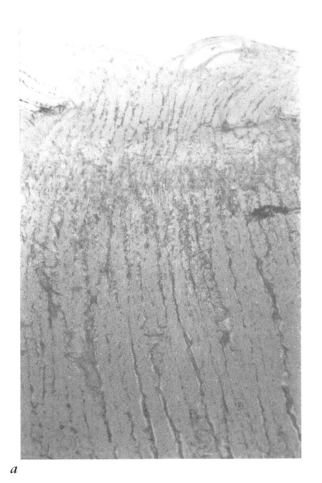

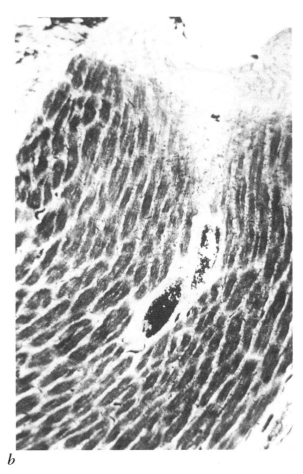

a *b*

Figure 3.5 *Histopathology of the optic nerve at the level of the lamina cribrosa. Note the difference in thickness between unmyelinated prelaminar nerve fibers and the myelinated post laminar fibers (a). Myelin stain demonstrating myelination of the retrolaminar optic nerve (b). (Courtesy of David Barsky MD).*

The intraorbital optic nerve is 25–30 mm long and extends from the eye to the orbital apex, a distance of 20–25 mm. This 6–8 mm of redundancy in the optic nerve length results in a sinuous course through the orbit allowing the optic nerve to move freely during eye movements. It also allows a considerable degree of proptosis to occur before there is significant visual dysfunction.

The intraorbital optic nerve is inseparable from the pia mater from which it obtains its blood supply. It is enveloped in arachnoid and surrounded by dura mater. The dura mater is continuous with the sclera at the posterior globe (Fig. 3.4) and fuses with the periorbita at the orbital apex, lining the optic canal. The subarachnoid space surrounding the intraorbital optic nerve freely communicates with the intracranial subarachnoid space through the optic canal (Figs 3.6 and 3.7). This allows for the free flow of spinal fluid from the brain to the optic nerve at the back of the eye. Elevated cerebrospinal fluid (CSF) pressure may be transmitted to the optic

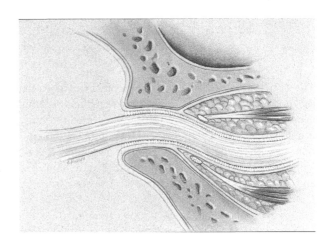

Figure 3.6 *Relationship of the intraorbital optic nerve to the orbital apex and optic canal. Note that the dura of the optic nerve becomes the dural lining of the optic canal.*

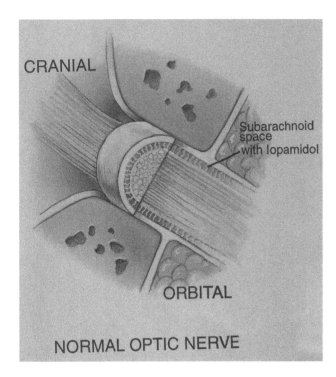

Figure 3.7 *The subarachnoid space of the optic nerve is continuous with the intracranial subarachnoid space.*

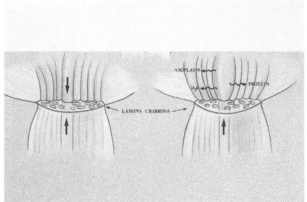

Figure 3.8 *Compression of the optic nerve fibers at the lamina cribrosa causes axoplasmic stasis, transudation of fluid and evolves to papilledema.*

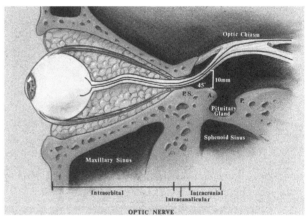

Figure 3.9 *Sagittal section demonstrating the intracranial optic nerves forming the optic chiasm.*

nerve causing papilledema and visual dysfunction by compressing optic nerve fibers at the lamina cribrosa (Fig. 3.8). At the orbital apex, the optic nerve is surrounded by the origins of the superior, inferior and medial rectus forming the annulus of Zinn. This close relationship between muscles and optic nerve accounts for the pain with eye motion present in patients with posterior optic nerve inflammation.

INTRACANALICULAR OPTIC NERVE

The optic nerve exits the orbit and enters the brain via the optic canal (Fig. 3.3). The intracanalicular optic nerve is 6–10 mm long and fitted tightly into the optic canal, with the dura adherent to the optic canal and continuous with the dura of the intraorbital optic nerve (Fig. 3.6). In the optic canal, the optic nerve is quite immobile and subject to injury by trauma and compression by radiologically silent lesions.

INTRACRANIAL OPTIC NERVE

Exiting the intracranial optic canal, the optic nerve loses its layer of dura mater and extends 10 mm posterior and

medial at a 45° incline to join the contralateral optic nerve and form the optic chiasm (Figs 3.3 and 3.9). The intracranial optic nerves are bound superiorly by the frontal lobes and the olfactory tracts of the brain, separated by the anterior cerebral and anterior communicating arteries (Fig. 3.10). The internal carotid artery lies lateral to each optic nerve and is often attached to it by the ophthalmic artery arising from the carotid and lying inferior and lateral to the optic nerve (Fig. 3.10). Medially, the posterior ethmoid air cells and sphenoid sinus border the optic nerve (Fig. 3.3). Inferior to the optic nerve lies the planum sphenoidale and the pituitary gland (Fig. 3.9). Infections, tumors and aneurysms of these intracranial structures may present as an isolated optic neuropathy or a chiasmal syndrome.

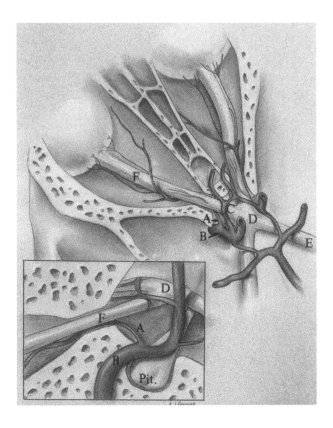

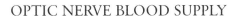

Figure 3.10 *Relationship of the optic nerve and chiasm to adjacent intracranial arteries. A, ophthalmic artery; B, int. carotid artery; C, anterior communicating artery; D, optic chiasm; E, optic tract; F, optic nerve.*

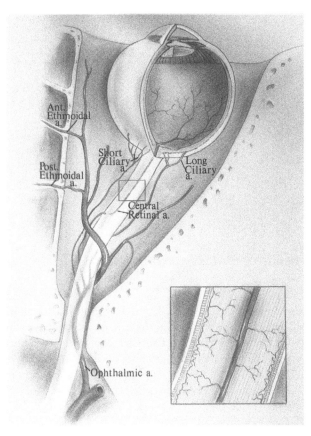

Figure 3.11 *Ophthalmic artery entering the orbit through the optic canal, passing inferior to the optic nerve.*

OPTIC NERVE BLOOD SUPPLY

The eye and optic nerve receive their blood supply from branches of the ophthalmic artery. The ophthalmic artery arises from the internal carotid artery lateral to the optic nerve. Passing inferior to the optic nerve, it enters the orbit through the optic foramen (Fig. 3.11). The central retinal artery arises from the ophthalmic artery and penetrates the optic nerves 6–12 mm posterior to the globe (Fig. 3.12). The major branch passes anteriorly to nourish the retina and a minor branch extends posteriorly through the optic nerve. Small, perforating branches nourish the central portions of the intraorbital optic nerve. As it enters the eye, the central retinal artery divides into major retinal branches. Capillaries derived from these branches nourish the nerve-fiber layer of the retina and the surface of the optic disc.

The short posterior ciliary arteries are the most significant blood supply to the optic nerve. These vessels nourish the choroid, prelaminar optic nerve, lamina cribrosa and form the pial plexus along the entire retrolaminar

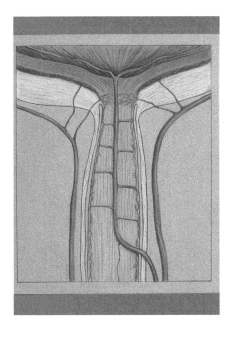

Figure 3.12 *Branches of the central retinal artery, the long and short ciliary arteries.*

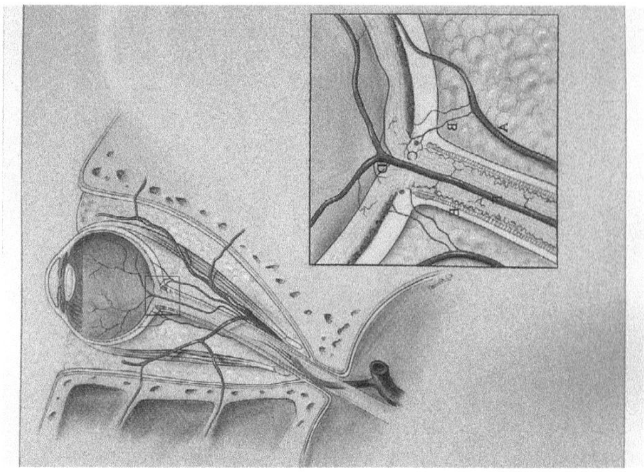

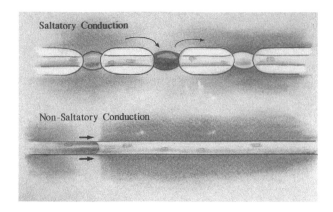

Figure 3.14 *Nerve conduction in a myelinated and unmyelinated axon.*

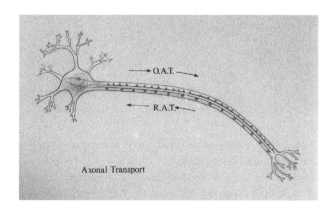

Figure 3.13 *Optic nerve and retinal blood supply.*

optic nerve (Figs 3.4 and 3.13). Compromise of a short ciliary artery may result in optic nerve head or peripapillary retinal infarction. Excessive damage to the short ciliary arteries may compromise optic nerve function. Obstruction of this blood supply is clinically significant in both arteritic and nonarteritic ischemic optic neuropathy.

MYELINATION

Myelination of the optic nerve posterior to the lamina cribrosa is accomplished by oligodendrocytes. Myelination insulates an axon, making impulse conduction more efficient. The impulse in a myelinated axon propagates by depolarizing from one node of Ranvier to the next, passing more rapidly than an action potential in an unmyelinated axon (Fig. 3.14). This conserves metabolic energy since the axon must repolarize only at the nodes of Ranvier and not along the entire length of the axon. Myelination is not necessary for vision but it makes it much more efficient. Newborn infants can see but their optic nerves are incompletely myelinated. Patients with demyelinating disease of their optic nerves have an increased latency on visually evoked potential testing, since the impulses are propagated by action potentials in demyelinated axons rather than in nodes of Ranvier in myelinated axons.

AXOPLASMIC TRANSPORT (FIG. 3.15)

Intracellular movement of molecules and organelles occurs in all cells. In neurons it is known as axoplasmic transport. Axoplasmic transport is an active process necessary for survival of the ganglion cell body and its

Figure 3.15 *Fast and slow axoplasmic transport.*

axon: it occurs in both rapid and slow phases. Nutrients, proteins and transmitters are transported orthograde from the ganglion cell to the axon synaptic terminal. This is rapid orthograde transport at a rate of 400 mm/day. Cytostructural elements are transported by slow orthograde transmission at a rate of 1–4 mm/day. Pinocytotic vesicles and lysosomes are transported retrograde from the synaptic terminal to the ganglion cell body at a rate of 200 mm/day. Retrograde axoplasmic transmission conveys information to the cell body about the metabolic state of the axon and synaptic function, allowing the cell body to modify amounts and types of substances manufactured for orthograde transport. Altered neuronal activity, axonal degeneration or trauma may modulate the retrograde signal to the neuron. This may be the mechanism inducing chromatolysis and destruction of the neuron after injury to the axon. The clinical correlation is loss of retinal ganglion cells 4–6 weeks after injury to the optic nerve axons. These are active transport mechanisms that are energy dependent and necessary for the survival and function of the ganglion cell and its axon. Papilledema and acute elevation of intraocular pressure may disrupt axoplasmic flow. Any process interfering with this energy-dependent process may impair it, including ischemia, compression, inflammation and toxins. Some believe that impaired axoplasmic flow may be the final common pathway for optic nerve dysfunction and damage.[1]

OPTIC NEUROPATHIES

Damage to the optic nerve results in an optic neuropathy accompanied by decreased visual function (subtle to obvious), dyschromatopsia and a relative afferent pupillary defect (RAPD). There are many causes of optic nerve dysfunction, some of which are eminently treatable and others that are not. Distinguishing between the two in a timely fashion and diagnosing the uncommon, but possibly treatable, cause of optic nerve dysfunction is the art and science of neuro-ophthalmology.

Evaluation, diagnosis and management of optic neuropathies is the essence of neuro-ophthalmology. Although the seasoned practitioner may trivialize the evaluation of another optic neuritis or ischemic optic neuropathy, a clinical disaster may be lurking right around the corner, and the unexpected must always be expected. Intervention may have dramatic results—be that dramatically bad or dramatically good.

CASE STUDY 1

A 40-year-old lady presented with decreased vision and pain with motion of her left eye. A computerized tomography (CT) scan and sinus x-rays were normal. Examination revealed a definite optic neuropathy with markedly decreased vision, a RAPD, and a normal ocular and fundus examination. Since the amount of pain was significantly greater and more sustained than usually encountered with optic neuritis, the CT scan of the brain and orbits was repeated, and she was started on oral prednisone with the diagnosis of idiopathic orbital inflammation affecting the optic nerve. She returned 3 days later with a totally normal repeat CT scan, visual acuity had improved to 20/20 in the affected eye, visual field had normalized and the RAPD was gone, as was the dyschromatopsia. After a round of self-praise, steroids were tapered and a happy patient went on her way. Two weeks later she called with recurrent orbital pain and visual loss. Since she was unable to come in for examination, steroids were increased and the pain improved. She returned 3 days later with total visual loss and a frozen globe. Yet another CT scan demonstrated some enlargement of the optic nerve, erosion of the optic canal and subtle mucosal thickening in the sphenoid sinus (Fig. 3.16). Biopsy demonstrated aspergillosis (Fig. 3.17), confirmed by culture. Her clinical condition deteriorated rapidly and she died 10 days later. Autopsy confirmed aspergillosis of her optic canal, orbital apex and sphenoid sinus (Fig. 3.18).

This patient was encountered over 20 years ago and the present author would probably treat a similar patient

Figure 3.16 *A CT scan demonstrating enlargement of the optic nerve, erosion of the optic canal and subtle mucosal thickening of the sphenoid sinus.*

Figure 3.17 *Biopsy of sphenoid sinus mucosa demonstrating Aspergillus hyphae confirmed by culture.*

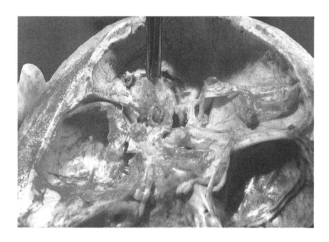

Figure 3.18 *Autopsy specimen demonstrating erosion of the optic canal, invasion and necrosis of the optic nerve by aspergillosis.*

in the same manner today, except more sophisticated imaging studies would probably be negative. Managing patients with optic neuropathies has always been, and remains, challenging. Twenty years later, a similar patient was referred for evaluation of painful diplopia and visual loss.

CASE STUDY 2

This lady was evaluated shortly after the present author presented the patient with aspergillosis at the International Neuro-Ophthalmologic Society meeting. One of the ranking senior neuro-ophthalmologists stated that, 'Treating optic neuropathies with corticosteroids repre-

sented a nervous doctor treating a nervous patient and was not science'.

This patient had the misfortune of being referred shortly after that meeting. A 28-year-old lady was referred with a swollen optic nerve and visual loss to counting fingers. Visual field was markedly constricted (Fig. 3.19a and b). CT scan was normal, as were serologies. No treatment was offered. She returned 1 month later with optic atrophy, and permanently decreased visual acuity and visual field (Fig. 3.20a and b). Timely corticosteroid therapy may have been sight saving. Patients with atypical optic neuritis should be fully evaluated, followed carefully and treated when the optic neuritis becomes atypical. Patients with typical optic neuritis may be reassured and observed. The clinician and patient must react and respond when typical optic neuritis becomes atypical.

CASE STUDY 3

A 67-year-old lady was referred with painful diplopia due to a partial third-nerve paresis. Magnetic resonance imaging (MRI) was normal. Visual function in the left eye was subjectively decreased, but this could not be confirmed with objective signs. She was not treated. She returned several weeks later, her third-nerve paresis partially resolved. She continued to complain of decreased vision. A trace RAPD was present. Visual acuity and field remained normal. Observation continued until her pain worsened and her visual function deteriorated. With evidence for progressive visual loss, repeat MRI was performed, demonstrating some subtle thickening and enhancement of the optic nerve at the orbital apex. She was treated with 80 mg prednisone daily with rapid resolution of her pain, diplopia and normalization of her

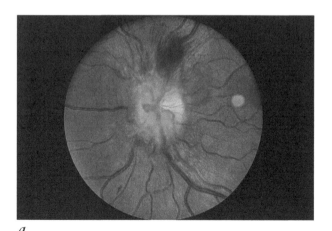

a

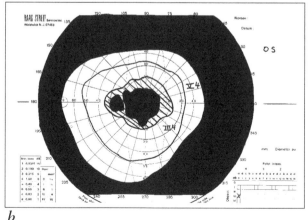

b

Figure 3.19 *Swollen optic disc (a) and central scotoma (b) in a patient with atypical optic neuritis.*

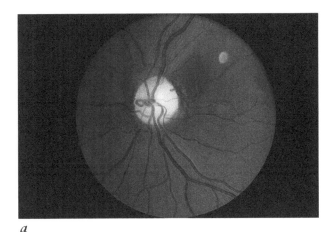

a

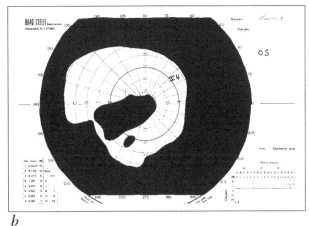

b

Figure 3.20 *Ensuing optic atrophy (a) and a dense central scotoma (b).*

visual function. Steroids were tapered and discontinued. Her visual function remained unimpaired.

This lady had apical idiopathic orbital inflammation causing pain, a partial third-nerve paresis and eventually an inflammatory optic neuropathy that improved dramatically and completely with corticosteroid therapy. Treatment was timely and effective in restoring visual function.

OPTIC ATROPHY

CLINICAL CAVEAT

Any patient presenting with non-glaucomatous optic atrophy without an obvious explanation requires a neuroimaging study.

Each optic nerve is composed of one million axons of retinal ganglion cells. Destruction of either the ganglion cell or its axon will cause pallor of the optic disc (optic atrophy). If an axon is damaged, its ganglion cell will autolyse causing loss of the retinal ganglion cell layer as seen in endstage glaucoma. This represents descending optic atrophy.

ASCENDING OPTIC ATROPHY

Analogously, if a retinal ganglion cell is destroyed, its axon will degenerate with resultant optic atrophy: this is ascending optic atrophy. Ascending optic atrophy is secondary to a primary retinal disorder destroying ganglion cells. Examples include central retinal artery occlusion (CRAO; Fig. 3.21), extensive macular lesions (Fig.

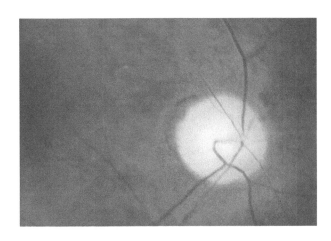

Figure 3.21 *Optic atrophy due to diffuse loss of retinal ganglion cells after central retinal artery occlusion.*

3.22), infiltration and destruction of ganglion cells (Tay-Sachs and Batten-Mayou diseases; Fig. 3.23) or diffuse retinal disease (retinitis pigmentosa; Fig. 3.24). There are a variety of metabolic (mucopolysaccharidoses, lipidoses) and degenerative neurologic diseases (Friedreichs's ataxia, spinocerebellar degeneration, Charcot-Marie-Tooth disease) associated with optic atrophy and visual loss. Detailed descriptions of these entities may be found elsewhere.[2]

Retinal causes of optic atrophy should be easy to diagnose once they are considered. A complete examination of the fundus, including the macula and peripheral retina, coupled with a timely use of the electroretinogram (ERG), fluorescein angiogram and retinal consultation, is usually diagnostic. The vast majority of retinal ganglion cells are in the macular region. A large macular

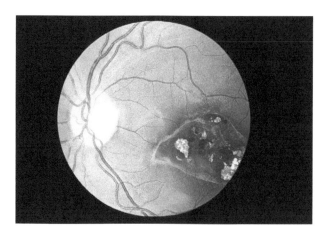

Figure 3.22 *Sector optic atrophy due to an extensive macular scar.*

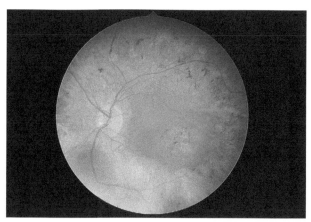

Figure 3.24 *Optic atrophy due to diffuse loss of retinal function in a patient with retinitis pigmentosa.*

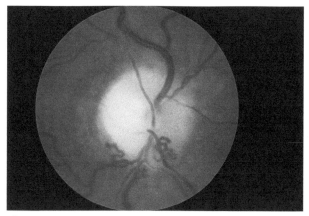

a

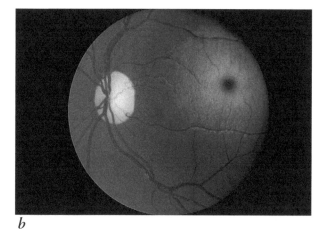

b

Figure 3.23 *Descending optic atrophy in a patient with chronic atrophic poapilledema due to neglected pseudotumour cerebri (a) Optic atrophy due to diffuse loss of retinal ganglion cells in a patient with Tay-Sachs disease (b).*

scar may cause optic atrophy, especially temporal pallor (Fig. 3.22). A normal-appearing optic nerve would be compatible with extensive panretinal photocoagulation sparing the macula (Fig. 3.25).

DESCENDING OPTIC ATROPHY

Any process that damages enough optic nerve axons will eventually cause optic atrophy and loss of retinal ganglion cells. The optic nerve may be transected in the deep orbit with total loss of vision, an amaurotic pupil and a totally normal-appearing optic disc (Fig. 3.26a). Over a

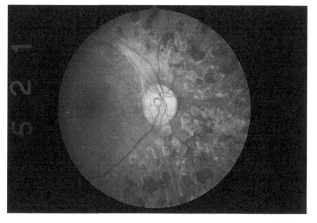

Figure 3.25 *Normal-appearing optic nerve after diffuse retinal damage sparing the macula after panretinal photocoagulation.*

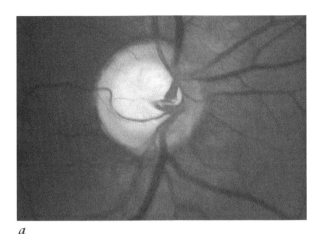 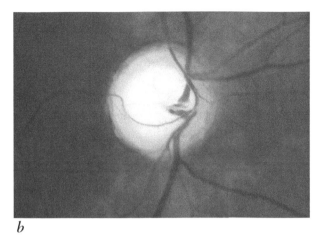

a *b*

Figure 3.26 *Appearance of the optic nerve immediately after a penetrating injury resulting in total visual loss (a). Optic atrophy develops over a 4–6-week period (b).*

4–6-week period, optic atrophy will develop (Fig. 3.26b). The more posterior the injury, the longer it takes for optic atrophy to occur. Any process—compression, trauma, demyelination, infarction or toxins affecting the visual pathways anterior to the lateral geniculate bodies—may cause descending optic atrophy. When confronted with a pale optic disc and no reliable history as to its cause, the ophthalmoscopic appearance of the optic nerve and fundus may be helpful in several ways. Obvious pathology in the macula may make the diagnosis of ascending optic atrophy clear and obviate the need for neuroimaging, directing the evaluation back to the retina where it belongs (Fig. 3.27). If the optic disc is pale and there is obvious attenuation of the retinal arterioles throughout the fundus (Fig. 3.28), this is diagnostic of an

old CRAO, and no further neuroradiologic evaluation is necessary. If the optic disc appears obviously glaucomatous with cupping and obliteration of the neuroretinal rim (Fig. 3.29), in conjunction with elevated intraocular pressure (IOP) and appropriate visual field changes, glaucoma may be diagnosed and treated, with no further evaluation necessary. On the other hand, if pallor of the neuroretinal rim accompanies the cupping, further evaluation is necessary (Figs 3.30 and 3.31). All other optic atrophy requires further evaluation to determine its etiology. Neuroimaging is readily available and should be utilized if the cause of the optic atrophy is not obvious. A baseline visual field should be obtained, remembering Dr J Lawton Smith's aphorism that the most important visual field obtained in evaluating an optic neuropathy is

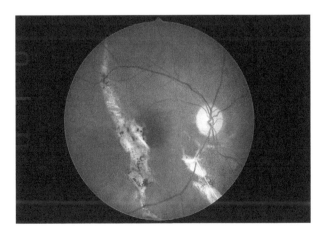
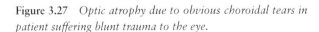

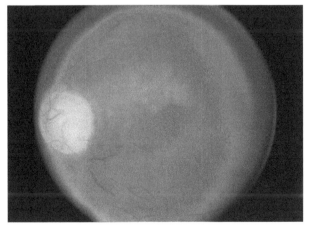

Figure 3.27 *Optic atrophy due to obvious choroidal tears in patient suffering blunt trauma to the eye.*

Figure 3.28 *Attenuated arterioles and optic atrophy in a patient with an antecedent CRAO.*

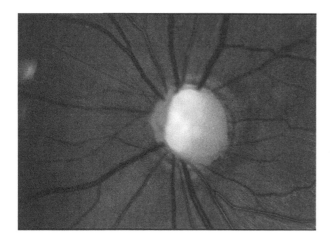

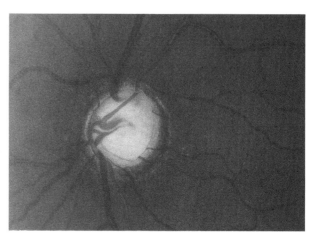

Figure 3.29 *Obvious glaucomatous optic atrophy with markedly enlarged cup-to-disc ratio and obliteration of the neuroretinal rim.*

Figure 3.30 *Pseudoglaucoma due to a compressive intracranial lesion. Enlarged cup-to-disc ratio is accompanied by pallor of the neuroretinal rim.*

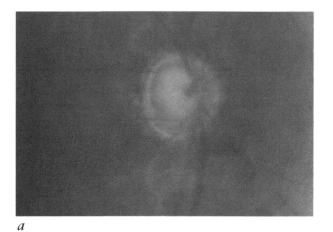

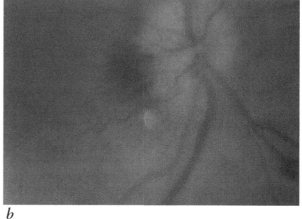

a   *b*

Figure 3.31 *Pseudoglaucoma with enlarged cup-to-disc ratio and neuroretinal rim pallor due to diffuse loss of optic nerve fibers in patient with giant cell arteritis (a). Appearance of the optic disc during the acute arteritic event the previous year (b).*

that of the normal eye. An MRI scan with gadolinium enhancement is the standard of care in the USA. If this is negative (review it yourself), repeat the visual field 1 month later. If it is improved or stable, you can be quite sure there is no progressive process occurring and the patient has a static optic neuropathy (antecedent demyelination, ischemia, trauma or congenital). If visual field loss progresses in the face of a normal MRI scan, consider one of the medical etiologies for optic atrophy (syphilis, Lyme disease or sarcoidosis; see below). Remember that 'chronic' optic neuritis does not exist. Progressive visual loss still demands an explanation. When confronted with optic atrophy and optociliary shunt vessels (Fig. 3.32) think in terms of compression by

meningioma or elevated intracranial pressure. If shunt vessels are more prominent than optic atrophy, consider a remote central retinal vein occlusion (Fig. 3.33).

GLAUCOMA

Glaucoma is the most common optic neuropathy seen in an ophthalmologist's practice and sometimes a perplexing and overdiagnosed entity when presenting in the neurologist's office. The diagnosis is not difficult when presented with an elevated IOP, arcuate visual field

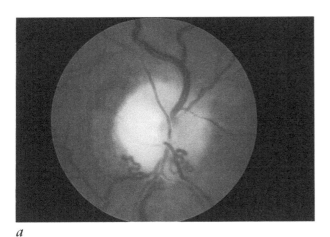

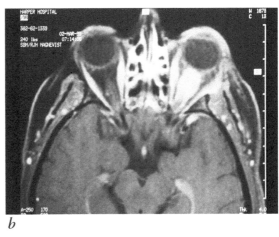

a   *b*

Figure 3.32 *Optic atrophy and optociliary shunt vessels (a) due to chronic compression of the optic nerve by an optic nerve sheath meningioma manifest as optic nerve enhancement on MRI scan (b).*

defects, a nasal step and an increased cup-to-disc ratio with obliteration of the neuroretinal rim (Fig. 3.34). The glaucomatous optic disc has a distinctive appearance. There is an increased cup-to-disc ratio (Figs 3.29 and 3.34), the neuroretinal rim may be thinned (Fig. 3.34) or obliterated (Fig. 3.29), but never pale. Pallor of the neuroretinal rim (Figs 3.30 and 3.31) indicates a non-glaucomatous process. Classic glaucomatous optic atrophy occurs in the presence of elevated intraocular pressure or a history of elevated IOP. Visual field defects are often distinctive and correlate with the appearance of the optic disc (Fig. 3.35).

LOW-TENSION GLAUCOMA (LTG)

LTG is a diagnosis of exclusion. If the optic disc appears glaucomatous but the IOP is normal, carefully examine the neuroretinal rim. If pallor is present, consider the pseudoglaucomas—compression, previous infarction, trauma, demyelination, toxins and syphilis.

LTG is indistinguishable from glaucoma due to an elevated IOP except for the pressure elevation in the latter. Many patients labeled with the moniker LTG probably have chronic open-angle glaucoma with unrecognized elevated IOP, a secondary glaucoma that has not been

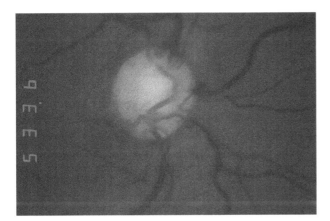

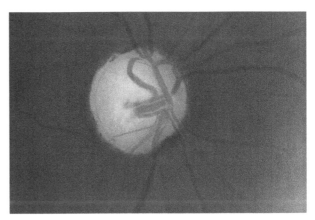

Figure 3.33 *Optociliary shunt vessels without obvious optic atrophy most likely due to a remote central retina vein occlusion.*

Figure 3.34 *Glaucomatous optic atrophy with an increased cup-to-disc ratio and thinning but no pallor of the neuroretinal rim.*

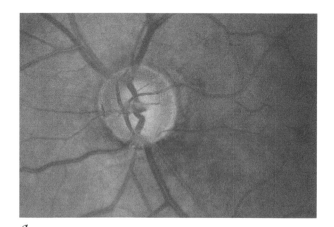
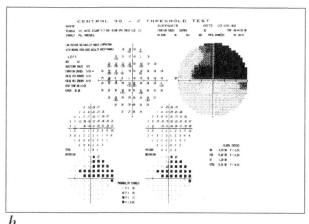

a   b

Figure 3.35   *Inferior notching of the optic disc (a) with a corresponding superior visual field defect (b).*

diagnosed, or burned-out glaucoma. There are some patients with glaucomatous-appearing optic nerves, visual field defects who have never had a documented IOP > 21 mmHg (Fig. 3.36). Also consider undetected diurnal variations in IOP and other causes of intermittent elevation of IOP—total inversion (head standing), subacute angle closure attacks or glaucomatocyclitic crisis.[3]

Since LTG is a diagnosis of exclusion, all of these patients should have an MRI scan to rule out a compressive lesion, and have repeated IOP measurements and sequential visual fields. Many patients have static, nonprogressive visual field defects often dense and closer to fixation than those found in comparable-appearing optic discs chronic open-angle glaucoma (Fig. 3.37). These optic discs may demonstrate focal atrophy and cupping accompanied by a peripapillary hemorrhage (Fig. 3.38). If there is no evidence for progressive visual field changes or changes in the appearance of the optic disc, these

patients may be safely followed with serial visual fields and optic disc photographs. If there is evidence for slow, relentless progression of visual field loss, central vision and color vision are often spared, differentiating LTG from other progressive optic neuropathies.

There are several theoretical etiologies for LTG. The present author favors an optic disc that for whatever reason cannot tolerate otherwise normal IOP, i.e. the normal pressure is more than the optic disc can tolerate. An ischemic infarction of the optic disc could account for the stable visual field defects evident in many of these patients, as well as the increased incidence of migraine headache and ischemic white matter changes present in patients with LTG. Another published theory suggested compression of the intracranial optic nerve by an enlarged carotid artery with a resultant optic neuropathy.[4]

If there is no evidence for progressive loss of visual field, the majority of patients with LTG may be observed

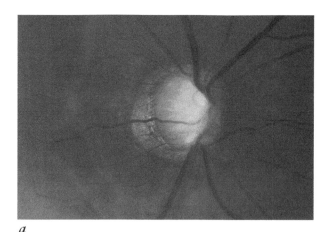
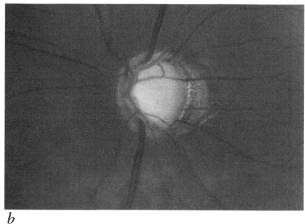

a   b

Figure 3.36   *LTG with enlarged cup-to-disc ratio, obliteration of the neuroretinal rim, and a never documented IOP > 20 mmHg.*

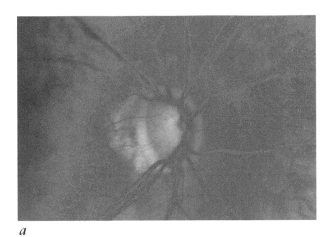

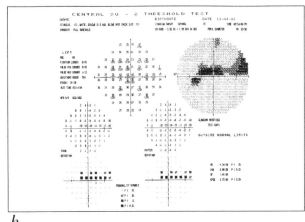

a *b*

Figure 3.37 *LTG with inferior optic disc notching (a) with a corresponding central visual field defect (b).*

without treatment. If there is progressive visual field loss, some intervention is necessary. Both optic nerve sheath decompression and glaucoma filtration surgery have their advocates. A more sensible approach would entail using one of the many glaucoma eye drops to lower the 'normal' IOP and see if that retards the visual field loss.

PSEUDOGLAUCOMA

Any optic neuropathy may cause an arcuate scotoma. The glaucomatous arcuate scotoma will be accompanied by visible notching of the neuroretinal rim (Figs 3.35 and 3.37). A swollen or normal-appearing optic disc may accompany the arcuate scotoma caused by other optic

neuropathies. Eventually, neuroretinal rim pallor will accompany the disc cupping (Fig. 3.31).

Pseudoglaucoma is acquired cupping of the optic disc with a non-glaucomatous etiology. Any cause of axonal attrition and death may result in optic disc cupping. Pallor of the neuroretinal rim (Fig. 3.31) most often accompanies increased cupping caused by compression, infarction, inflammation and trauma. The presence of pallor distinguishes these conditions from glaucomatous optic disc cupping (Fig. 3.39). In glaucoma the neuroretinal rim may become obliterated (Fig. 3.29) but pallor is not evident (Fig. 3.34). Visual loss is often not proportional to the appearance of the optic disc (Fig. 3.40). The patient in Fig. 3.40 was referred for evaluation of glaucoma due to his asymmetric cup-to-disc ratio. Visual acuity and field were markedly decreased in the right eye,

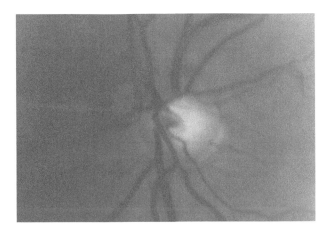

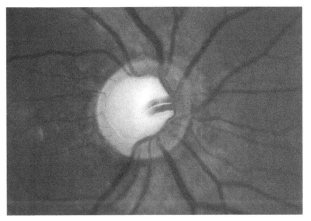

Figure 3.38 *Peripapillary hemorrhage in a patient with optic disc notching may indicate decompensation of the optic nerve head or be due to an unrelated posterior vitreous detachment.*

Figure 3.39 *Pallor of the neuroretinal rim due to a traumatic optic neuropathy superimposed upon pre-existent glaucomatous cupping.*

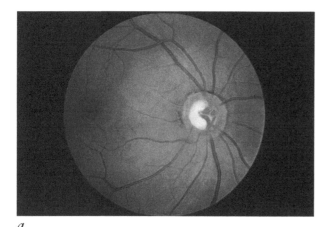

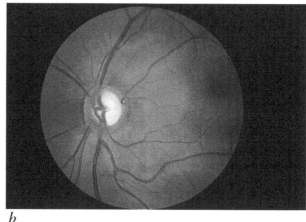

a   *b*

Figure 3.40 *Asymmetric cup-to-disc ratio out of proportion to the patient's visual loss and RAPD.*

out of proportion to the degree of disc cupping. A CT scan demonstrated a large meningioma compressing both optic nerves (Fig. 3.41).

Myopic optic discs may appear glaucomatous (Fig. 3.42). Axial myopes tend to have a higher incidence of glaucoma and ocular hypertension. Myopia is also more common in patients with open-angle glaucoma. Myopic discs should be suspected of being glaucomatous.[5]

Optic pits are defects of the neural retinal rim with discrete, sharp margins (Fig. 3.43a), which are usually distinct from the disc margin and cup. They are usually unilateral (88%) and often located inferotemporally. Their location and distinct, sharp margins distinguish them from glaucomatous cupping: they may also be accompanied by a serous detachment of the macula (Fig. 3.43b).

Tilted optic discs arise from the optic nerve entering the eye at an oblique angle, leaving a scleral crescent and a tilted-appearing optic disc (Fig. 3.44). These are common in high myopes and may be accompanied by bitemporal visual field defects attached to the blind spot. These visual field defects do not respect the vertical midline and the cause is obvious if you think of it. They should not be confused with a bitemporal hemianopia due to chiasmal compression.

Colobomas of the optic disc are congenital abnormalities, non-progressive and often bilateral. They result from failure of embryonic fetal tissue to fuse and are often accompanied by colobomas of the retina, choroid and inferior iris (Fig. 3.45).

The enlarged optic disc with a central staphylomatous depression present in the morning glory optic disc

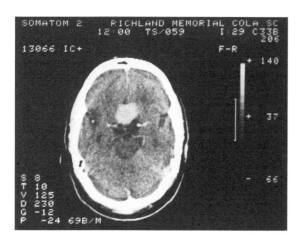

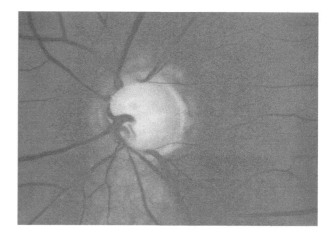

Figure 3.41 *A CT scan demonstrating a suprasellar meningioma.*

Figure 3.42 *Tilted myopic optic disc may be associated with or mistaken for glaucomatous cupping.*

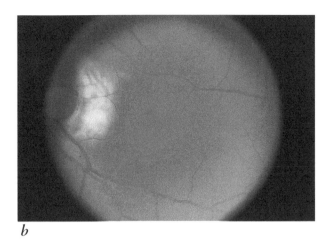

a

b

c

Figure 3.43 *Large optic pit (a) with associated serous detachment of the macula (b); and a smaller optic pit (c).*

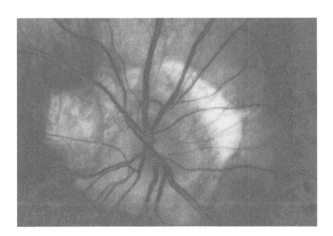

Figure 3.44 *Tilted optic disc with scleral crescent in a highly myopic eye.*

(Fig. 3.46) may be mistaken for glaucoma. This enlarged optic disc, surrounded by a halo of pigment with retinal blood vessels radially looped over its edges, has a distinct clinical appearance (Fig. 3.46). These eyes usually have very poor visual function.

Dysthyroid orbitopathy may mimic glaucoma. These patients often have elevated IOP due to elevated orbital pressure caused by enlarged muscles and orbital fat compressing the globe and its venous blood flow. The simple diagnostic key is that when patients are asked to elevate their eyes, IOP will rise > 4 mmHg. This sign is diagnostic of a restrictive orbitopathy. A tight inferior rectus muscle tethers the eye and IOP rises as the patient attempts to elevate it. In the uncommon situation when the inferior rectus is normal and the medial rectus is the only muscle involved, abducting the eye will cause a similar elevation of intraocular pressure. It is important

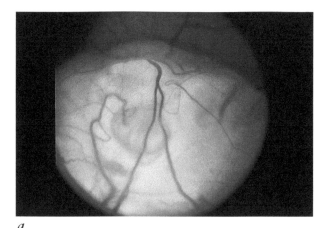
a

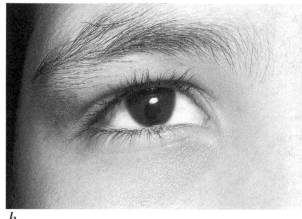
b

Figure 3.45 *Colobomatous optic disc (a) associated with an iris coloboma (b).*

to realize that this elevated pressure rarely causes cupping of the optic disc or discernible visual field defects.[6]

IOP elevation due to dysthyroid orbitopathy rarely needs to be treated and even more rarely needs aggressive treatment. The patient in Fig. 3.47a was being treated by a glaucoma specialist with pilocarpine, Timoptic and systemic acetazolamide, and had undergone two laser trabeculoplasties in attempts to lower his IOP, which caused neither significant field changes nor disc cupping (Fig. 3.47b and c). Prior to trabeculectomy, the present author was asked to render a second opinion. Orbital decompression was performed (Fig. 3.47d), IOP normalized and glaucoma medications discontinued. The patient, with obvious stigmata of thyroid eye disease (Fig. 3.48a) whose CT scan is depicted in Fig. 3.48b, actually underwent cataract extraction with trabeculec-

tomy to treat visual loss and elevated IOP caused by severe dysthyroid orbitopathy.

Caveats to help distinguish pseudoglaucoma from glaucoma include visual loss not proportional to the appearance of the optic disc, pallor of the neuroretinal rim, atypical visual field defects (respecting the vertical midline, central or centro-cecal), and rapid onset or progression of visual loss. These are not characteristic of glaucoma and should alert the clinician to look elsewhere for the correct etiology.

HEREDITARY OPTIC NEUROPATHIES

Awareness of these entities theoretically should allow the clinician to avoid expensive and time-consuming imaging studies; but in reality, in our medico-legal quagmire, most of these patients are imaged regardless of the clinical picture. These patients have visual loss due to optic nerve dysfunction. It may be mild or profound, is untreatable, and there are a variety of inheritance patterns.

LEBER'S HEREDITARY OPTIC NEUROPATHY (LHON)

This should not be confused with Leber's congenital amaurosis—blindness due to diffuse photoreceptor dysfunction occurring in infants. Patients with LHON present with subacute sequential visual loss in their second or third decade of life, and 80–90% are males. Inheritance is maternal via cytoplasmic mitochondrial DNA.

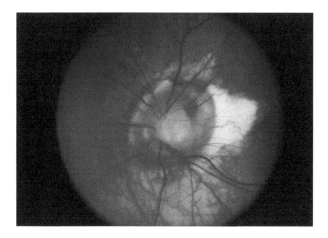

Figure 3.46 *Megalopapilla.*

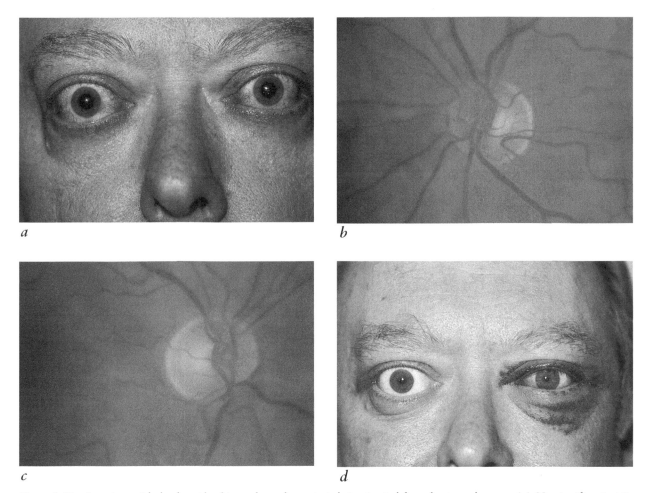

a

b

c

d

Figure 3.47 *A patient with dysthyroid orbitopathy and proptosis being treated for refractory glaucoma (a). No significant optic disc cupping is evident (b and c) in spite of an IOP > 30 mmHg. Appearance after orbital decompression resolved his pressure elevation (d).*

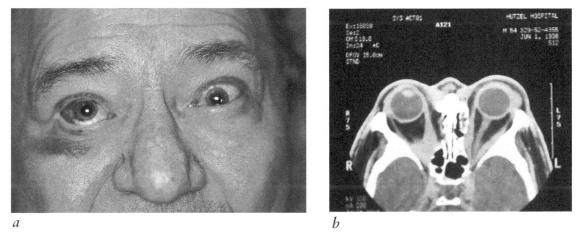

a

b

Figure 3.48 *A patient with stigmata of thyroid eye disease (lid retraction and motility restriction) (a). A CT scan demonstrates asymmetric enlargement of the extraocular muscles (b).*

Case study

A 38-year-old man presented with visual loss in his left eye. Except for vision decreased to 20/200, dyschromatopsia, a central scotoma and a RAPD, examination was normal (Figs 3.49 and 3.50). Neuroimaging was normal and a course of intravenous corticosteroids did not improve his vision. Two months later he returned with visual loss in his right eye and underwent a similar examination (Fig. 3.51). Another course of intravenous corticosteroids was not helpful. He remained 20/200 in both eyes with dense central scotomas verified by Goldmann perimetry (Fig. 3.52). Fundus examination now demonstrated a slice of temporal pallor on each optic disc compatible with the central scotomas (Fig. 3.53). Blood samples were sent for genetic testing and both 14484 and 11778 mutations were negative.

One eye is initially involved followed several months later by the second eye. Simultaneous, bilateral involvement may commonly occur. Visual loss ranges from 20/200 to 5/200, accompanied by dyschromatopsia. Visual fields demonstrate a central or centro-cecal scotoma (Figs 3.51 and 3.52). Peripheral visual fields remain intact. Early fundus appearances are said to be diagnostic, especially if seen in the preclinical state. There is a pseudo-edema of the peripapillary nerve fiber layer surrounded by circumpapillary, telangiectatic microangiopathy (Fig. 3.54). This typical fundus appearance may be very helpful when present or obvious. Practically, however, when confronted with a patient with bilateral sequential visual loss, unless it is very obvious, LHON remains a diagnosis of exclusion that can often only be verified by polymerase chain reaction testing of the mitochondrial DNA. There is no effective treatment for LHON.

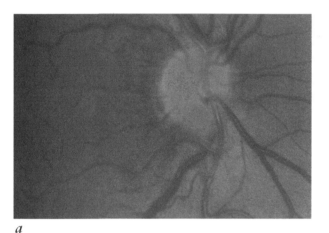

a

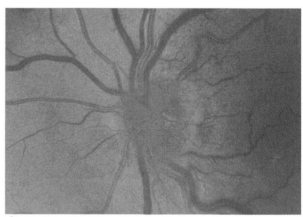

b

Figure 3.49 *Normal, crowded optic discs.*

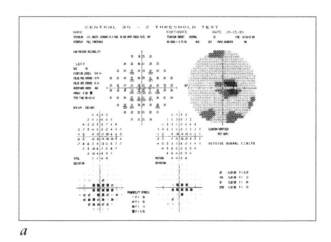

a

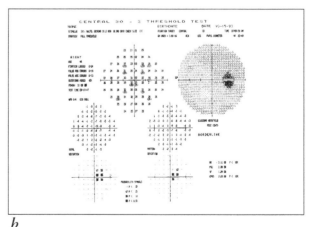

b

Figure 3.50 *Visual fields demonstrating a central scotoma in the left eye (a), the right visual field is normal (b).*

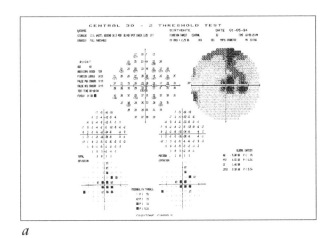
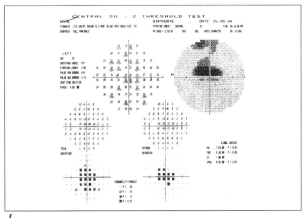

Figure 3.51 *Visual fields demonstrating central scotomas in both eyes.*

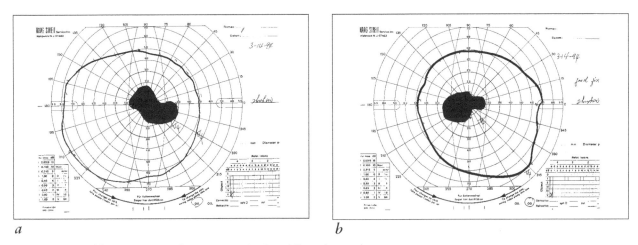

Figure 3.52 *Goldman perimetry demonstrates absolute, bilateral central scotomas.*

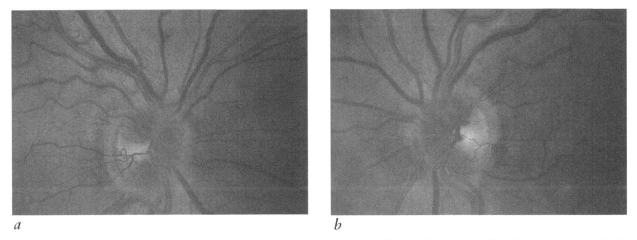

Figure 3.53 *Optic discs now demonstrate a bit of temporal pallor compatible with the visual field defects. Compare with the initial optic disc appearance in Fig. 3.51.*

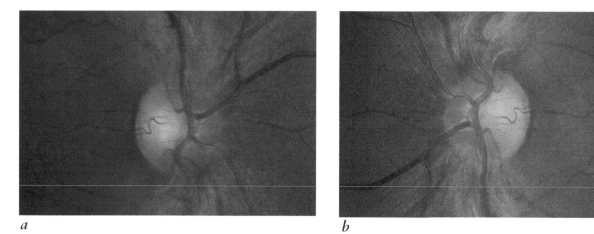

a   *b*

Figure 3.54 *Leber's optic neuropathy with pseudopapilledema of the peripapillary nerve fiber layer and circumpapillary, telangiectatic microangiopathy.*

Spontaneous improvement may occur more commonly in patients with the 14484 mutation than those with the 11778 mutation.[7]

Environmental factors may play a role in initiating or worsening visual loss in those patients with a genetic predisposition to LHON. Family history and the typical fundus appearance can identify these patients. They should be advised to avoid environmental toxins, cigarette smoke (cyanide) and alcohol.[8]

DOMINANT OPTIC ATROPHY

Dominant optic atrophy, originally described by Kjer,[9] presents in children towards the end of their first decade.

Visual loss is bilateral, and is often asymmetric and mild, ranging from 20/20 to 20/200. Forty percent of patients have visual acuity of 20/60 or better. Visual fields demonstrate central or central-cecal scotomas and there is distinctive blue–yellow dyschromatopsia. Optic discs often have a distinct sector of pallor but diffuse atrophy may be present (Fig. 3.55). As the name implies, it is dominantly inherited, but with variable expression. Visual loss may often be asymptomatic.[10] Examination of both parents may be very helpful in making the diagnosis, but this is often done after negative MRI. The risk of missing a treatable, compressive lesion in a child with mild to moderate visual function is too great to make this a diagnosis of anything but exclusion.

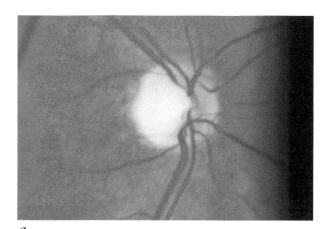

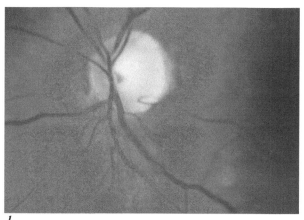

a   *b*

Figure 3.55 *A patient with dominant optic atrophy. Diffuse atrophy of the right optic disc (a) and sector atrophy on the left (b).*

RECESSIVE OPTIC ATROPHY

Recessive optic atrophy causes severe visual loss, accompanied by nystagmus, in children between the ages of 2 and 4. There is often a history of consanguinity. Optic discs are diffusely pale with attenuated blood vessels. Differentiation from childhood blindness caused by Leber's congenital amaurosis (diffuse photoreceptor dysfunction) may be accomplished with an ERG.

COMPRESSIVE OPTIC NEUROPATHIES

As mentioned in the chapter on visual loss, decreased vision due to optic nerve dysfunction must be differentiated from other causes of visual loss (refractive, subtle media opacities, maculopathies, monofixation syndrome and bilateral visual loss due to posterior visual pathway lesions). Before delving into the esoteric optic neuropathies that neuro-ophthalmologists thrive on, and that comprehensive ophthalmologists and neurologists never see or do not recognize, we must be aware of treatable optic neuropathies that will be encountered in our daily practices.

DYSTHYROID OPTIC NEUROPATHY

Thyroid eye disease is a great imitator and may mimic other disorders. It is a treatable cause of optic nerve dysfunction. Manifestations may be obvious (Fig. 3.56) or quite subtle (Fig. 3.48). Thinking of the diagnosis, looking for subtle eyelid signs and obtaining the appropriate imaging studies (CT of orbits) minimizes diagnostic errors, allowing diagnosis and treatment before visual loss is permanent. CT scan findings that positively correlate with dysthyroid optic neuropathy include: crowding of the optic nerve by enlarged extraocular muscles at the orbital apex, prolapsed orbital fat and a muscle index > 50%.[11] Patients with dysthyroid orbitopathy may have subtle or obvious optic neuropathy. The present author had followed the patient in Fig. 3.60 for over 10 years, performing a levator recession 7 years prior to correction of upper eyelid retraction. After an absence of 3–4 years, she returned to the office complaining of vague visual symptoms: there were no localizing neuro-ophthalmic signs. Fundus examination demonstrated some mottled retinal pigment epithelium and visual fields were thought to be nonlocalizing (Fig. 3.57a). A fluorescein angiogram was unproductive and she returned in 3 weeks still complaining that her vision was not right in

the left eye. Visual field changes progressed (Fig. 3.57b and c) and a RAPD was detected. A CT scan demonstrated enlargement of the extraocular muscles at the orbital apex (Fig. 3.58). Medial apical orbital decompression through an external ethmoidectomy was curative (Fig. 3.59).

This case represents subtle and overlooked compressive optic neuropathy in a patient with known but forgotten dysthyroid orbitopathy. In retrospect, the key to earlier diagnosis is the temporal flare of the upper eyelids (Fig. 3.60) and the previous history of thyroid disease. The mechanism of visual loss in dysthyroid optic neuropathy is compression of the optic nerve at the orbital apex by enlarged extraocular muscles (Fig. 3.61a and b). There are scattered reports of dysthyroid optic neuropathy with normal-sized extraocular muscles caused by stretching of the optic nerve,[12] but these cases are quite uncommon. The present author has seen maybe two cases in 20 years of subspecialty practice.

Since the optic neuropathy is caused by compression of the optic nerve at the orbital apex, treatment must entail either shrinking the extraocular muscles or expanding the orbit to allow the extraocular muscles to prolapse into the sinus and relieve the pressure upon the optic nerve (Fig. 3.59). This actually requires removal of the medial orbital wall. The back wall of the maxillary sinus usually is located 10 mm from the orbital apex; therefore, removing the floor of the orbit will not relieve the apical orbital compression and the resultant optic neuropathy. The lady in Fig. 3.62 underwent bilateral orbital decompressions through a fornix incision without improvement in her visual function. She sought a second opinion. Visual acuity was 20/40 right eye (OD)

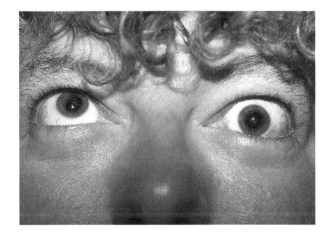

Figure 3.56 *Obvious stigmata of dysthyroid orbitopathy: proptosis, upgaze restriction and marked upper eyelid retraction.*

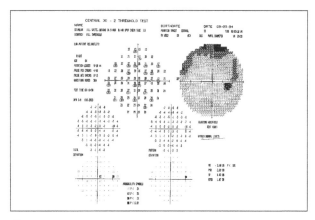

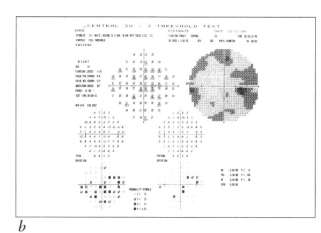

a

b

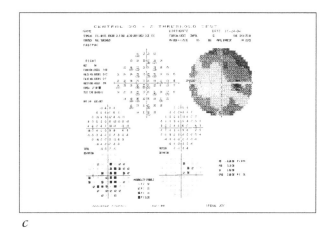

c

Figure 3.57 *Progressive visual field changes in a patient with vague visual complaints.*

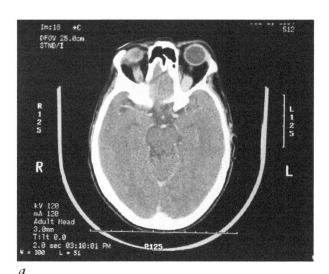

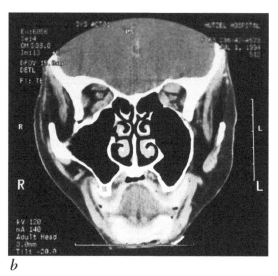

a

b

Figure 3.58 *A CT scan demonstrates enlargement of the extraocular muscles at the orbital apex: axial (a) and coronal (b).*

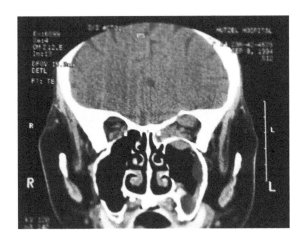

Figure 3.59 *A coronal CT scan after apical orbital decompression via external ethmoidectomy.*

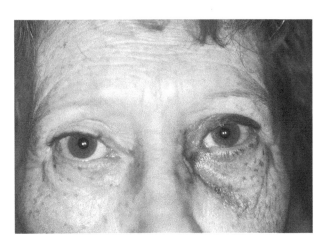

Figure 3.60 *Temporal flare of the upper eyelids and a history of thyroid orbitopathy made the diagnosis obvious.*

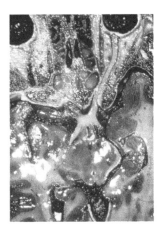

a

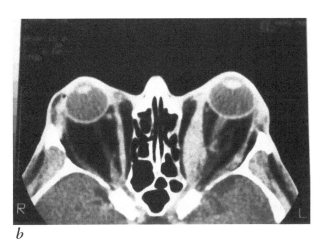

b

Figure 3.61 *Axial cadaver section though the orbital apex demonstrates the proximity of the medial rectus muscle to the optic nerve (a). A CT scan demonstrates an enlarged medial rectus muscle compressing the optic nerve at the orbital apex (b).*

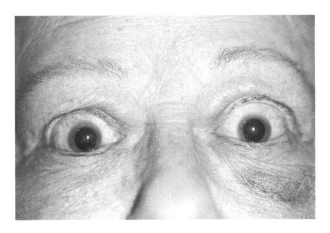

Figure 3.62 *Patient with residual optic neuropathy after orbital floor decompression.*

and 20/400 left eye (OS). She had an obvious RAPD in the left eye. A repeat CT scan demonstrated an excellent decompression of the orbital floors but only partial removal of the medial wall of the right orbit and failure to remove the medial wall of the left orbit (Fig. 3.63). She underwent a medial orbital decompression through an external ethmoidectomy on the left orbit (Fig. 3.64). The medial orbital wall and periorbita was intact. The bone was removed and the periorbita incised under direct visualization. The day after surgery, vision had improved to 20/25 in the left eye and there was now an obvious relative afferent defect in the right eye. A similar procedure was performed on the right side with significant improvement in visual function. The lesson: when decompressing the orbit for dysthyroid optic neuropathy, the medial orbital wall must be removed and the

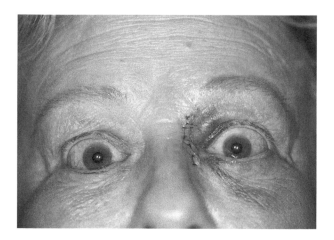

Figure 3.63   *A CT scan demonstrating an intact left medial orbital wall and partial removal of the right medial orbital wall.*

Figure 3.64   *A patient after undergoing left external ethmoidectomy and apical orbital decompression.*

periorbita incised. This is best done under direct visualization either endoscopically or via external ethmoidectomy. It is difficult if not impossible to completely remove the medial wall and incise the medial periorbita through an inferior orbital incision. If the compressive optic neuropathy is caused by compression of the optic nerve by an enlarged medial rectus muscle, removal of the entire orbital floor will not remove the compression. If the back wall of the maxillary sinus is located 10 mm anterior to the orbital apex, it is impossible to decompress the orbital apex by removal of the orbital floor.

There is no consensus as to the appropriate treatment for patients with dysthyroid optic neuropathy. There are vocal advocates of systemic corticosteroids, external beam irradiation of the orbital apex and surgical decompression of the orbital apex. Common sense and not emotion should guide decision-making. Whatever treatment is chosen it must either shrink the extraocular muscles or allow them to expand into the sinuses. Corticosteroids will shrink extraocular muscles, as they treat the acute orbital inflammation, so are a good first-line treatment for acute congested dysthyroid orbitopathy with optic nerve compression. Dosage should be adequate (80 mg prednisone) to suppress the orbital inflammation and prolonged enough to keep it suppressed. A standard regimen would be prednisone 80 mg/day for 2 weeks, 60 mg/day for 2 weeks, 40 mg/day for 2 weeks, 20 mg/day for 2 weeks and 10 mg/day for 2 weeks. Zantac 150 mg twice daily is offered for ulcer prophylaxis. This regimen is almost always complicated by steroid side effects, ranging from gastric ulceration, to psychosis, to acne and Cushingoid features.

There is a place for treatment with external beam irradiation to the orbital apex. It may be quite effective, but

you are taking your risks down the road instead of upfront as with surgical decompression. There are published and anecdotal cases of severe radiation complications after treatment with ostensibly safe amounts of irradiation. There are vocative advocates for irradiation treatment, but most of them are not surgeons. There are recent data questioning whether there is any role for external beam irradiation in treating dysthyroid orbitopathy.[13]

The patient in Fig. 3.65 was a 55-year-old man with severe dysthyroid optic neuropathy and visual loss to counting fingers in his left eye. He had been adequately treated with both steroids and irradiation to no avail. A CT scan demonstrated marked enlargement of his extraocular muscles on the left side with a resultant compressive optic neuropathy (Fig. 3.66). He underwent

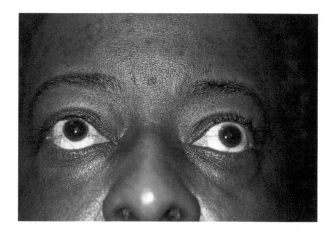

Figure 3.65   *Sensory exotropia secondary to profound visual loss in a patient with severe dysthyroid optic neuropathy.*

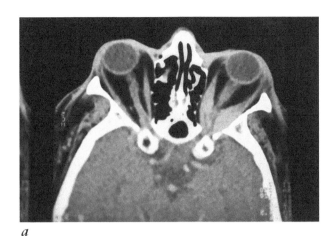
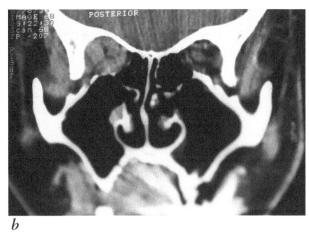

a   *b*

Figure 3.66 *Axial (a) and coronal (b) CT scans demonstrating markedly enlarged extraocular muscles on the left side.*

medial orbital decompression through an external ethmoidectomy with normalization of visual function. He returned 18 months later with severe visual loss due to radiation retinopathy.

Common sense should dictate what treatment to offer a patient with dysthyroid optic neuropathy and visual loss. A frail, elderly patient is not a good candidate for corticosteroid treatment and irradiation or surgery would be a better choice. A young, attractive lady with unsightly proptosis might better be served by an orbital decompression than by long-term corticosteroid treatment. A patient with marginal optic nerve compression and acute orbital congestion is an excellent candidate for a course of corticosteroids. The bottom line is that none of these treatments mitigate against using another. Orbital decompression can certainly be performed after irradiation therapy, and steroids can be used at any time. The present author prefers to take risks upfront and judiciously treats patients with acute congestive orbitopathy with a course of steroids and offers orbital decompression to those patients with significant optic nerve compression. Irradiation therapy is reserved for patients who fail to respond to an ADEQUATE orbital decompression as confirmed by the absence of the medial orbital wall and herniation of the medial rectus muscle into the ethmoid sinus on a postoperative CT scan (Fig. 3.59).

ORBITAL TUMORS

Compression of the optic nerve by an encapsulated orbital tumor is a very treatable cause of visual dysfunction. A patient with a large tumor compressing the optic nerve may present with visual obscurations (transient blackouts of vision lasting seconds), a swollen optic disc and mild or obvious proptosis. If an orbital etiology is considered and the orbit imaged, this is not a difficult diagnosis. MR scans may be very helpful in differentiating a mass evident on a CT scan from the optic nerve (Fig. 3.67), which may be beneficial when planning surgery. The surgical approach chosen should keep the tumor between the surgeon's instruments and the optic nerve. The tumor imaged in Fig. 3.68 should be approached via a lateral orbitotomy, since it lies between the optic nerve and the lateral orbital wall. The tumor in Fig. 3.69 should be approached medially, since the optic nerve lies lateral to the tumor as verified by a MR scan. These patients were referred for evaluation of a swollen optic disc and visual obscurations.

Apical orbital lesions may present with more subtle, slowly progressive visual loss and a normal or mildly atrophic optic nerve. A CT scan may demonstrate a diffuse apical orbital mass (Fig. 3.69a), which upon MR scanning is noted to be well encapsulated and totally resectable (Fig. 3.69b). These lesions are much better imaged with today's MRI scans (Fig. 3.70).

Tumors, inflammation and infection originating in the sphenoid or ethmoid sinuses may cause optic nerve dysfunction by direct involvement in either the posterior ethmoid or sphenoid sinus sphenoid sinusitis. The lateral wall of the sphenoid (medial wall of the optic canal; Fig. 3.61) may be very thin or absent in a number of patients, allowing inflammation or infection in these sinuses to directly influence optic nerve function (Fig. 3.71).

INTRACRANIAL TUMORS

The unforgivable sin in neuro-ophthalmology is missing the treatable compressive intracranial mass that is causing

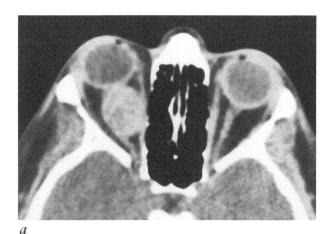
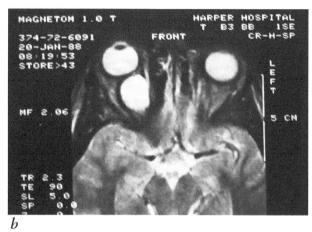

a　　　　　　　　　　　　　　　　　　　*b*

Figure 3.67　*A CT scan demonstrating a large, orbital mass medial to the optic nerve (a). An MRI scan clearly differentiates the mass from the adjacent optic nerve (b).*

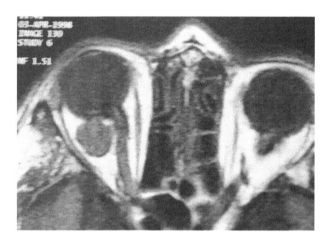

Figure 3.68　*An MRI scan demonstrating an encapsulated orbital tumor lateral to the optic nerve.*

slowly progressive or for that matter rapid visual loss. Children may be especially challenging. You cannot image every child with a headache but all too often these children 'slip through the cracks' and irreparable visual loss, optic atrophy and expensive litigation result.

A 6-year-old girl presented to her pediatrician with headache, nausea and vomiting. A flu-like illness was diagnosed and the girl sent home with appropriate supportive treatment. Visual acuity on that day was documented at 20/20. Six months later, the child returned for an earache and was treated with oral antibiotics. Visual acuity was documented at 20/20 OD and 20/40 OS. She was referred to an optometrist who could not correct her vision better than 20/40 and 20/60 with any lenses. She saw another optometrist, had visual acuity of 20/100 and 20/200, and was referred to an ophthalmologist. His

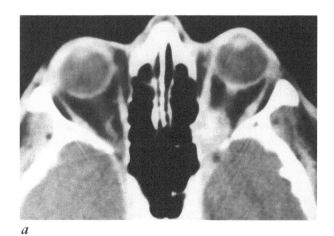
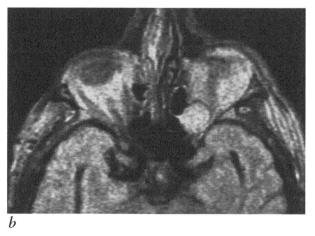

a　　　　　　　　　　　　　　　　　　　*b*

Figure 3.69　*A CT scan demonstrates a diffuse apical orbital mass (a). A first-generation MRI scan demonstrates a distinct encapsulated orbital mass (b).*

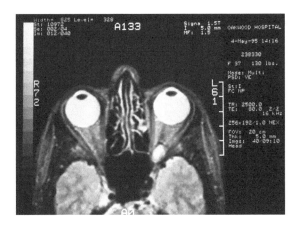

Figure 3.70 *Small apical orbital mass clearly demonstrated with MRI.*

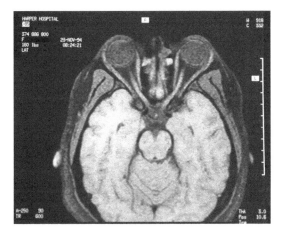

Figure 3.71 *Axial MRI scan demonstrating relationship between the optic nerve and the sphenoethmoid sinuses.*

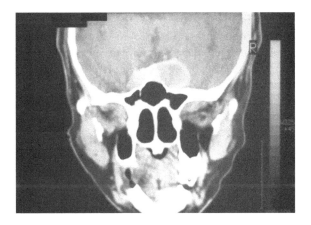

Figure 3.72 *Large craniopharyngioma causing bilateral blindness.*

examination demonstrated a mild hyperopic refractive error (+1.25). A diagnosis of bilateral amblyopia was made and glasses prescribed. Several months later the child presented to the local emergency room with headache, double vision, nausea and vomiting. A physician actually looked at her fundus and noted optic atrophy. A pediatric ophthalmologist documented very poor visual acuity in both eyes and a sixth-nerve paresis. A CT scan demonstrated a large suprasellar mass, which at surgery proved to be a craniopharyngioma (Fig. 3.72). No useful vision returned. The child is blind and litigation is pending.

This is not an isolated case. The present author has rarely seen children with craniopharyngiomas diagnosed in a timely fashion. Visual prognosis is directly related to the size of the tumor at the time of diagnosis. Early diagnosis may be vision saving. These missed diagnoses transcend socioeconomics. Although some segments of the population may be less demanding of an explanation, it is amazing how many parents do not listen to their children's complaints of visual dysfunction and listen to the doctor's erroneous diagnosis.

The little girl aforementioned was in and out of her Health Maintenance Organization (HMO) and the local children's hospital with headache, nausea, vomiting and vague visual complaints. The diagnosis of sinusitis was repeatedly made. A CT scan was not ordered until finally a set of sinus x-rays demonstrated suprasellar calcifications. The CT scan when obtained demonstrated a large suprasellar mass (Fig. 3.72).

A 10-year-old boy was followed all summer for a sinus infection thought to be causing his headaches. Headaches that were so bad that a CT scan was obtained to rule out a fresh subarachnoid hemorrhage, which was read as negative. (A CT scan looking for fresh blood is done without contrast and concentrated on the base of the brain.) Symptoms continued and he complained of decreased vision is his left eye. A bit of pallor of the left optic disc was noted and he was referred for an opinion. Visual acuity was 20/20 in the right eye and hand motions only in the left eye. There was an obvious left RAPD and pallor of the left optic disc (Fig. 3.73). An MRI scan demonstrated a massive mass extending from the sphenoid sinus and compressing the optic chiasm (Fig. 3.74). Surgery demonstrated a large cystic mass that was drained. Vision did not improve in the left eye.

These patients and others have tragic and preventable visual loss. You cannot order a CT scan on every child with a headache and sinusitis, but you can look for a RAPD, check visual acuity and perform a visual field if the child is old enough.

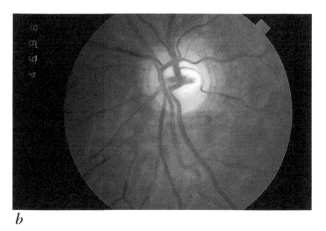

Figure 3.73 *The fundus demonstrating an increased cup-to-disc ratio and mild pallor of the left optic disc.*

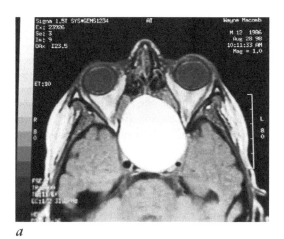

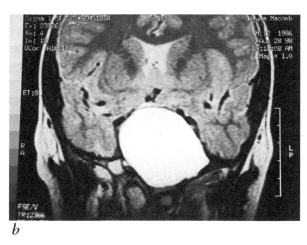

Figure 3.74 *MRI scans—axial (a) and coronal (b)—demonstrate a large, cystic mass compressing the optic chiasm.*

OPTIC NERVE SHEATH MENINGIOMAS [14–16]

Meningiomas are benign neoplasms that arise from the meningothelial cells of the meninges. Histopathology demonstrates patterns of whorls and sheets of meningothelial cells (Fig. 3.75). The optic nerve may be compressed by meningiomas confined to the optic nerve itself or by orbital extension of intracranial tumors. Slowly progressive, relentless visual loss may be accompanied by proptosis and extraocular motility dysfunction (Fig. 3.76). Patients may present with slowly progressive visual loss and optic atrophy with optociliary shunt vessels (Fig. 3.77), or with visual obscurations due to optic disc swelling, excellent visual acuity and subtle visual field changes (Fig. 3.78) that remain stable for years without significant progression (Fig. 3.79).

Other patients may present with vague visual symptoms, non-specific visual field changes and near-normal-appearing optic discs (Fig. 3.80). MRI scans demonstrate the abnormal enhancement of the entire optic nerve sheath (Fig. 3.80c).

Primary optic nerve sheath meningiomas are rarely resectable tumors. These patients present with visual dysfunction, an RAPD and a normal, swollen or atrophic optic disc (Figs 3.76–3.80). An MRI scan may be diagnostic (Fig. 3.81) if it is obtained with gadolinium enhancement. An unenhanced scan may appear somewhat normal with equivocal enlargement of the optic nerve (Fig. 3.81a). Both the intracranial and the intraorbital extent of the meningioma can be delineated with fat-suppressed gadolinium-enhanced MRI scans (Fig. 3.81b). Only enhanced MRI scans can delineate intracanalicular extension of an optic nerve sheath meningioma.

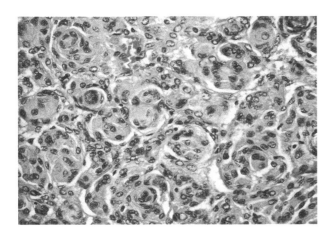

Figure 3.75 *Histopathology demonstrates whorls of meningothelial cells and calcified psammoma bodies.*

There have been reports over the years of surgical resection of optic nerve sheath meningiomas with preservation and actual improvement in vision.[15] These are really the exception rather than the rule and visual loss continues to progress in most of these patients. When considering any form of treatment, remember that the natural history of the disease may allow maintenance of good visual function for many years (Figs 3.78 and 3.79) especially in male patients.

The following patient represents the classic presentation and course of an optic nerve sheath meningioma. She was seen and underwent surgery in 1978 when the present author was Dr John S Kennerdell's fellow. She was referred for evaluation of a swollen optic disc and mild visual dysfunction. Visual acuity was 20/25 in the involved eye with mild dyschromatopsia. Her optic disc was very swollen (Fig. 3.82a) and her visual field was

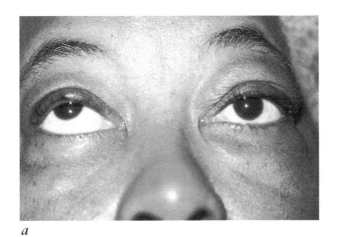

a

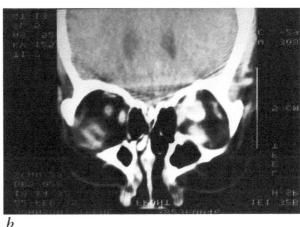

b

Figure 3.76 *A patient with proptosis, upgaze restriction (a), due to a calcified optic nerve sheath meningioma evident on CT scan (b).*

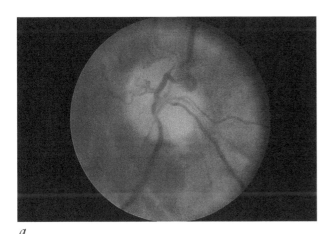

a

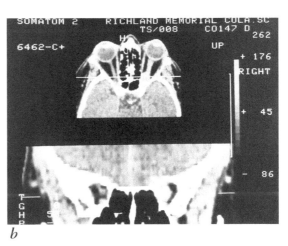

b

Figure 3.77 *A patient followed for several years with 'chronic' optic neuritis presented with optic atrophy and optociliary shunt vessels (a). A CT scan demonstrated an apical orbital meningioma (b).*

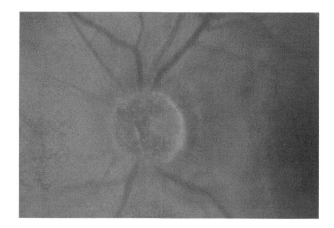

a

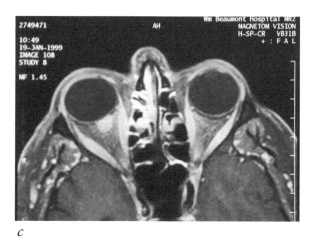

b   *c*

Figure 3.78 *Optic disc swelling (a), subtle visual field changes (b) and enhancement of the retrobulbar optic nerve on MRI (c).*

minimally impaired (Fig. 3.82b). A CT scan demonstrated an enlarged optic nerve (Fig. 3.82c). Meningioma was suspected but in view of her excellent visual function she was observed. Over a 2-month period visual fields progressively and rapidly deteriorated (Fig. 3.83a–c). This sequence of visual field loss, with the marked peripheral constriction and the sparing of central vision, is the hallmark of optic nerve sheath meningioma. In the face of the rapidly progressive loss of useful vision, she underwent excision of the meningioma via an extended lateral orbitotomy. The optic nerve sheath was enlarged and distended (Fig. 3.84). When incised, a friable tumor mass was surrounding and compressing the optic nerve (Fig. 3.85). This was microsurgically removed with restoration of visual function (Fig. 3.86a and b) and resolution of optic disc swelling (Fig. 3.87). Over the next few years, optic atrophy relentlessly ensued (Fig. 3.88) and she lost vision in the eye in spite of subsequent radiation therapy.

Most authorities, including the present author, manage these patients very conservatively. If the tumor is confined to the optic nerve sheath on a gadolinium-enhanced MRI scan and the visual function is good, observation with serial visual fields and fundus examinations is appropriate (Figs 3.78 and 3.79). This patient was followed conservatively for over 10 years with no significant decrease in visual function. MRI scans may be obtained once or twice a year. If there is significant intracranial involvement (Fig. 3.89), the patient should have a neurosurgical opinion. If the visual function is good, the present author defers surgery to the neurosurgeon and does not operate on the intraorbital optic nerve. There is literature supporting careful removal of the roof of the optic canal to help decompress the optic nerve and prolong useful vision.

If visual function progressively deteriorates and the MRI scan is consistent with a perioptic meningioma (Fig. 3.84), irradiation of the involved optic nerve is a

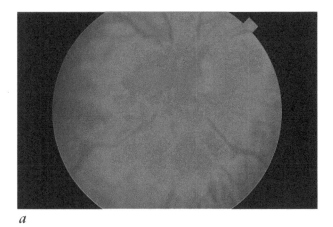

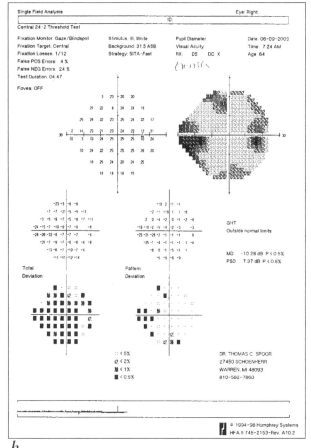

Figure 3.79 *The same patient as in Fig. 3.78 10 years later.*

viable option. Excellent results, actually reversing visual loss with three-dimensional conformational radiation therapy, have recently been reported.[16,17] With today's MRI imaging, many radiation oncologists are willing to irradiate the patient without a histopathologic diagnosis. This is fine for the patient but when you have a spectacular result, as in this patient (see Fig. 3.93), you cannot be certain that you are treating a perioptic meningioma or some form of radiosensitive orbital inflammation mimicking meningioma on a MRI scan.

Three-dimensional conformational radiation therapy has been reported to be effective in controlling growth and actually improving vision in some patients with optic nerve sheath meningiomas.[16,17] Enthusiasm for treatment should be tempered by the natural history of these tumors.[18] Many patients have stable, good visual function for years after initial diagnosis. Treatment should be reserved for those patients with documented progressive or initially significant visual loss.[18]

A patient with a blind, proptotic eye (Fig. 3.90) may benefit from total resection of the meningioma. This is best accomplished via a craniotomy and superior orbitotomy. Prior to manipulation of the optic nerve and its tumor, it should be severed anterior to the chiasm to avoid trauma to the chiasm and a significant temporal visual field defect in the sighted eye. After the optic nerve is severed and the roof to the optic canal removed, the nerve and tumor may be safely dissected anteriorly into the orbit and severed behind the globe and totally removed.

The lady in Fig. 3.90 had excessive manipulation of the involved optic nerve prior to removal and had an unexpected temporal visual field defect after surgery. Fortunately it was due to chiasmal edema and cleared completely within a week, but there were two very worried surgeons checking her visual fields that week.

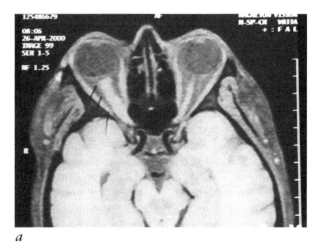

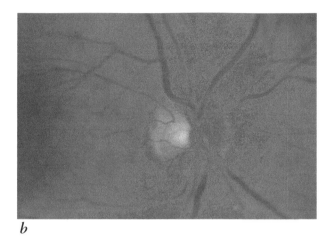

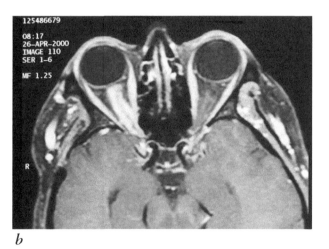

Figure 3.80 *Normal-appearing optic discs (a and b). An MRI scan clearly shows an enhanced optic nerve lesion (c).*

Figure 3.81 *Optic nerve sheath meningioma demonstrating mild enlargement of the optic nerve on unenhanced MRI (a). Gadolinium-enhanced MRI demonstrates diffuse enhancement surrounding the optic nerve (b) almost pathognomonic of a perioptic meningioma.*

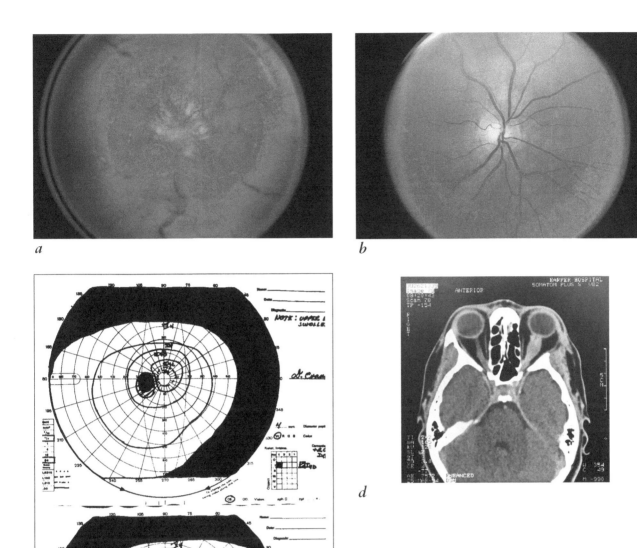

Figure 3.82 *Significant swelling of the right optic disc (a) and a normal-appearing left optic disc (b) in a patient with an optic nerve sheath meningioma. Visual fields demonstrate mild enlargement of the blind spot in the right eye and a normal left eye (c). A CT scan demonstrates a markedly enlarged optic nerve (d).*

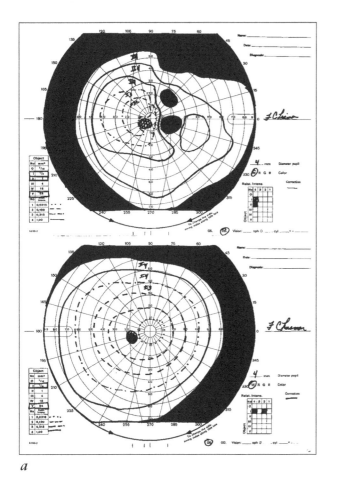

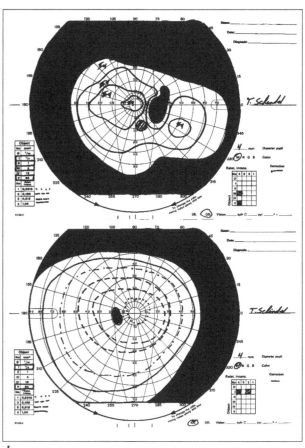

a

b

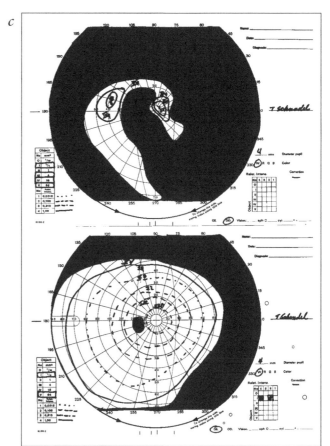

c

Figure 3.83 *Progressive deterioration of the visual fields over a 2-month interval.*

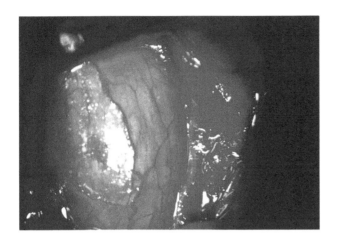

Figure 3.84 *Surgical view of a markedly distended optic nerve sheath.*

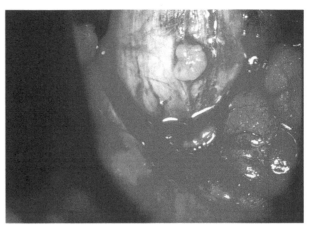

Figure 3.85 *Presentation of soft, friable meningioma after incision of the optic nerve sheath.*

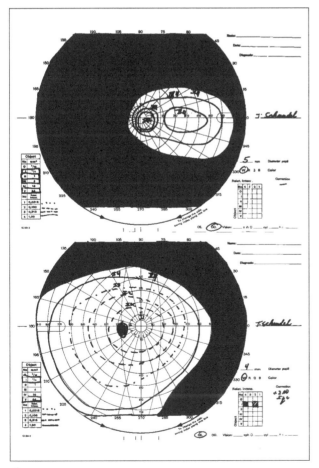

a

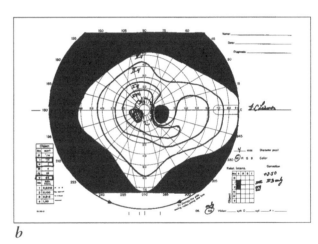

b

Figure 3.86 *Improvement immediately after (a) and 3 weeks after surgical excision (b). Compare with Fig. 3.83c (the immediate preoperative visual field).*

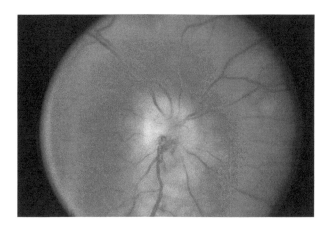

Figure 3.87 *Partial resolution of optic disc swelling 3 weeks after surgery.*

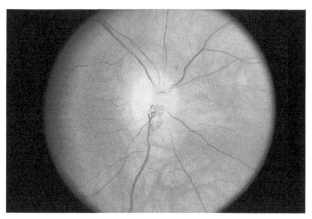

Figure 3.88 *Very evident optic atrophy and optociliary shunt vessels 2 months after surgery.*

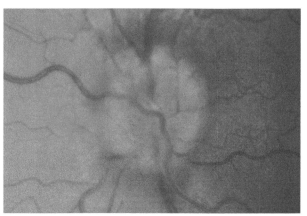

a

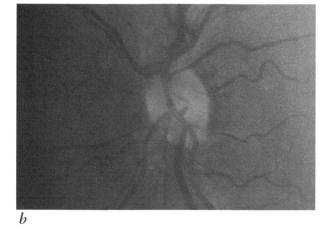

b

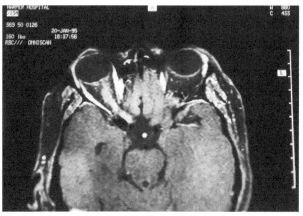

c

Figure 3.89 *A patient referred with optic disc swelling and visual loss (a and b). Enhanced MRI demonstrates an optic nerve sheath meningioma with evidence for intracranial extension (c).*

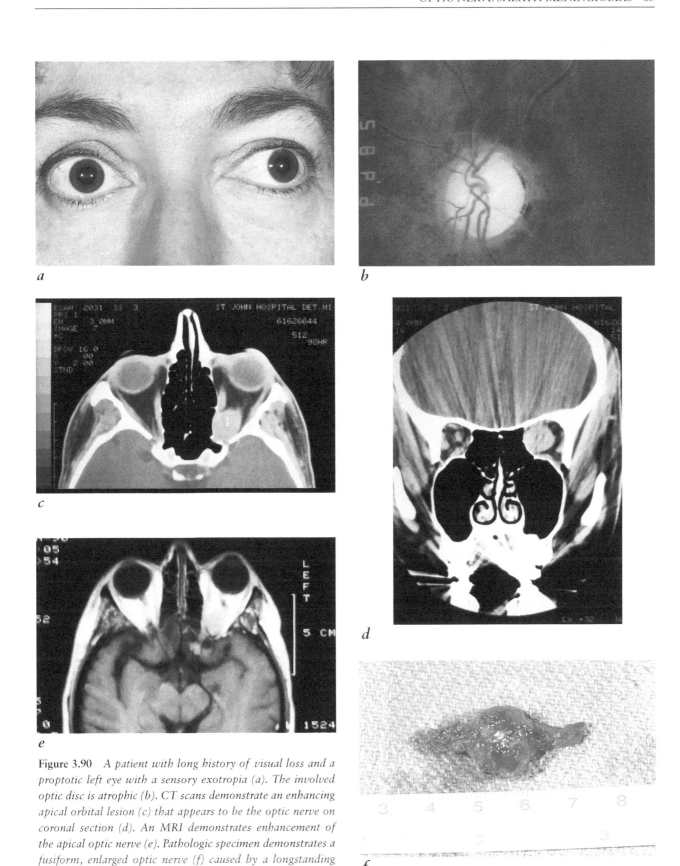

Figure 3.90 *A patient with long history of visual loss and a proptotic left eye with a sensory exotropia (a). The involved optic disc is atrophic (b). CT scans demonstrate an enhancing apical orbital lesion (c) that appears to be the optic nerve on coronal section (d). An MRI demonstrates enhancement of the apical optic nerve (e). Pathologic specimen demonstrates a fusiform, enlarged optic nerve (f) caused by a longstanding meningioma.*

OPTIC NERVE GLIOMAS[19]

Gliomas of the anterior visual pathways are the most common tumors of the central nervous system, accounting for 2% of all gliomas and 5% of childhood gliomas. They occur most commonly in the first two decades of life. Sixty-five percent occur in the first decade and 90% occur before 20 years of age. Gliomas account for 65% of all intrinsic optic nerve tumors. Involvement of the intraorbital optic nerve is most common (47%), followed by the intracranial optic nerve (26%). Intracranial and chiasmal involvement occur in 12 and 5% of gliomas that affect the optic chiasm, respectively.

Patients present with exophthalmos, decreased visual function and dyschromatopsia accompanied by a RAPD (Fig. 3.91). The optic disc may appear swollen, normal or atrophic. MRI scanning demonstrates intrinsic enlargement of the optic nerve (Fig. 3.92). The presence and extent of the glioma is best demonstrated by MRI.

If visual function is good, isolated intraorbital optic nerve gliomas may be followed with serial visual fields and MRI scans every 6–12 months to detect potential intracranial extension. If vision is poor, and exophthalmos is excessive and unsightly, the lesion may be excised via craniotomy and superior orbitotomy. If there is evidence for intracranial extension of a glioma originally confined to the orbit, it should be removed to prevent chiasmal, hypothalamic or third ventricle involvement.

Frequently, optic nerve gliomas are found in association with neurofibromatosis type 1, which is present in

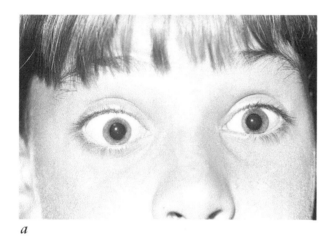
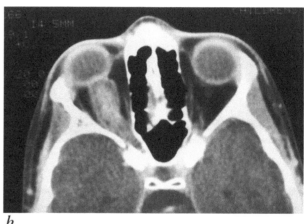

a

b

Figure 3.91 *A patient with an optic nerve glioma presenting with painless proptosis and visual loss (a). A CT scan demonstrates enlargement of the optic nerve extending to the orbital apex (b).*

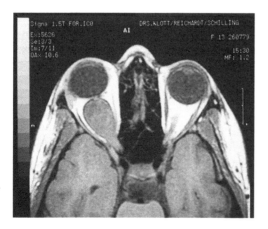
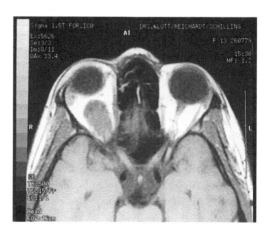

a

b

Figure 3.92 *Optic nerve gliomas. MRI demonstrating enlargement of the right optic nerve (a), with no evidence for intracranial involvement (b).*

25% of patients with optic nerve gliomas. Optic nerve gliomas are present in 15% of patients with neurofibromatosis.

Optic nerve gliomas are true neoplasms with an early growth spurt often followed by years of stability. Visual prognosis is poor but, if confined to the optic nerve, long-term survival is excellent. If the optic chiasm, hypothalamus or third ventricle is involved, prognosis for life diminishes. If the hypothalamus is involved, mortality increases to > 50%. There is no proven, effective treatment for optic nerve gliomas[20] and spontaneous regression may occur.[21]

MALIGNANT OPTIC NERVE GLIOMAS

Malignant gliomas of the optic nerve and anterior visual pathways are rare. Patients present with rapidly progressive, painful visual loss accompanied by signs of an optic neuropathy. Initial visual loss may be unilateral or bilateral (chiasmal involvement). Rapid progression to bilateral blindness and death are constant features. Depending upon the original location of the tumor, visual loss may be accompanied by diplopia, proptosis or venous stasis retinopathy. The optic disc may appear normal, swollen or atrophic.

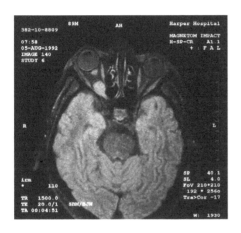

a

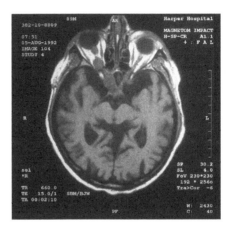

b

Figure 3.93 *Malignant optic nerve glioma. An MRI demonstrates enlargement of the apical optic nerve (a), with obvious intracranial extension (b).*

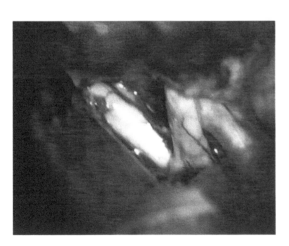

Figure 3.94 *View of the optic nerves and chiasm through the operating microscope. Note the flattening and pallor of the left optic nerve compared with the more normal-appearing right optic nerve, with pial blood vessels evident.*

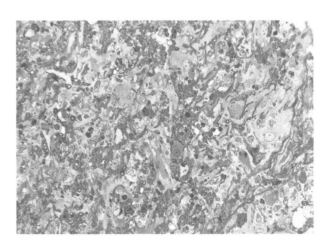

Figure 3.95 *Biopsy specimen from the left optic nerve demonstrating bizarre, atypical malignant astrocytes separating disrupted myelin sheaths (toluidine blue, 250×).*

Imaging studies demonstrate enlargement of the involved optic nerves or chiasm (Fig. 3.93). Diagnosis of this devastating disease should be confirmed by biopsy of the involved optic nerve (Fig. 3.94). Biopsy specimens demonstrate bizarre, atypical malignant astrocytes separating disrupted myelin sheaths (Fig. 3.95). There is no effective treatment for malignant optic nerve gliomas. Bilateral blindness ensues within 6–8 weeks and death follows within 6–9 months of the initial symptoms.[5]

REFERENCES

1. Morrison JC. Anatomy and physiology of the optic nerve. In: (Kline LB, ed) Optic Nerve Disorders. (American Academy of Ophthalmology and Palace Press: San Francisco, 1996) 1:1–20.

2. Hoyt Miller NR. Walsh and Hoyt's Clinical neuro-ophthalmology. Williams and Wilkins: Baltimore, 1982.

3. Gittinger JW, Miller NR, Keltner J, Burde RM. Clinical challenges glaucomatous cupping-sine glaucoma. *Survey Ophthalmol* 1981; **25**:383–9.

4. Stroman GA, Stewart WC, Golnick C et al. MRI in patients with low tension glaucoma. *Arch Ophthalmol* 1995; **113**:168–72.

5. Spoor TC, Kennerdell JS, Martinez J. Malignant gliomas of the optic pathways. *Am J Ophthalmol* 1980; **89**:284–90.

6. Cockerham KP, Pal C, Jani B et al. The prevalence and implications of ocular hypertension and glaucoma in thyroid associated orbitopathy. *Ophthalmology* 1997; **104**:914–17.

7. Newman NJ, Lott MT, Wallace DC. Clinical characteristics and pedigree of Leber's hereditary optic neuropathy with the 11778 mutation. *Am J Ophthalmol* 1991; **111**:750–62.

8. Johns DR, Smith KH, Savino PJ et al. Leber's hereditary optic neuropathy: clinical characteristics of the 15257 mutation. *Ophthalmology* 1993; **100**:981–6.

9. Kjer P. Infantile optic atrophy with dominant mode inheritance: a clinical and genetic study of 19 Danish families. *Acta Ophthalmol* 1959; **54**:1–46.

10. Votruba M, Fitzke FW, Holder GE et al. Clinical features from affected individuals from 21 pedigrees with dominant optic atrophy. *Arch Ophthalmol* 1998; **116**:793–800.

11. Giaconio JA, Kazim M, Rho T et al. CT scan evidence of dysthyroid optic neuropathy. *Ophthalmol Plast Reconst Surg* 2002; **18**:177–82.

12. Anderson RL, Tweeten JP, Patrinely JR et al. Dysthyroid optic neuropathy without extraocular muscle enlargement. *Ophthalmol Surg* 1989; **20**:568–74.

13. Gorum C, Garrity JA, Fatourechi V et al. A prospective, randomized, double blind placebo controlled study of orbital radiotherapy for Graves' orbitopathy. *Ophthalmology* 2001; **108**:525–34.

14. Dutton JJ. Optic nerve sheath meningiomas. *Surv Ophthalmol* 1992; **37**:167–83.

15. Kennerdell JS, Maroon JC, Malton M et al. The management of optic nerve sheath meningiomas. *Am J Ophthalmol* 1998; **106**:450–7.

16. Moyer PD, Golnik KC, Breneman J. Treatment of optic nerve sheath meningiomas with 3-dimensional conformal radiation. *Am J Ophthalmol* 2000; **129**: 694–6.

17. Narayan S, Cornblath WT, Sandler HM et al. Preliminary visual outcomes after 3 dimensional conformational radiation therapy for optic nerve sheath meningioma. *Int J Rad Oncol Biol Phts* 2003; **56**:5376–543.

18. Egan RA, Lessell S. A contribution to the natural history of optic nerve sheath meningiomas. *Arch Ophthalmol* 2002; **20**:1505–8.

19. Dutton JJ. Gliomas of the anterior visual pathways. *Surv Ophthalmol* 1994; **38**:427–52.

20. Listernick R, Darling C, Greenwald M et al. Optic pathway tumors in children: the effect of neurofibromatosis type 1 on the clinical manifestations and natural history. *J Pediatr* 1995; **127**:718–22.

21. Passo CF, Hoyt CS, Lesser RL et al. Spontaneous regression of optic nerve gliomas documented by serial neuroimaging. *Arch Ophthalmol* 2001; **119**:516–19.

Chapter 4   Optic neuritis

Optic neuritis, primary demyelination of the optic nerve, is the best-studied optic nerve disorder due to the efforts of the Optic Neuritis Treatment Trial (ONTT). The ONTT prospectively followed a cohort of 448 patients presenting to a variety of medical centers with optic neuritis and visual loss. Patients were divided into three groups: no treatment (placebo), oral prednisone 80 mg/day and 3 days of intravenous methylprednisolone 250 mg four times daily followed by 11 days of prednisone 80 mg/day.[1-4]

CHARACTERISTICS

The prospective data obtained in this study can be applied to a larger cohort of patients. Seventy-seven percent of the patients were female, the average age was 32 years and 85% of the patients were white. Optic neuritis is a disease primarily of white females of northern European ancestry. It is uncommon in those of southern European, African and Asian descent. In these patients, be attuned to the differential diagnosis for atypical optic neuritis (see below).

In patients with typical optic neuritis, visual loss occurs over 1–2 weeks accompanied by dyschromatopsia and a relative afferent pupillary defect (RAPD). Orbital pain with eye movement occurs 3–5 days before the onset of visual loss in 92% of patients and the pain rarely lasts > 7 days. If pain lasts > 7 days, consider the diagnosis of atypical optic neuritis.

Visual acuity loss ranges from 20/20 to no light perception (NLP). Ten percent of patients in the ONTT had 20/20 vision, 25% had visual acuity ranging from 20/25 to 20/40, 29% from 20/50 to 20/190 and 36% had visual acuities of 20/200 to NLP. All patients had defective color vision (dyschromatopsia). This could often be solicited subjectively by comparing color saturation perceived by the affected and unaffected eyes.

Visual field defects were present in almost all patients. Diffuse defects were present in 45% of cases and localized defects in 55%. Localized defects were divided into altitudinal (29%), three quadrant (14%) and central or centro-cecal (16%). Mild optic disc swelling was present in about one-third of the patients. Less than 5% of patients had any evidence for retinal inflammation—vitreous cells, phlebitis or exudates. If these are present, think in terms of atypical optic neuritis or neuroretinitis.

EVALUATION

No lab tests, computerized tomography (CT) scans, cerebrospinal fluid (CSF) studies or x-rays were of any predictive value in treating or prognosticating patients presenting with typical optic neuritis. Magnetic resonance imaging (MRI) scans were helpful in predicting which patients would eventually develop multiple sclerosis (MS) and may be helpful in prognosticating visual recovery in some patients. MRI abnormalities in these patients consisted of plaques in the white matter (Figs 4.1 and 4.2) due to a breakdown of the blood–brain barrier. These plaques located in periventricular and subcortical white matter and in the pons are T2 hyperintense (Fig. 4.1) and, if active, are enhanced on T1

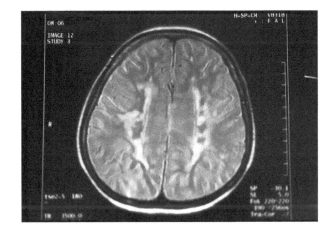

Figure 4.1 *An MRI scan demonstrating hyperintense periventricular and subcortical white matter plaques evident on T2 images.*

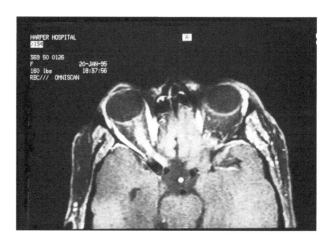

Figure 4.2 *An MRI scan demonstrating gadolinium enhancing periventricular and subcortical white matter plaques on T1 images.*

Figure 4.3 *An MRI scan demonstrating diffuse enhancement of the entire optic nerve in a patient with optic neuritis and severe visual loss.*

images (Fig. 4.2). Fifty-nine percent of ONTT patients with normal neurologic histories had abnormal MRI scans containing three or more plaques: 49% of the study patients had normal MRI scans. After 5 years, 51% of patients with abnormal MRI scans developed MS, while only 16% of patients with a normal MRI scan did.

After 10 years, risk profiles for developing MS have been described for this cohort of patients.[5,6] Patients with an initial normal MRI scan—no demyelinating plaques—had a 22% risk of developing MS 10 years after their episode of optic neuritis. Patients with one or more abnormal lesions on their initial MRI scan had a 56% risk of developing clinical MS after 10 years. The overall risk of developing MS after typical optic neuritis was 38%. Other demographic and clinical features mitigating against developing MS include: male gender, optic disc swelling, peripapillary hemorrhages, exudates initial vision of NLP and absence of pain (atypical features; see Atypical optic neuritis below).

Utilizing more sophisticated MR imaging of the optic nerves (fat suppression) in patients with optic neuritis, 80% will have abnormal enhancement of their optic nerves. Patients with extensive optic nerve enhancement (Fig. 4.3) or optic canal enhancement have a worse visual prognosis than those with anterior to mid-orbital enhancement. As mentioned previously, the enhancement is due to disruption of the blood–brain barrier. With recovery of visual function and restoration of the blood–brain barrier, the enhancement is no longer evident.

TREATMENT

Treatment has no effect on the ultimate visual or neurologic outcomes in patients with typical optic neuritis. Patients treated with intravenous steroids recovered vision more rapidly but there was no difference after 1 year. Patients with abnormal MR imaging and treated with intravenous steroids had a lesser incidence of MS development after 2 years, but the benefit had disappeared at a 3-year follow-up.

Patients treated with oral prednisone had an increased rate of recurrence of optic neuritis throughout the study. This was an important finding since the standard of care for most physicians treating patients with optic neuritis prior to the ONTT was oral prednisone. This practice has since been abandoned. Most patients recover with or without treatment. Patients with more severe initial visual loss have a poorer prognosis for visual recovery, but most still resolve.

OPTIC NEURITIS IN CHILDREN

Optic neuritis in children has not been prospectively studied. It does appear to be a bit different to adult optic neuritis. Bilateral involvement and optic disc edema occur in 50–75% of children (Fig. 4.4). Some series report

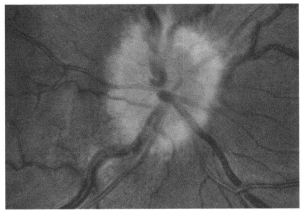

a

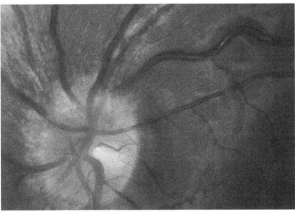

b

Figure 4.4 *Bilateral papillitis in a child with optic neuritis (a) and severe bilateral visual loss (b).*

significant improvement in visual function with > 80% of patients returning to 20/20 vision when treated with high-dose intravenous methylprednisolone. Others report more dismal results with 70% of patients attaining 20/200 or worse visual acuity. MS eventually develops in 10–50% of patients.[7,8]

OPTIC NEURITIS IN THE ELDERLY

Although the present author no longer considers a patient over 50 years of age as elderly, optic neuritis seems to have a different course in older patients. Optic neuropathies in most patients over 50 years of age result from non-arteritic anterior ischemic optic neuropathy (NAION) and have a typical clinical presentation and course (see below). Older patients with visual loss, optic

nerve dysfunction and a normal-appearing optic disc whose visual function improves with time do not have NAION but optic neuritis of the elderly.

The clinical picture is similar to optic neuritis, with rapid visual loss and eventual, predictable recovery. Reviewing 14 patients over 50 years of age with optic neuritis, Jacobson et al[9] found that 78% recovered visual acuity of 20/30 or better, 43% developed recurrent optic neuritis and 21% developed MS. Systemic steroids are of little benefit and may cause significant complications in this age group.[9,10]

NEURORETINITIS

Patients with neuroretinitis present in a similar fashion to those with typical optic neuritis but develop macular exudates 1–2 weeks later. This often occurs after a systemic viral infection (50%) and there is no increased risk for developing MS. Neuroretinitis typically occurs in patients aged 10–50 years. There is no sexual predilection. Vitreous cells are present in > 90% of patients. Macular exudation results from leakage of fluid from the optic disc capillaries. Lipid deposited into the outer plexiform layer of Henle results in the typical stellate appearance (Fig. 4.5). Lipid deposition in the macula is a non-specific finding that may occur with any cause of optic disc swelling. Patients with neuroretinitis have the typical clinical picture of visual loss followed by the development of the macular exudation. Unlike optic neuritis, where systemic evaluation is rarely necessary, patients with neuroretinitis should be evaluated for specific causes: cat-scratch fever (*Bartonella henselai*), syphilis, Lyme disease and toxoplasmosis. This serologic evaluation may be very productive and identify a treatable cause for the patient's visual loss.

Patients with neuroretinitis do not have the same high risk of developing MS as do patients with optic neuritis.[5,11]

ATYPICAL OPTIC NEURITIS AND SYSTEMIC DISEASE CAUSES OF OPTIC NEURITIS

This is an area where the neuro-ophthalmologist's expertise can really make a difference in salvaging a patient's vision. If a patient with typical optic neuritis does not show improvement after 1–2 weeks, suspect an

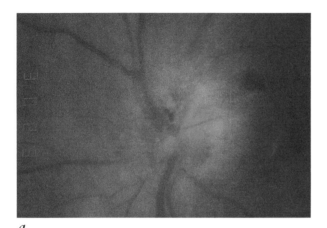

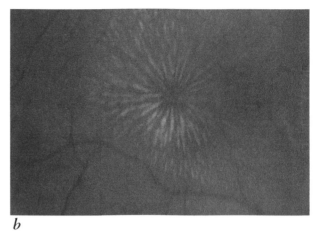

a   *b*

Figure 4.5   *Neuroretinitis: optic disc swelling and stellate maculopathy due to lipid deposits in the outer plexiform layer of the retina.*

atypical optic neuritis due to a systemic disease affecting the optic nerve. Whereas a full systemic evaluation is not terribly useful in patients with typical optic neuritis, it is essential in patients with an atypical presentation.

AUTOIMMUNE OPTIC NEUROPATHIES

Atypical optic neuropathies may be the result of auto-immune diseases. This is not a difficult diagnosis in a patient with a known autoimmune disease presenting with acute visual loss due to an optic neuropathy; however, it is more equivocal in a patient with atypical optic neuritis and borderline or equivocal serologies. It is important to differentiate an autoimmune optic neuritis from demyelinating optic neuritis. The former may be very responsive to systemic corticosteroids and visual function may not improve without them, whereas treatment with systemic steroids has little effect on the eventual visual outcome in patients with typical, demyelinating optic neuritis.[12]

SYSTEMIC LUPUS ERYTHEMATOSUS (SLE)[13]

A 42-year-old lady hospitalized with an acute cerebritis due to SLE was seen as a routine courtesy consult and had a normal neuro-ophthalmologic examination. Two days later she had totally lost vision in the left eye and developed a right sixth-nerve palsy. The left pupil was amaurotic and fundus examination was normal. She was treated with 250 mg methylprednisolone every 6 hours with no response after 24 hours. This was increased to 500 mg every 6 hours, resulting in a prompt improvement

in visual function. Three days later, visual acuity had returned to 20/20 in the left eye. Steroids were decreased and tapered and she maintained excellent vision until her death 2 years later.

The present author believes that many patients with atypical optic neuritis have an autoimmune optic neuritis. Who are these patients? The patient who has manifestations of typical optic neuritis but fails to improve or actually has progressive deterioration in vision over a 2-week period. These patients deserve a complete neuro-ophthalmic evaluation, as well as all the appropriate serologic tests for autoimmune diseases as well as syphilis and sarcoidosis. Unfortunately, the serologic tests for autoimmune disease are rarely definitive enough to make a formal diagnosis of SLE or any other autoimmune disease. Do not rely on the equivocations of the rheumatology consultant. Treat the patient with intravenous megadose steroids for 3 days and then with prednisone 80 mg/day and taper as rapidly as the patient's response allows. Atypical optic neuritis requires aggressive evaluation and treatment. Failure to treat aggressively may result in irreversible visual loss.

Shortly after presenting the previously described patient with optic neuritis due to aspergillosis at the International Neuro-ophthalmology Society and taking a verbal beating from his more senior colleagues, the present author returned to his academic practice somewhat humbled and reticent to treat optic neuritis with high-dose, or indeed any dose of, corticosteroids.

A 34-year-old lady was referred with visual loss and a swollen optic disc. Remembering the admonition that treating an optic neuropathy with corticosteroids represented a nervous doctor treating a nervous patient and was not science, no treatment was offered. Visual function never improved and optic atrophy ensued (see Figs

3.19 and 3.20). That was the last patient with atypical optic neuritis that this author has failed to treat with corticosteroids. Observe typical optic neuritis: evaluate and treat atypical optic neuritis. When a patient with typical optic neuritis does not improve after 2 weeks, it becomes atypical optic neuritis and requires a full evaluation and treatment with intravenous corticosteroids—250–500 mg methylprednisolone every 6 hours for 3 days followed by a tapering course of oral prednisone.[13]

SARCOIDOSIS

Sarcoidosis is more common than most clinicians believe and ranks with syphilis as one of the great imitators in neuro-ophthalmology. When there is no other cause for an afferent or an efferent neuro-ophthalmologic problem, this diagnosis should be considered. Diagnosis is based upon clinical suspicion and biopsy proof. Lacrimal gland biopsy may provide a rapid and easy method to establish the diagnosis prior to initiating treatment. Chest x-ray and biopsy via bronchoscopy or mediastinoscopy may also be diagnostic. Angiotensin-converting enzyme (ACE) levels are obtained with impunity but usually only elevated in the presence of obvious pulmonary disease. A tissue diagnosis is very helpful and often easily obtainable. In a recent series of patients with pulmonary sarcoidosis, 32 of 123 (26%) had neurologic involvement including cranial nerve palsies (59%) and papilledema (6%).[14]

A 32-year-old lady was referred with an anterior orbital mass (Fig. 4.6a) and rapidly decreased vision secondary to an optic neuropathy. Visual acuity in the right eye was decreased to 20/400 and the visual field vas severely depressed (Fig. 4.6b). There was a RAPD and the optic disc was swollen (Fig. 4.6c). The visual function in the left eye was normal. The anterior orbital mass was biopsied that day, and obvious non-caseating granulomas were present. Treatment with oral prednisone 80 mg/day resulted in rapid restoration of visual function and optic disc appearance (Fig. 4.7). This lady was fortunate in that an easily accessible orbital mass accompanied her optic neuropathy. Sarcoidosis was immediately considered and treatment was promptly initiated.

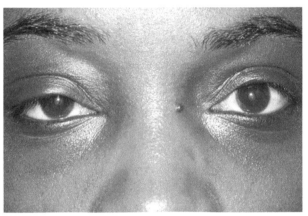

a

b

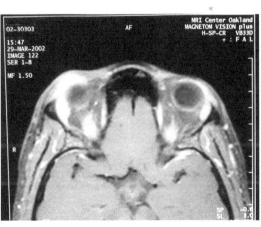

c

Figure 4.6 *A patient with sarcoidosis presenting with an anterior orbital mass and marked visual field loss (a), visual loss and a swollen optic disc (b). An MRI scan demonstrating enhancement of lacrimal gland and eyelid (c).*

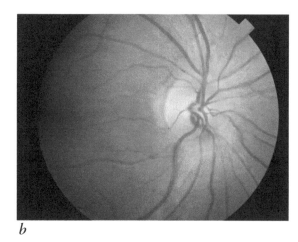

a

b

Figure 4.7 *Resolution of orbital inflammation (a), normalization of visual field and optic disc edema (b) after treatment with systemic corticosteroids.*

A 24-year-old man was referred with visual loss and a swollen optic disc (Fig. 4.8). An MRI scan demonstrated enlargement and enhancement of the optic nerve and extraocular muscles (Fig. 4.9). Visual loss was relentless. A chest x-ray demonstrated hilar adenopathy and mediastinoscopy confirmed the diagnosis of sarcoidosis. Visual function and the appearance of the optic disc normalized (Fig. 4.10) after treatment with systemic corticosteroids.

If diagnosis is delayed, visual loss can be relentless and total. A 28-year-old man presented to the eye clinic with decreased vision and a visual field defect in his right eye (Fig. 4.11). He was sent for a CT scan and was lost to follow-up. He returned 2 months later with total loss of vision in his right eye and optic atrophy (Fig. 4.12). A CT scan demonstrated erosion of his optic canal (Fig. 4.13) and some scattered enhancing plaques on the surface of the brain. Neurosurgical exploration revealed erosion of his optic canal and intracanalicular optic nerve by non-caseating granulomas.[15,16]

SYPHILIS[17–20]

Dr J Lawton Smith popularized neuro-ophthalmologic manifestations of syphilis a generation ago. He was vilified by some in the ophthalmologic establishment for his unorthodox thinking but did alert some of us with more open minds to the ophthalmologic manifestations and ubiquitous nature of the great imitator. In spite of demonstrations of spirochetes in the aqueous humor, CSF and the almost epidemic nature of Fluorescent Treponemal Antibody Absorption (FTA-ABS) reactivity in some populations, syphilis believers were considered

almost cult-like until the appearance of the human immunodeficiency virus (HIV) and the acquired immune deficiency syndrome (AIDS) epidemic. Syphilis then became very popular and mainstream as it efficiently infected those immune-compromised individuals. Spirochetes are ubiquitous and the diagnosis of syphilis should be considered in any patient with recurrent iritis/vitritis (Fig. 4.14), atypical optic neuropathy, non-rhegmatogenous retinal detachments (Fig. 4.15), chorioretinitis (Figs 4.16 and 4.17) without an obvious etiology and any HIV-compromised patient. An FTA-ABS test is easy to obtain and is often positive in the presence of a non-reactive Venereal Disease Research Lab (VDRL).[20] Once accurately diagnosed, syphilis is very treatable with a variety of penicillin regimens.

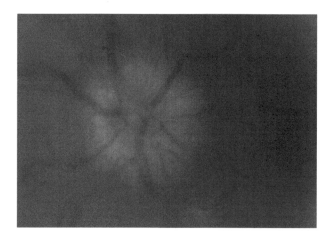

Figure 4.8 *Optic disc swelling in a patient with sarcoidosis.*

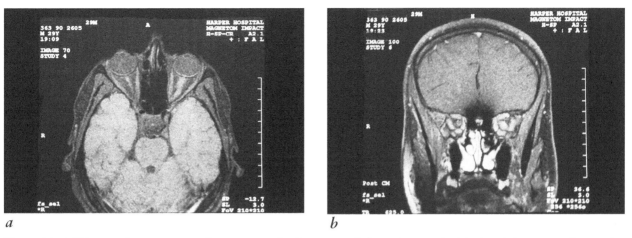

Figure 4.9 *MRI scans demonstrating enhancement and enlargement of the optic nerve (axial, a) and the extraocular muscles (coronal, b).*

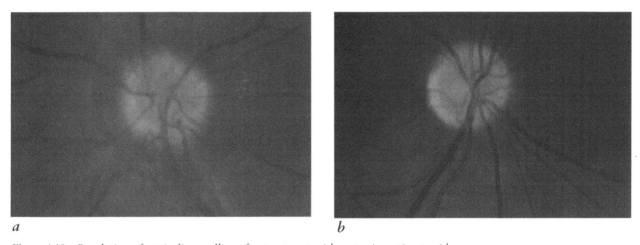

Figure 4.10 *Resolution of optic disc swelling after treatment with systemic corticosteroids.*

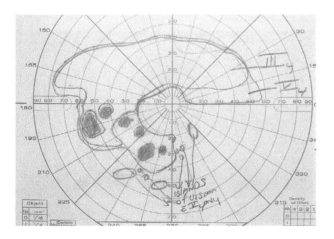

Figure 4.11 *Inferior visual field defect demonstrated by Goldman perimetry.*

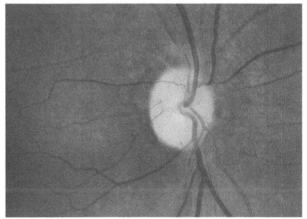

Figure 4.12 *Optic atrophy accompanying total visual loss.*

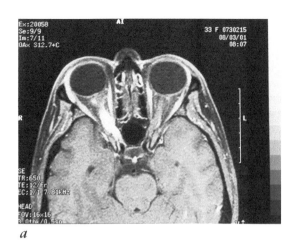

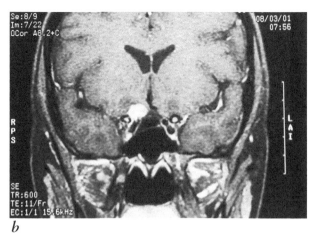

a   *b*

Figure 4.13   *MRI scans demonstrating an enhancing optic nerve mass with intracranial extension by eroding through the optic canal: axial (a) and coronal (b).*

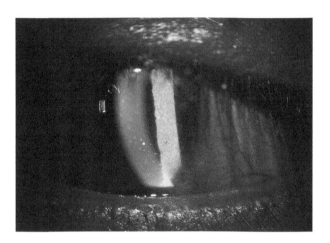

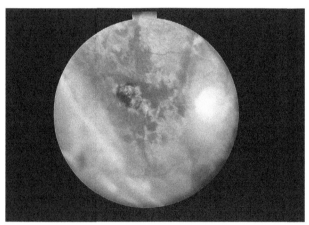

Figure 4.14   *Recurrent iritis/vitritis as a manifestation of syphilis.*

Figure 4.15   *Non-rhegmatogenous retinal detachment and chorioretinitis in ocular syphilis.*

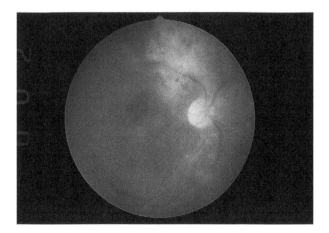

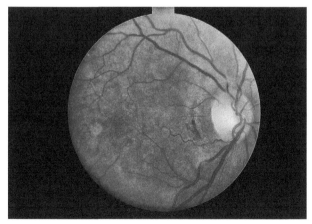

Figure 4.16   *Acute chorioretinitis in secondary syphilis.*

Figure 4.17   *Chronic chorioretinitis in late ocular syphilis.*

HIV OPTIC NEUROPATHIES

Patients with HIV disease may be inflicted with a variety of optic neuropathies. HIV may primarily infect the optic nerve presenting as 'typical' optic neuritis with pain on eye movement and a normal-appearing optic disc or slowly progressive visual loss. Unlike optic neuritis, this does not spontaneously improve after several weeks and quickly becomes an atypical optic neuritis and the diagnosis becomes obvious when it is considered.

Cryptococcal meningitis may cause an optic neuropathy with acute, devastating visual loss in HIV patients. The fungus may directly invade the nerve, cause an adhesive arachnoiditis, or compromise the optic nerve via markedly elevated intracranial pressure. An HIV-infected patient (Fig. 4.18) presenting with papilledema should be considered to have cryptococcal meningitis until proven otherwise. The intracranial pressure may be markedly elevated, and visual loss may be rapid and devastating. Optic nerve sheath decompression (ONSD) may be sight saving (Fig. 4.19). The present author considers this to be the single best indication for ONSD. Other organisms including toxoplasmosis, aspergillus, mycobacterium and syphilis can cause a similar clinical picture.

Cytomegalic inclusion virus (CMV), although usually causing a retinitis with hemorrhagic necrosis of the retina (Fig. 4.20), involves the optic nerve head in about 4% of infected patients (Fig. 4.21). Likewise, herpes simplex virus, although usually causing an acute retinal necrosis syndrome, may infect the optic nerve with a resultant optic neuritis.[21]

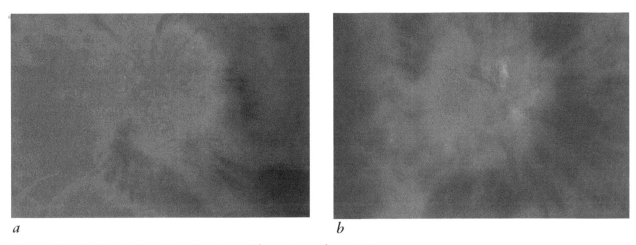

a   *b*

Figure 4.18   *Florid optic disc edema in patient with cryptococcal meningitis.*

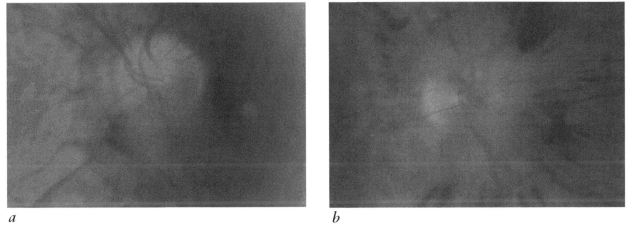

a   *b*

Figure 4.19   *Marked reduction in optic disc edema 3 weeks after bilateral ONSD.*

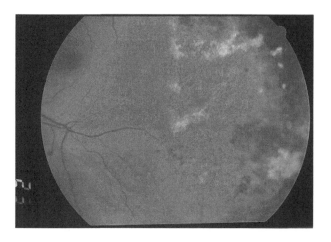

Figure 4.20 *CMV retinitis.*

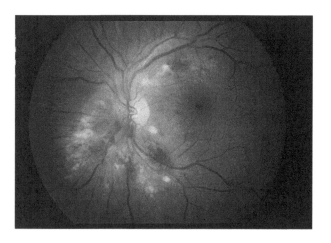

Figure 4.21 *CMV retinitis with optic nerve involvement.*

LYME DISEASE

Optic neuritis is an uncommon manifestation of Lyme disease and is probably overdiagnosed by including patients with optic neuritis and ischemic optic neuropathy based only on a positive Lyme serology. To accurately attribute an optic neuropathy to a Lyme disease etiology, there should be a history of exposure to a tick bite, subsequent erythema migrans and positive Lyme titers in serum and CSF confirmed by Western blot testing. The fundus picture is that of a neuroretinitis with retina and optic nerve involvement often accompanied by an iritis.[22]

CAT-SCRATCH FEVER

Patients with cat-scratch fever have had a recent viral illness with fever and sometimes very significant lymphadenopathy. Patients may develop optic disc swelling and visual loss followed by neuroretinitis. Cat-scratch fever is considered self-limiting and resolves spontaneously. Like some others,[23] the present author treats patients with visual dysfunction, neuroretinitis and positive Bartonella titers with a short course of doxycycline or azithromycin in an attempt to shorten the clinical course and prevent permanent visual dysfunction (Fig. 4.22).

NUTRITIONAL/TOXIC OPTIC NEUROPATHIES

The characteristics of nutritional and toxic optic neuropathies are gradual, painless, progressive and always bilateral visual loss, accompanied by dyschromatopsia and centro-cecal visual field defects. Due to the bilaterality, a RAPD may not be readily apparent but light-near dissociation of the pupils will be evident. The pupils will react more briskly at near than they do to light due to the optic nerve dysfunction. The optic discs will initially appear normal. Optic atrophy will ensue. These entities need to be differentiated from the hereditary optic neuropathies, retinopathies and non-organic visual dysfunction.

DEFICIENCIES[24]

Deficiency states result from malnutrition, malabsorption or epidemic starvation, often in conjunction with a toxin, although a rare cause of optic neuropathy, vitamin B12 deficiency has been well studied due to its role in pernicious anemia and associated neurologic deficits. The hallmarks of vitamin B12 deficiency are a megaloblastic anemia, subacute degeneration of the spinal cord and peripheral neuropathy with decreased deep tendon reflexes. Vitamin B12 deficiency is usually the result of malabsorption due to gastrectomy or removal of the proximal ileum. True deficiency is rare but may occur in a strict vegan. Treatment is with parenteral vitamin B12.

Tobacco–Alcohol Amblyopia

Tobacco–alcohol amblyopia, or the more politically correct nutritional amblyopia, is a nutritional deficiency

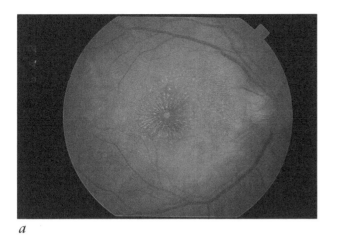

a

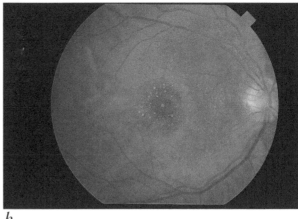

b

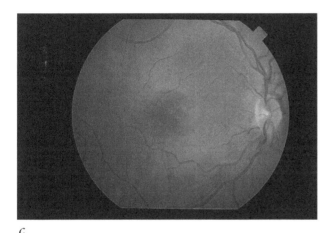

c

Figure 4.22 *Cat-scratch neuroretinitis (a), improvement evident 3 weeks after treatment with azithromycin (b), total resolution 6 weeks after treatment (c).*

state exacerbated by the toxic effects of alcohol or tobacco. There have been some intriguing reports postulating a genetic predisposition resulting from a mitochondrial DNA deficiency as in Leber's hereditary optic neuropathy (LHON).[25] Since neither tobacco nor alcohol is toxic to the anterior visual pathways, there must be some nutritional basis for this disorder, exacerbated by the cyanide in tobacco smoke. Regardless of etiology, it does exist and is a potentially reversible cause of visual loss. Patients have the usual painless, progressive, bilateral loss of central vision. In the present author's experience, all patients smelled of alcohol in the office and had a history of heavy smoking and drinking that prompted the diagnosis. A recent patient complained that everything he saw appeared green. Vision was mildly impaired and bilateral central scotomas were evident on visual fields (Fig. 4.23): optic discs were normal. Although acute fundus changes of peripapillary dilated vessels and hemorrhages have been reported, the optic discs usually are normal. Supplemental B vitamins and parenteral B12 normalized visual function even though the patient still smelled of alcohol when he visited the office.

TOXINS

Methanol and ethylene glycol

Unlike the slow progressive visual loss caused by other toxins, methanol and ethylene glycol cause a rapid, often non-reversible, bilateral visual loss with optic disc swelling indistinguishable from papilledema. Visual loss may be profound even after ingesting small amounts. Patients are often comatose with metabolic acidosis. Symptoms occur 12–48 hours after ingestion. Visual function rarely improves. Treatment of the underlying acidosis and intravenous ethanol to compete with the methanol may be life saving but is rarely sight saving. Methanol toxicity is the best studied, based on the classic study of 320 prisoners who ingested methanol-spiked moonshine whiskey.[26]

Ethambutol, now largely obsolete for treating tuberculosis, causes a dose-related optic neuropathy in patients taking > 15 mg/kg/day. The visual field loss may be central or peripheral, or may mimic chiasmal defects. It is largely reversible, although there are some documented

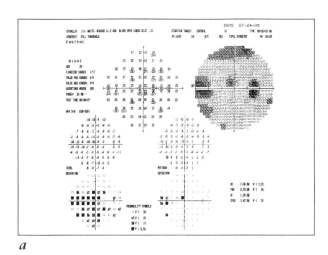
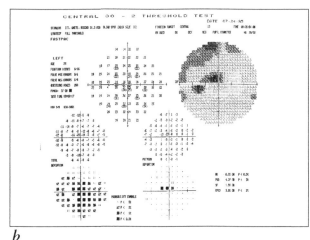

a   *b*

Figure 4.23   *Bilateral central scotomas from nutritional amblyopia.*

cases where visual loss continued to progress after the drug was discontinued.[27]

The antiarrythmic agent amiodarone, well known for causing a universal but clinically inconsequential keratopathy, may rarely cause a significant optic neuropathy. The clinical presentation may mimic NAION and in some instances may actually be NAION, since patients taking amiodarone have similar vasculopathic risk factors as patients with NAION. However, there is a subgroup of patients with insidious, bilateral visual loss occurring over several months. Their visual loss is usually less severe than patients with NAION and may improve after discontinuing the medication.[28]

A variety of anti-neoplastic agents are well known to cause optic neuropathies. These include vincristine, methotrexate and cisplatin. More will be described as more aggressive chemotherapeutic regimens keep these patients alive and functioning longer. Other commonly encountered medications with well-recognized optic neuropathies include disulfiram (Antabuse), used for treating alcoholism, and isoniazid (INH), a common treatment for tuberculosis.

PEARL: Toxic optic neuropathies are always bilateral. Except for methanol and ethylene glycol (see above), visual loss is insidious, slow and progressive.

CANCER-RELATED OPTIC NEUROPATHIES

If a patient with an underlying malignancy presents with a neuro-ophthalmologic or orbital problem, it is due to the malignancy until proven otherwise. This aphorism will prevent you from making a number of stupid mistakes.

CARCINOMATOUS MENINGITIS

These patients are usually very ill from their underlying malignancy, and are often in terminal stages of lung or breast carcinoma. The tumor has metastasized to the meninges. Patients may have acute or chronic progressive visual loss. Optic discs may appear normal or swollen depending upon the site of involvement. There may be associated cranial neuropathies, most commonly cranial nerves three and six are involved but five, seven and eight may also be affected. MRI scans may initially be normal but eventually the optic nerve will appear thickened and enhance with contrast. Diagnosis is confirmed by detecting carcinomatous cells and elevated protein in the CSF. It may take several lumbar punctures to obtain a positive result. Corticosteroids and radiation therapy may help prolong visual function.

OPTIC NERVE METASTASIS

Breast, lung, stomach and pancreatic carcinoma may metastasize to the optic nerve, although orbital and choroidal involvement is much more common. This is uncommon and presents as visual loss accompanied by a visible mass invading the optic nerve head (Fig. 4.24). Compression of the vasculature may cause a central retinal vein or artery occlusion (CRVO and CRAO, respectively). Patients with more posterior optic nerve involvement may present with visual loss and a normal-appearing optic disc. Imaging studies demonstrate

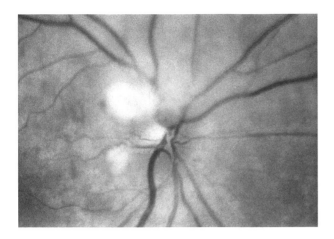

Figure 4.24 *Adenocarcinoma of lung metastatic to optic nerve head.*

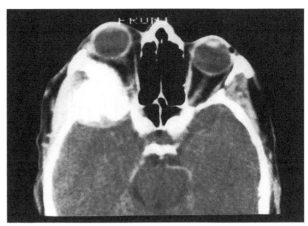

Figure 4.25 *Osteoblastic metastasis from prostatic carcinoma may cause a compressive optic neuropathy.*

fusiform enlargement of the optic nerve or compression of the optic canal from osteoblastic bony metastasis seen in prostatic carcinoma (Fig. 4.25). Treatment of the underlying malignancy and adjunct radiation therapy may help prolong visual function.

LYMPHOMA AND LEUKEMIA

Lymphomatous meningitis may directly invade the optic nerve via the pial septa, or an enlarging orbital mass may cause a compressive optic neuropathy. Leukemia causes an optic neuropathy by directly infiltrating the optic nerve. Imaging studies demonstrate an enlarged optic nerve (Fig. 4.26). Visual loss is often sudden and progressive (Fig. 4.27), and it is often, but not always, accompanied by

uveal and retinal involvement. Treatment of the underlying disease and adjunctive radiation therapy may help prolong useful visual function.

PARANEOPLASTIC OPTIC NEUROPATHY

Paraneoplastic optic neuropathy is much rarer than paraneoplastic retinopathy and may occur as a remote manifestation of lung carcinoma. As with the retinal disease, an antibody formed against a tumor antigen cross reacts with a host antigen (optic nerve) causing an optic neuritis-type syndrome that may respond transiently to corticosteroids. History of an underlying malignancy is crucial to making this diagnosis, although it may occur in patients not yet diagnosed with lung cancer.

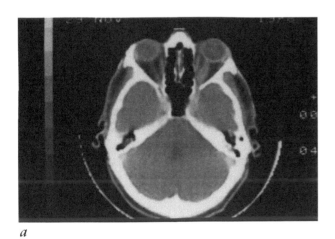

a

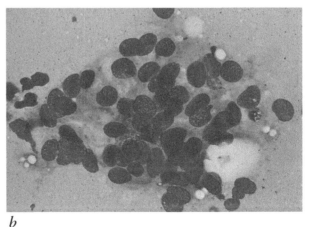

b

Figure 4.26 *A CT scan demonstrating isolated enlargement of the optic nerve (a) due to leukemic infiltration (b).*

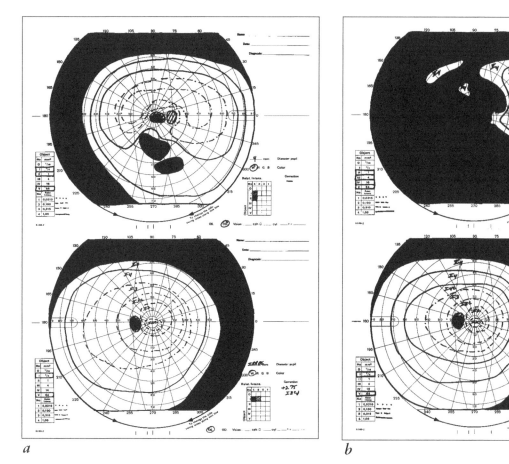

a   *b*

Figure 4.27   *Visual field defect (a) in a patient with leukemic infiltration of the optic nerve (see Fig. 4.26), progressing over a 3-week period (b) obviating useful vision.*

RADIATION OPTIC NEUROPATHY

Acute, painless visual loss occurring 12–18 months after irradiation for head and neck malignancies is the hallmark of radiation optic neuropathy. The optic chiasm may also be involved. These patients present with bilateral visual loss. Radiation has damaged the glial and vascular endothelial cells resulting in a microvasculopathy and an occlusive endarteritis-causing ischemia of the optic nerve head. This may be accompanied or preceded by evidence for radiation retinopathy (Fig. 4.28). Visual loss progresses over weeks to months and must be distinguished from visual loss caused by tumor recurrence. MRI scans may demonstrate focal enhancement in mildly enlarged optic nerves.

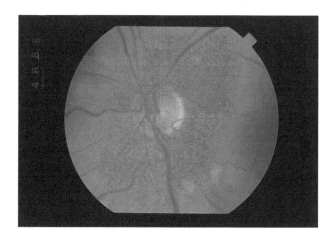

Figure 4.28   *Radiation retinopathy preceding radiation-induced optic neuropathy.*

REFERENCES

1. Beck RW, Cleary PA, Anderson MM et al. A randomized, controlled trial of corticosteroids in the treatment of acute optic neuritis. *N Engl J Med* 1992; **326**:581–6.
2. Beck RW. The optic neuritis treatment trial. Three year follow up results. *Arch Ophthalmol* 1995; **113**:136–7.
3. Optic neuritis study group. The five year risk of MS after acute optic neuritis: experience in the Optic Neuritis Treatment Trial. *Neurology* 1997; **49**:1404–13.
4. Beck RW, Cleary PA, Trobe JD et al. The effect of corticosteroids for acute optic neuritis on the subsequent development of multiple sclerosis. *N Engl J Med* 1993; **329**:1764–9.
5. Beck RW, Trobe JR, Moke PS et al. High and low risk profiles for developing MS within 10 years after optic neuritis. Experience of the ONTT. *Arch Ophthalmol* 2003; **121**:944–9.
6. Levin LA, Lessell S. Optic neuritis and multiple sclerosis. *Arch Ophthalmol* 2003; **121**:1039–40.
7. Farris BK, Pickard DJ. Bilateral postinfectious optic neuritis and intravenous steroid therapy in children. *Ophthalmology* 1990; **97**:339–45.
8. Brady KM, Brar AS, Lee AG et al. Optic neuritis in children: clinical features and visual outcome. *J AAPOS* 1999; **3**:98–103.
9. Jacobson DM, Thompson HS, Corbett JJ. Optic neuritis in the elderly. *Neurology* 1988; **38**:1834–7.
10. Slavin ML, Liebergall DA. Acute unilateral visual loss in the elderly due to retrobulbar optic neuropathy. *Surv Ophthalmol* 1996; **41**:261–7.
11. Maitland CG, Miller NR. Neuroretinitis. *Arch Ophthalmol* 1984; **102**:1146–50.
12. Kupersmith MJ, Burde RM, Warren FA et al. Autoimmune optic neuropathy: evaluation and treatment. *J Neurol Neurosurg Psychiatr* 1988; **51**:1381–6.
13. Lessell S. The neuro-ophthalmology of systemic lupus erythematosus. *Doc Ophthalmol* 1979; **47**:13–42.
14. Allen RK, Sellars RE, Sandstrom PA. A prospective study of 32 patients with neurosarcoidosis. *Sarcoidosis Vasc Diffuse Lung Dis* 2003; **20**:118–25.
15. Beardsley TL, Brown SVL, Sydnor CF et al. Eleven cases of sarcoidosis of the optic nerve. *Am J Ophthalmol* 1984; **97**:62–77.
16. Beck AD, Newman NJ, Grossniklaus HE et al. Optic nerve enlargement and chronic visual loss. *Surv Ophthalmol* 1994; **38**:555–6.
17. Folk JC, Weingeist TA, Corbett JJ et al. Syphilitic neuroretinitis. *Am J Ophthalmol* 1983; **95**:480–6.
18. Johns BR, Tierney M, Felsusteion D. Alteration in the natural history of neurosyphilis by the concurrent infection with the human immunodeficiency virus. *N Engl J Med* 1987; **316**:1569–72.
19. McLeish WM, Pulido JS, Holland S et al. The ocular manifestations of syphilis in the human immunodeficiency virus type-1 infected host. *Ophthalmology* 1990; **97**:196–203.
20. Spoor TC, Ramocki JM, Nesi FA, Sorsher M. Ocular syphilis—1986. Prevalence of FTA-ABS reactivity and cerebrospinal fluid findings. *J Clin Neuro-Ophthalmol* 1987; **4**:191–7.
21. Winward KE, Hamed LM, Glaser JS. The spectrum of optic nerve disease in human immunodeficiency virus infection. *Am J Ophthalmol* 1989; **107**:373–80.
22. Balcer LJ, Winterkorn JM, Galetta SL. Neuroophthalmologic manifestations of Lyme disease. *J Neuro-Ophthalmol* 1997; **108**:108–21.
23. Reed JB, Scales DK, Wong MT. Bartonella henselae neuroretinitis in cat scratch disease. Diagnosis, management and sequelae. *Ophthalmology* 1998; **105**:459–66.
24. Lessell S. Nutritional amblyopia. *J Neuro-Ophthalmol* 1998; **18**:106–11.
25. Rizzo JF, Lessell S. Tobacco amblyopia. *Am J Ophthalmol* 1993; **116**:84–7.
26. Benton CD, Calhoun FP. The ocular effects of methyl alcohol poisoning. Report of a catastrophe involving 320 persons. *Trans Am Acad Ophthalmol Otolaryngol* 1952; **56**:875–85.
27. DeVita EG, Miao M, Sadun AA. Optic neuropathy in ethambutol-treated renal tuberculosis. *J Clin Neuro-Ophthalmol* 1987; **7**:77–86.
28. Nazarian SM, Jay WM. Bilateral optic neuropathy associated with amiodarone therapy. *J Clin Neuro-Ophthalmol* 1988; **8**:25–8.

Chapter 5   The swollen optic disc

Compression of the optic nerves with or without decreased visual function may result from increased intracranial pressure (ICP). There may be an identifiable cause of the increased ICP (i.e. brain tumor) or it may be idiopathic pseudo-tumor cerebri. The optic nerves may not actually be swollen but appear swollen due to an anatomic variant—pseudopapilledema. The optic nerve may also appear swollen because the eye is hypotonous, allowing the ICP to exceed the intraocular pressure (IOP) (Fig. 5.1). Inflammation of the optic nerve itself may result in optic disc swelling, most always accompanied by decreased visual function (papillitis: see Chapter 4).

PSEUDOPAPILLEDEMA

HYPEROPIA

Hyperopic eyes may have crowded optic discs that on casual examination may appear swollen (Fig. 5.2). Differentiation is cost-effectively accomplished by detecting the degree of hyperopia with a cycloplegic refraction. Additionally, there will be no evidence for peripapillary nerve fiber layer hemorrhage or infarction. The peripapillary nerve fiber layer will not be swollen and spontaneous venous pulsations may be evident. Hyperopic pseudopapilledema is rarely an issue with adults but may be perplexing with children, especially if they are too young to carefully examine in the office environment.

BURIED OPTIC DISC DRUSEN

Buried optic disc drusen are a common cause of pseudopapilledema, especially in children. Careful examination is often difficult to impossible with a squirming, screaming child; however, when possible, this diagnosis can often be made by careful fundus examination (Fig. 5.3). Diagnosis may be confirmed by demonstrating calcification in the optic nerve on ultrasonography (Fig. 5.4). Drusen may also be readily apparent on a computerized tomography (CT) scan.

TILTED OPTIC DISCS

The temporal portion of the optic disc may appear swollen in myopic patients with tilted optic discs (Fig. 5.5). This is of no pathologic significance.

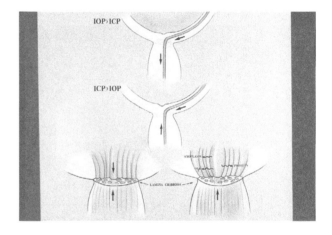

Figure 5.1 *Relationship between IOP and ICP at the lamina cribrosa. IOP normally exceeds ICP, augmenting the flow of axoplasm from the eye towards the brain (above). As ICP exceeds IOP, axoplasm obstipates and the optic disc swells.*

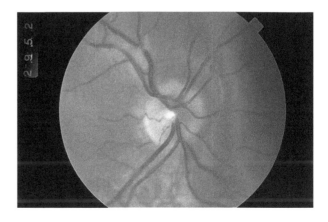

Figure 5.2 *Pseudopapilledema in a hyperopic child.*

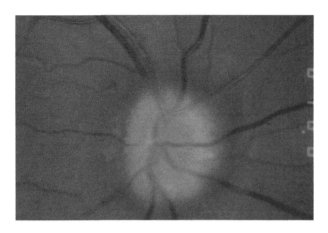

Figure 5.3 *Buried optic disc drusen.*

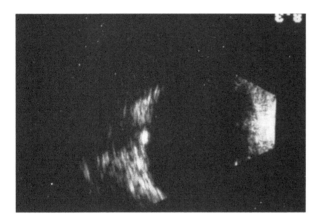

Figure 5.4 *B-scan ultrasonography with reduced gain demonstrates a brightly refractile optic disc drusen.*

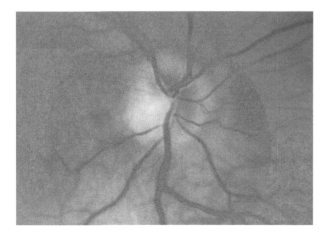

Figure 5.5 *Pseudopapilledema due to a tilted, myopic optic disc.*

Pseudopapilledema is often a perplexing diagnosis. The clinician is afraid of not diagnosing true papilledema and ordering the appropriate studies. Excessive imaging studies are often ordered for patients with pseudo-papilledema. A more confident and informed clinician may be comfortable enough to photograph the fundus and observe the patient in order to detect any significant changes. The knee-jerk response remains to see an atypical (often normal) optic disc and order a plethora of imaging studies, which often are totally unnecessary, except for physician protection in this increasingly litigious society.

The clinician must also differentiate true optic disc swelling due to elevated ICP from optic disc anomalies, papillitis and ischemic optic neuropathy. This is not always easy! Even experienced clinicians may have a difficult time distinguishing true papilledema from pseudopapilledema. The presence of spontaneous venous pulsations may be very helpful, indicating that ICP is < 200 mm cerebrospinal fluid (CSF). Patients with pseudopapilledema rarely, if ever, have evidence for peripapillary hemorrhages, exudates, distended retinal veins or choroidal stria. These are often present in patients with true papilledema.

Differentiating papilledema due to increased ICP from papillitis, ischemic optic neuropathy or other causes of true optic disc swelling is impossible by observation alone. The optic disc must be evaluated in the clinical context of the patient. True papilledema is most always bilateral but may be very asymmetric (Fig. 5.6). Visual function and visual fields are usually normal except for an enlarged blind spot. Patients with papillitis have decreased visual function, an obvious relative afferent pupillary defect (RAPD) and an abnormal visual field. Optic disc swelling is usually unilateral. Patients with non-arteritic anterior ischemic optic neuropathy (NAION) often have sector swelling of their optic discs (Fig. 5.7), an obvious RAPD and a distinctive visual field defect. This is usually unilateral but may occur bilaterally, especially after major surgical procedures. In these cases, the disc swelling is pallid, visual loss is often dramatic and the diagnosis is obvious in the presenting clinical context (Fig. 5.8). Having a little bit of papilledema is like being a little bit pregnant—the optic disc is swollen or it is not. If the discs are swollen due to increased ICP, the diagnosis is brain tumor until proven otherwise by negative neuroimaging. The diagnosis of papilledema requires prompt neuroimaging to rule out an expanding intracranial mass lesion (Figs 5.9 and 5.10).

The patient in Fig. 5.9 was being followed for hypertensive retinopathy when the referring physician became concerned about the atypical appearance of her optic discs. A CT scan demonstrated a large, enhancing mass

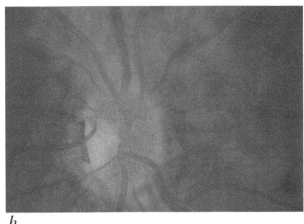

a   *b*

Figure 5.6   *Asymmetric papilledema in a patient with pseudotumor cerebri.*

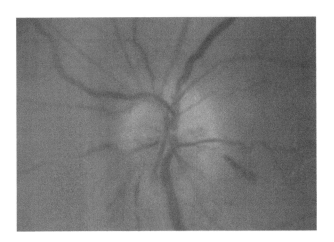

Figure 5.7 *Sector optic disc swelling and splinter hemorrhages in typical non-arteritic anterior ischemic optic neuropathy.*

compressing the ventricles with resultant papilledema (Fig. 5.10).

PAPILLEDEMA

Papilledema may be obvious (Fig. 5.11), subtle (Fig. 5.9) or pseudopapilledema (Figs 5.2 and 5.3). It may also rarely be unilateral or more commonly asymmetric (Fig. 5.6). Patients may also have markedly elevated ICP and normal-appearing optic discs (Fig. 5.12). Optic discs that have resolved papilledema may not swell again, even in the presence of markedly elevated ICP and the absence of discernible optic atrophy.

True papilledema due to elevated ICP must be differentiated from optic disc swelling secondary to inflammation,

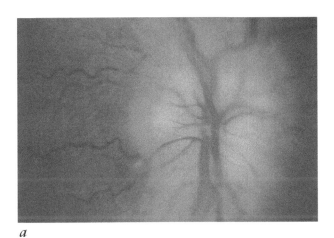

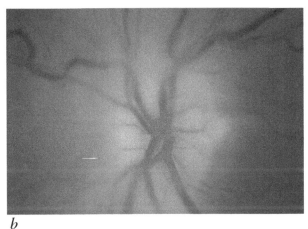

a   *b*

Figure 5.8   *Pallid optic disc edema in patient with bilateral postsurgical ischemic optic neuropathy.*

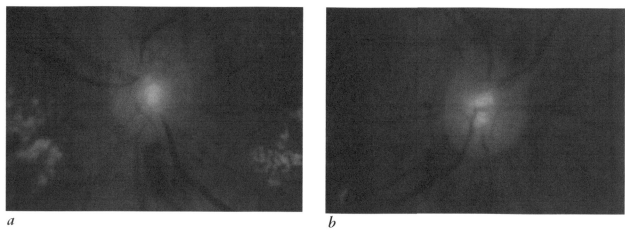

a   *b*

Figure 5.9   *Subtle optic disc swelling in a patient with elevated ICP due to brain tumor.*

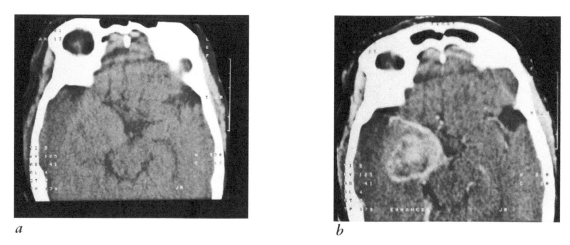

a   *b*

Figure 5.10   *CT scans demonstrating contrast-enhancing mass effacing the ventricular system: without (a) and with (b) contrast enhancement.*

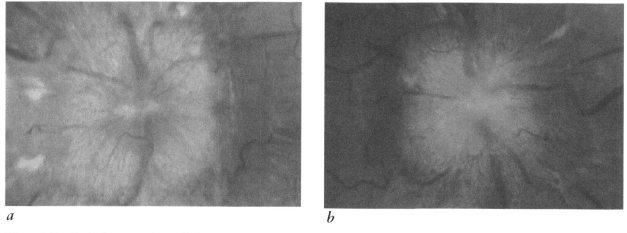

a   *b*

Figure 5.11   *Typical symmetric papilledema.*

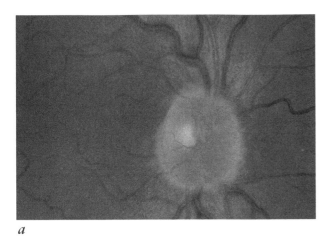
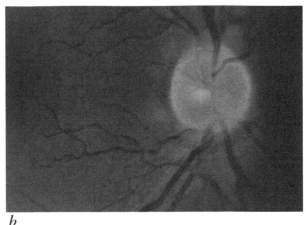

a   *b*

Figure 5.12 *Patient with PTC, ICP > 600 mm CSF and normal-appearing optic discs.*

infarction, compression and hypotony (Fig. 5.13). If considered, the diagnosis of hypotony should be obvious upon checking the IOP and taking a history. Disc swelling occurs when ICP > IOP. Although elevated ICP is a much more common etiology, decreased IOP should always be considered (Fig. 5.1).

Optic disc swelling (papillitis) caused by inflammation, infarction and compression is usually unilateral and accompanied by evidence for optic nerve dysfunction, i.e. decreased visual acuity, visual field defects, dyschromatopsia and a RAPD. Papilledema is usually bilateral, although it may be unilateral or very asymmetric (Fig. 5.6). Disc swelling may be obvious (Fig. 5.11) or subtle (Fig. 5.9). Visual function is initially normal but may deteriorate rapidly in the face of markedly elevated ICP and a compromised ischemic optic nerve head (Fig. 5.14).

PATHOGENESIS OF PAPILLEDEMA

The subarachnoid space of the optic nerve sheath is continuous with the intracranial subarachnoid space. The potential fluid-filled space extends from the back of the eye through the optic canal into the intracranial subarachnoid space. Elevated ICP is transmitted from the intracranial subarachnoid space to the retrobulbar optic nerve (Figs 5.15 and 5.16). The elevated ICP compresses the optic nerve fibers, causing stasis of both rapid and slow axoplasmic flow at the lamina cribrosa. The compressed axons swell, and there is subsequent leakage of water, protein and other axoplasmic contents into the extracellular space of the prelaminar optic nerve (Fig. 5.17).

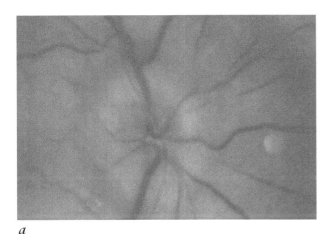
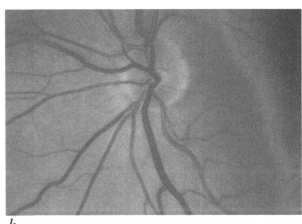

a   *b*

Figure 5.13 *Optic disc swelling due to chronic hypotony OD. Left optic disc is normal.*

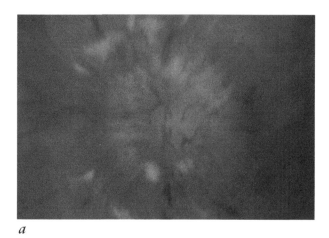

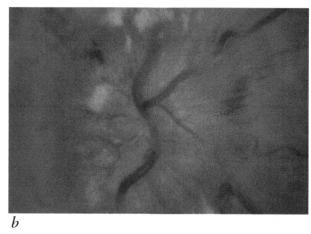

a   *b*

Figure 5.14 *Severe ischemic papilledema is a harbinger of a poor visual outcome.*

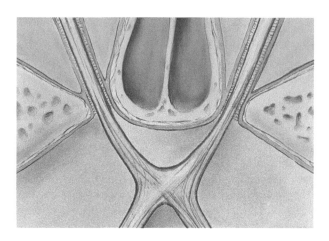

Figure 5.15 *Communication between the intracranial subarachnoid space (blue) and the optic nerve via the optic canal.*

Obstruction of slow axoplasmic flow is a pressure-related phenomenon. The tissue pressure on an intra-ocular portion of an optic nerve axon is determined by IOP: the pressure upon an intraorbital axon is governed by ICP. These two pressure compartments are separated by the lamina cribrosa (Fig. 5.17). Normally, IOP > ICP and axoplasm flows from the eye towards the brain. If ICP > IOP, this pressure gradient reverses and retards the flow of axoplasm down the axon at the lamina cribrosa. The axons of the optic nerve head anterior to the lamina cribrosa become swollen and distended by axoplasm. The obstipated axoplasm causes the axons to swell, leaking their contents into the prelaminar optic disc. This increases the osmotic pressure of the extracellular spaces of the optic disc resulting in further exudation of fluid and optic disc swelling.

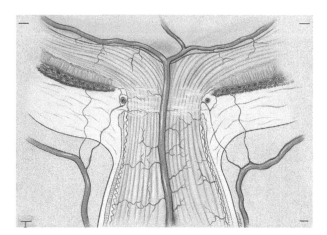

Figure 5.16 *Relationship between CSF and the optic nerve at the lamina cribrosa.*

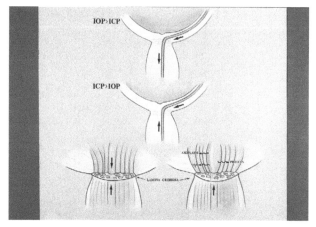

Figure 5.17 *Relationship between IOP and ICP at the lamina cribrosa.*

Papilledema is primarily a mechanical event resulting from obstruction of slow axoplasmic flow.[1] The vascular changes—venous stasis, capillary dilatation and obstruction, nerve fiber layer infarction and vascular telangiectasia on the optic disc—are secondary.[2]

STAGES OF PAPILLEDEMA

EARLY PAPILLEDEMA

An early sign of papilledema is blurring of the inferior and superior optic disc margins—the regions where nerve fibers are most dense (Fig. 5.18a–c). The optic disc is best viewed at the slit lamp with a 78- or 90-diopter lens, or with an indirect ophthalmoscope and a 14-diopter lens. Other early signs of papilledema include optic disc hyperemia due to capillary dilatation along the optic disc surface (Fig. 5.18c) and peripapillary nerve fiber layer hemorrhages (Fig. 5.19). In questionable cases, the presence of a hemorrhage confirms the diagnosis. These hemorrhages result from rupture of distended capillaries.

FULLY DEVELOPED PAPILLEDEMA

As papilledema becomes fully developed, the optic disc margin is blurred by the opaque nerve fiber layer, the retinal vessels become engorged, the optic disc is elevated above the surface of the retina, and infarcts appear on the surface of the disc and peripapillary retina (Fig. 5.20). Circumferential folds in the peripapillary retina (Paton's lines) may appear, possibly caused by a distended optic nerve sheath pressing upon the back of the eye (Fig. 5.21).

If true papilledema is present, neuroimaging must be obtained expeditiously to rule out an expanding intracranial mass (Figs 5.9 and 5.10). If no mass is present, the diagnosis of pseudotumor cerebri (PTC) should be considered and a lumbar puncture obtained to document elevated ICP and otherwise normal CSF studies. Elevated

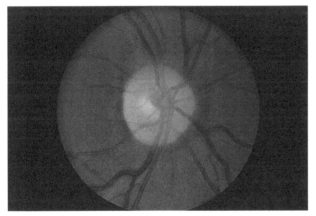

a

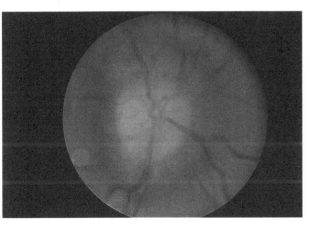

b

c

Figure 5.18 *Development of papilledema. Optic disc appears normal with just a hint of swelling of the nerve fiber layer at the superior pole (a). Nerve fiber layer swelling progresses and is evident at both the superior and inferior pole of the optic disc (b). Nerve fiber layer swelling is obvious, accompanied by disc hyperemia due to dilatation of capillaries (c).*

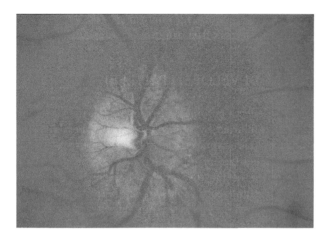

Figure 5.19 *Optic disc hyperemia, capillary dilatation and a single nerve fiber layer hemorrhage in developing papilledema.*

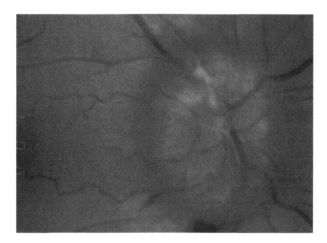

Figure 5.20 *Optic disc elevation with nerve fiber layer infarctions and distention of retinal veins in fully developed papilledema.*

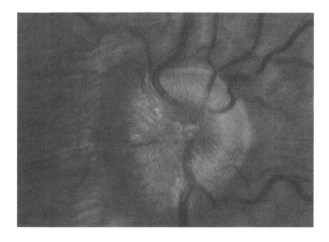

Figure 5.21 *Choroidal striae in papilledema.*

ICP, normal imaging excepting small ventricles and some pressure-related findings,[3,4] and no localizing signs excepting a sixth-nerve paresis, fulfill Dandy's criteria for the diagnosis of PTC.

Since Dandy's time other signs have been associated with PTC including fourth- and seventh-nerve paresis, tinnitus and vascular noises.[5,6] These are uncommon but evident if your cohort of PTC patients is large enough.

RESOLUTION OF PAPILLEDEMA

Fully developed papilledema (Fig. 5.22a) may take 6–8 weeks to resolve after normalization of ICP or a successful optic nerve sheath decompression. Retinal venous distention and optic disc capillary dilatation are first to regress (Fig. 5.22b), followed by disc hyperemia and elevation (Fig. 5.22c). Blurring of the optic disc margin and clouding of the peripapillary retina are the last to resolve (Fig. 5.23a–c). If ICP is normalized quickly, optic disc swelling will resolve with minimal damage to axons and the disc may appear normal (Fig. 5.22c), possibly leaving a high-water mark of pigmentation in the peripapillary retina and residual choroidal stria. If significant axonal damage has occurred, papilledema will resolve into optic atrophy with visual dysfunction (Fig. 5.24a–c). It is important to remember that once an optic disc has swollen, swelling may never again be obvious in spite of markedly elevated ICP. This is common knowledge when optic atrophy is present but may also occur with normal-appearing optic discs.[7]

Visual function in patients with early and fully developed papilledema is normal. If papilledema is not resolved in a timely fashion, optic nerve axons die with resultant diminished visual function and optic atrophy (Fig. 5.24). The degree of hemorrhage, exudation and venous engorgement has little value in prognosticating eventual visual function. However, severe optic disc swelling accompanied by extensive infarctions and attenuated arterioles has a poor prognosis often resulting in optic atrophy and severe visual dysfunction (Figs 5.25 and 5.26).

CHRONIC PAPILLEDEMA

With longstanding papilledema, there is slow resolution of hemorrhages and exudates, and rounding of the optic disc margin into a characteristic champagne cork shape (Fig. 5.27). Hard exudates on the optic disc may form drusen-like bodies, indicating that optic disc swelling has been present for at least several months. The presence of optic atrophy with or without optociliary shunt vessels

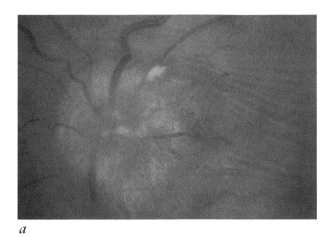

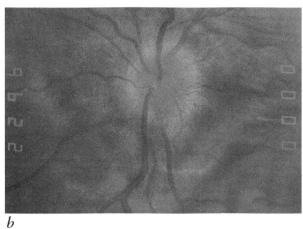

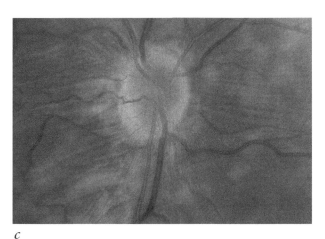

Figure 5.22 *Resolution of fully developed papilledema (a) with a normal-appearing optic disc (b) and residual choroidal striae (c).*

(Fig. 5.28) indicates that there has been a significant loss of axons and carries a poor prognosis for visual recovery.

HYPERTENSION AND PAPILLEDEMA

Obese patients with PTC and papilledema may also be hypertensive. This adds a degree of visual morbidity but may result in severe visual morbidity if the difference between hypertensive optic disc swelling and severe papilledema is not recognized and the blood pressure is lowered precipitously, infarcting the compromised optic disc. Fig. 5.29a–c represents grade 4 hypertensive retinopathy with optic disc swelling. The optic disc swelling is not as severe as that seen in patients with papilledema due to PTC who are also hypertensive (Fig. 5.30). There are also other signs of hypertensive retinopathy not evident in the patient with papilledema due to PTC. Aggressive treatment of this patient's coincidental hypertension prior to lowering

the CSF pressure resulted in rapid infarction of the optic nerve head and bilateral blindness, turning a functional individual into a relatively dysfunctional, dependent individual (Fig. 5.31).

PSEUDOTUMOR CEREBRI (PTC)

Most patients present with complaints of headache, diplopia due to a sixth-nerve paresis and obscurations of vision. Obscurations are momentary blackouts of vision (literally lasting seconds) due to optic nerve head swelling and axoplasmic stasis. Visual function may be normal or the visual field may be compromised. Loss of central vision is an ominous sign and indicates that the optic nerve compression has been too extensive and too long. Bilateral optic disc swelling is usually present (Fig. 5.32), although it may be very asymmetric (Fig. 5.33) or

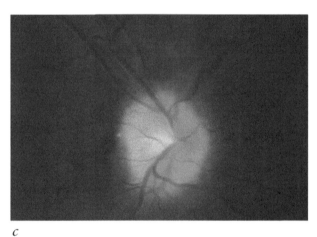

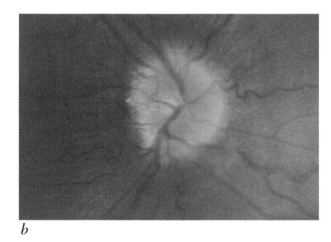

Figure 5.23 *Resolution of fully developed papilledema (a and b) with residual blurring of the optic disc margin (c).*

totally absent (Fig. 5.12) in spite of markedly elevated ICP. Optic disc swelling may be subtle or very obvious. Excessive optic disc swelling is often associated with markedly elevated ICP (Fig. 5.32). Patients with long-standing PTC may have optic atrophy with optociliary shunt vessels (Fig. 5.34) or chronic atrophic papilledema (Figs 5.35 and 5.36). Patients with optic atrophy or optociliary shunt vessels have a poor visual prognosis (Fig. 5.37).

PTC most commonly occurs in obese females in their childbearing years. It may also occur in males and may have a poorer visual prognosis. Pediatric PTC is more common than commonly realized,[8,9] and has no association with obesity and equal sexual predilection. Tetracycline ingestion or venous sinus thrombosis may be causative but the etiology is often unknown. ICP elevation and visual loss may be severe and require expeditious, definitive treatment.

CASE STUDY

A 16-year-old obese boy was referred with severe headache and rapidly deteriorating visual function due to pseudotumor cerebri with an ICP > 550 mm CSF. Visual acuity was 20/50 right eye (OD), 20/70 left eye (OS), pupils were sluggish and visual fields were severely compromised (Fig. 5.38). Fundus examination revealed severe ischemic papilledema with macular exudates (Fig. 5.39).

Child or adult, patients presenting with markedly elevated ICP (> 500 mm CSF), high-grade papilledema and visual loss are at risk of severe visual loss. This is 'malignant' PTC, and these patients have a very real risk of blindness in spite of aggressive and expeditious treatment. Treatment should consist of intravenous steroids and acetazolamide, expeditious optic nerve sheath decompression and, if necessary, a neurosurgical shunting procedure. Every effort should be made to decrease

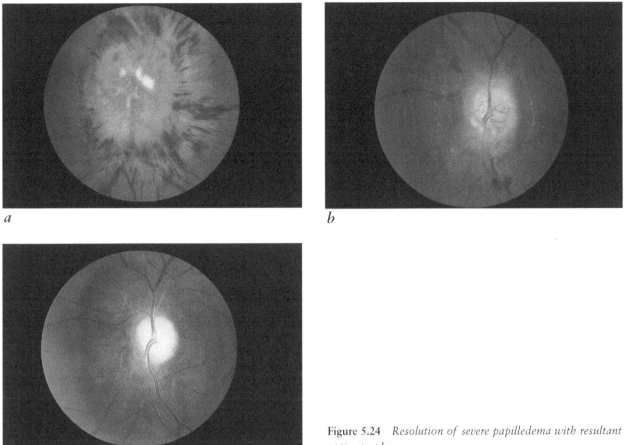

a

b

c

Figure 5.24 *Resolution of severe papilledema with resultant optic atrophy.*

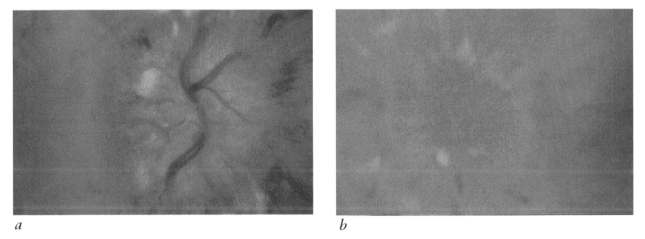

a

b

Figure 5.25 *Severe, ischemic papilledema in a patient with PTC.*

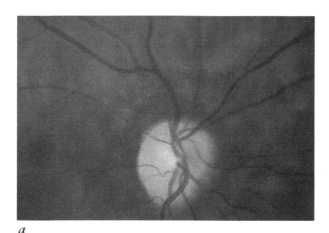

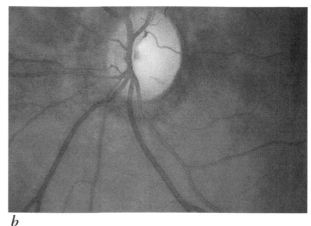

a   *b*

Figure 5.26   *Optic atrophy results after resolution of papilledema.*

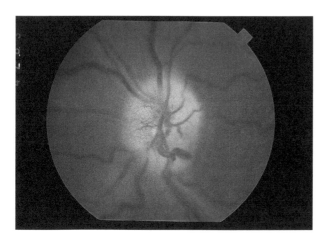

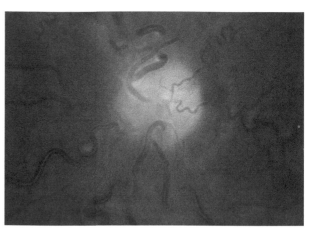

Figure 5.27   *Chronic atrophic papilledema in a patient with neglected PTC.*

Figure 5.28   *Optic atrophy and optociliary shunt vessels in endstage PTC.*

the ICP and relieve optic nerve compression, both medically and surgically.

The patient just described was admitted to the hospital, intravenous methylprednisolone 500 mg and acetazolamide 500 mg were administered and continued every 6 hours. An optic nerve sheath fenestration procedure was done sequentially on each eye and a neurosurgical opinion obtained to consider a thecoperitoneal shunting procedure. Aggressive, prompt treatment may be sight saving. In the present author's series of 35 patients with pediatric PTC, only one required a neurosurgical shunting procedure. This was done for intractable headache due to an ICP > 550 mm CSF, in spite of normal visual function 1 year after bilateral optic nerve sheath fenestrations.

Optic disc swelling promptly subsided (Fig. 5.40), and visual fields and acuity improved. Oral prednisone (80 mg/day) was continued for 6 weeks, as was acetazolamide (500 mg sequel daily). Six months later, visual acuity had returned to 20/25 both eyes (OU), visual fields were markedly improved (Fig. 5.41) and the fundus appearance normalized excepting some residual maculopathy (Fig. 5.42). After visual function was stabilized, a strict weight loss regimen was initiated. In many patients, weight reduction ≥ 10% is the most significant treatment for PTC.[10]

Unfortunately visual loss from optic nerve compression often occurs before an effective weight loss regimen can be implemented. Blind and thin is little better than blind and fat! The basic premise when treating patients

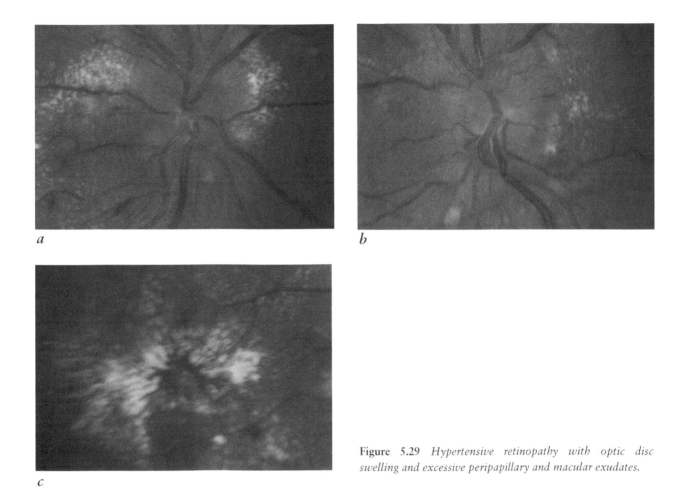

a

b

c

Figure 5.29 *Hypertensive retinopathy with optic disc swelling and excessive peripapillary and macular exudates.*

a

b

Figure 5.30 *Chronic, atrophic papilledema in a patient with PTC and coincident hypertension.*

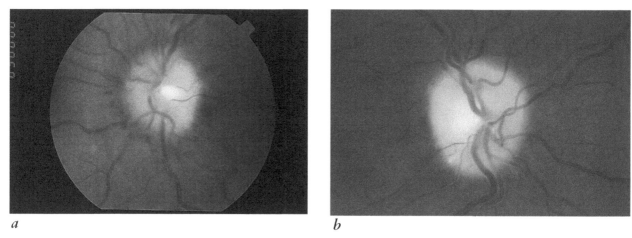

a   *b*

Figure 5.31   *Optic atrophy due to infarction of the optic discs after aggressive lowering of blood pressure without treating the markedly elevated ICP.*

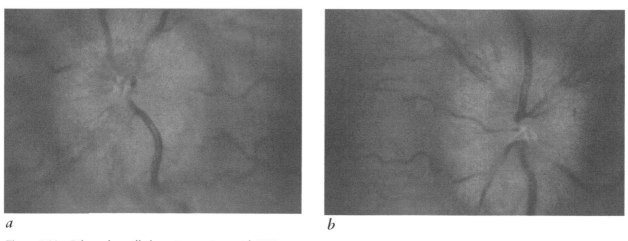

a   *b*

Figure 5.32   *Bilateral papilledema in a patient with PTC.*

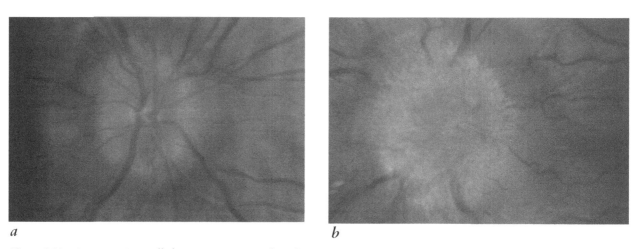

a   *b*

Figure 5.33   *Asymmetric papilledema in a patient with PTC.*

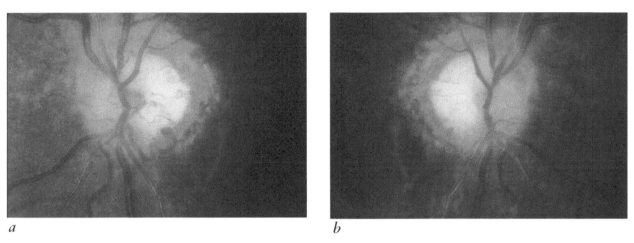

a   *b*

Figure 5.34   *Bilateral optic atrophy with optociliary shunt vessel on the right optic disc.*

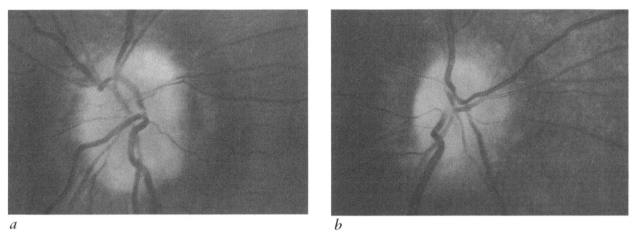

a   *b*

Figure 5.35   *Longstanding PTC with bilateral optic atrophy, peripapillary 'high water marks' from previous optic disc swelling and secondary optic disc drusen.*

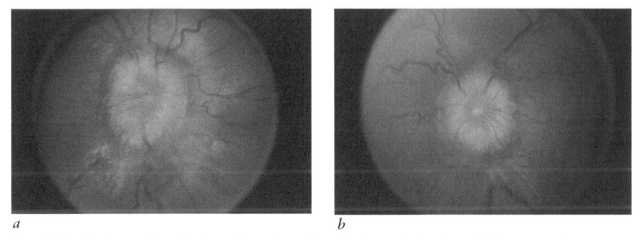

a   *b*

Figure 5.36   *Chronic atrophic papilledema with rounding of the optic disc margin into the typical champagne-cork appearance.*

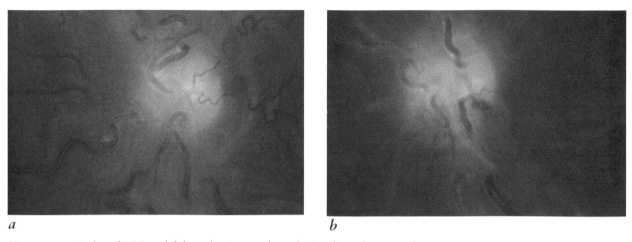

a   *b*

Figure 5.37   *Neglected PTC with bilateral optic atrophy and optociliary shunt vessels.*

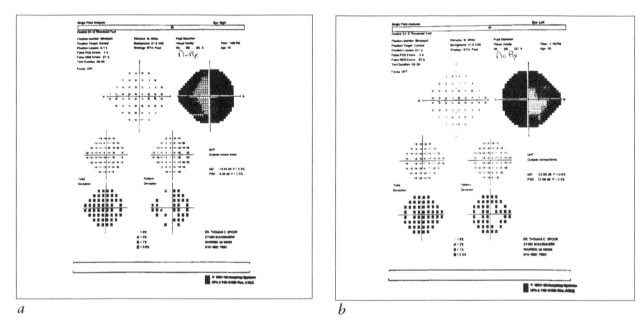

a   *b*

Figure 5.38   *Severely compromised visual fields in a patient with severe pediatric PTC.*

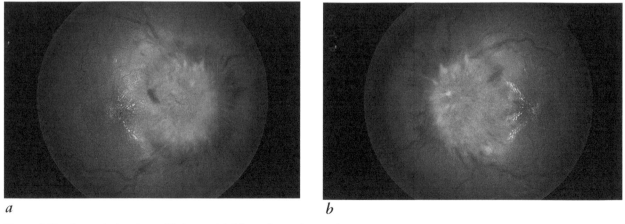

a   *b*

Figure 5.39   *Severe ischemic papilledema with bilateral macular exudates.*

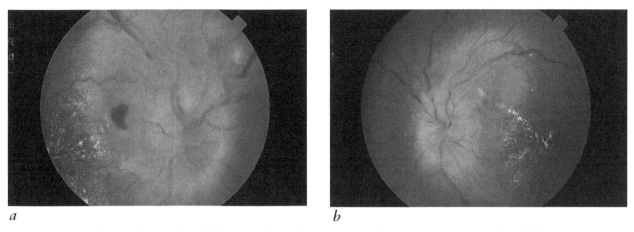

Figure 5.40 *Marked resolution of papilledema 10 days after treatment with systemic corticosteroids and bilateral optic nerve sheath fenestrations.*

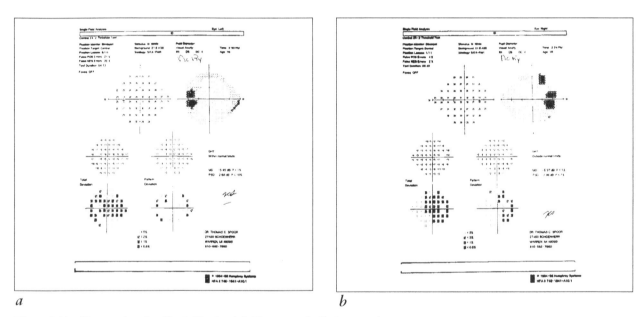

Figure 5.41 *Six months after Fig. 5.40, visual fields are markedly improved.*

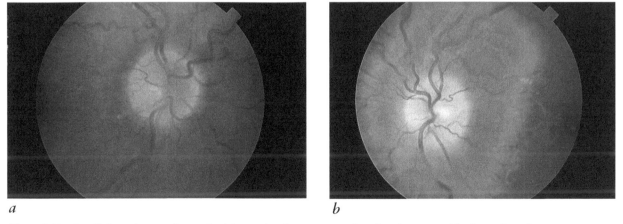

Figure 5.42 *Papilledema has totally resolved 6 months after treatment but there is some residual maculopathy.*

with PTC is to maintain and preserve visual function, everything else is secondary. The first priority is to relieve optic nerve compression. This may be accomplished medically or surgically, but in the present author's opinion, is rarely pursued with sufficient vigor.

If a patient has sufficient visual dysfunction secondary to optic nerve compression from elevated ICP, the pressure must be relieved. Surgically, this may be accomplished by optic nerve sheath decompression or by a thecoperitoneal shunting procedure. Neurosurgical shunting procedures may result in rapid visual loss due to changing pressure gradients across an already compromised optic nerve.[11] Patients awake from their shunting procedure with markedly decreased visual function and no apparent explanation. Medically, high-dose intravenous corticosteroids and acetazolamide may be equally effective.[12] Severe, progressive visual loss requires aggressive treatment, be it medical or surgical.

Optic nerve sheath decompression can and should be performed under local, infiltrative anesthesia in a non-traumatic fashion. The present author has performed > 1000 of these procedures; and with sufficient experience, complications should be minimal and surgical results uniformly excellent. The following technique has evolved over the past 15 years and continues to do so.[13]

TECHNIQUE

Optic nerve sheath decompression is now performed on an outpatient basis with a short-acting, local infiltrative anesthetic (1% xylocaine with hyaluronidase). After an appropriate level of intravenous sedation is attained, a small amount of local anesthetic is injected into the lateral canthal region to anesthetize the facial nerve. A speculum is placed, and 1 ml of local anesthetic is injected beneath the conjunctiva (Fig. 5.43). A 360° conjunctival peritomy is performed (Fig. 5.44), and Tenon's space is entered between the inferior and medial rectus with blunt Wescott scissors (Fig. 5.45). Two or 3 ml of anesthetic are then infiltrated into the retrobulbar Tenon's space with a 20-gauge angiocatheter (Fig. 5.46). If properly placed, the globe will protrude forward and the pupil will rapidly dilate (Fig. 5.47). This technique provides excellent anesthesia and analgesia with none of the risks of retrobulbar or peribulbar injections. Orbital pressure is not elevated, since the solution rapidly dissipates and there is never a closed space.

The medial rectus muscle is then isolated, and a 6-0 Vicryl suture is passed through its insertion. The muscle is disinserted from the globe and sutures placed at the superior and inferior ends of the muscle's insertion. They are looped through the insertion and locked. The

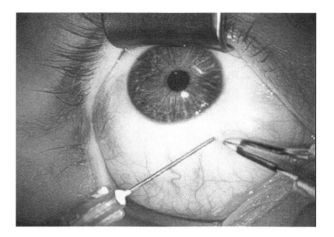

Figure 5.43 *A small amount of local anesthetic is injected beneath the conjunctiva.*

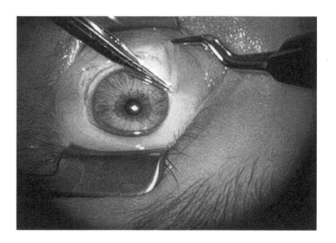

Figure 5.44 *A 360° conjunctival peritomy is performed.*

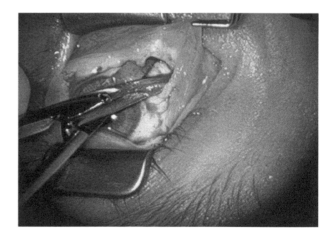

Figure 5.45 *A tunnel is formed between the inferior and medial recti with Wescott scissors.*

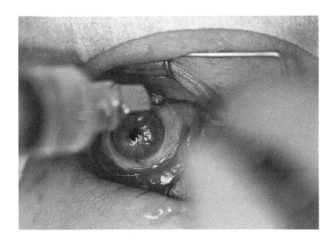

Figure 5.46 *Anesthetic is instilled into the peribulbar space with a blunt cannula.*

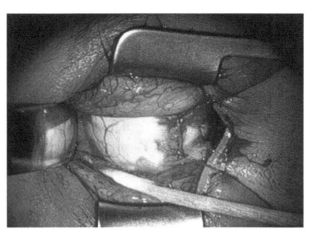

Figure 5.48 *Traction sutures clamped to the surgical drape abduct the eye, while the medial rectus complex is retracted with a Sewall retractor.*

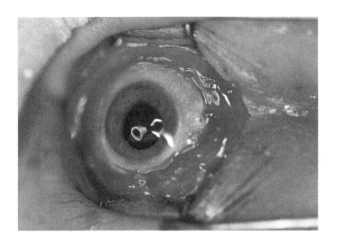

Figure 5.47 *The pupil immediately dilates, indicating that the appropriate degree of anesthesia and analgesia has been obtained.*

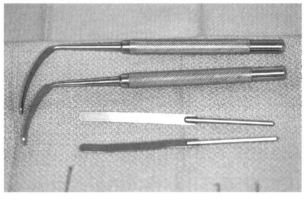

Figure 5.49 *Sewall retractors (above) and small blade retractors (below) may be helpful in retracting orbital fat.*

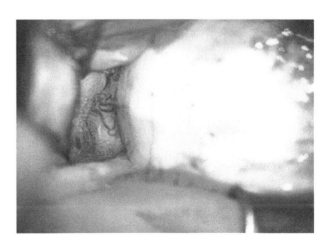

Figure 5.50 *An optic nerve sheath distended with CSF exposed at its juncture with the globe.*

sutures' placement allows the surgeon to abduct the globe in a controlled fashion. As the globe is abducted by clamping the sutures to the surgical drapes, the medial rectus muscle is retracted with a Sewall retractor (this is a basic ENT instrument used as a retractor during ethmoid sinus surgery) (Figs 5.48 and 5.49). This allows excellent exposure for the optic nerve as it exits the globe (Fig. 5.50). Orbital fat is packed away with moist neurosurgical cottonoids, exposing the optic nerve sheath and its overlying vessels and nerves (Figs 5.50 and 5.51). After reflecting the vessels and nerves with a nerve hook, the optic nerve sheath is incised with a sharp blade (Fig. 5.52). This is often accompanied by a large gush of CSF

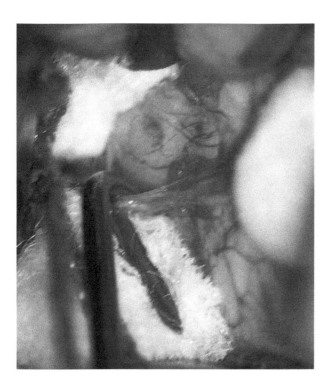

Figure 5.51 *Orbital fat is retracted with neurosurgical cottonoids, enhancing exposure of the optic nerve sheath.*

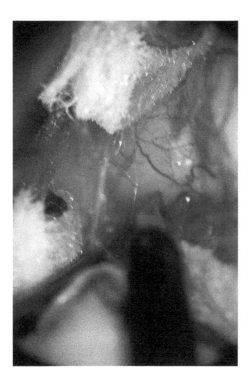

Figure 5.52 *Incision into the optic nerve sheath with a Superblade.*

from the incision site and the nerve is rapidly decompressed. Traction is released and, after a brief respite, the nerve again exposed. A blunt nerve hook (Fig. 5.53) is placed into the incision in the nerve sheath, traction is applied and it is elevated from the underlying optic nerve (Fig. 5.54). A vitreoretinal scissors (Greishaber or DORC; Fig. 5.55) is used to incise the nerve sheath as posteriorly as possible (Fig. 5.56). This completes the operation and very effectively decompresses the optic nerve. The operative site is inspected for bleeding—there should be none. The medial rectus is reinserted on the globe, usually recessed 1–2 mm. The conjunctiva is closed with several sutures with buried knots. The key points in performing a complication-free optic nerve sheath decompression are avoiding excessive manipulation of the globe and only allowing 60–90 seconds of continuous traction at any time. Adhering to these guidelines allows the surgeon to perform the procedure without complications.

PTC: WHO TO TREAT/HOW TO TREAT?

Patients with PTC and normal visual function may be observed or treated with acetazolamide (500 mg sequels bid) if their headaches are symptomatic. Many practitioners offer systemic steroids and repeat lumbar punctures. Systemic steroids have a tendency to make a fat patient fatter. Repeated lumbar punctures lead to non-compliance. Most patients do not like having a lumbar puncture performed repeatedly and have a tendency to avoid the office visit. This lack of compliance may lead to severe visual dysfunction due to chronic atrophic papilledema and optic atrophy (Figs 5.34–5.37).

Patients with markedly elevated ICP (> 500 mm CSF), significant loss of visual field or decreased visual acuity and ischemic papilledema (Fig. 5.39) need to be treated quickly and aggressively. The present author treats immediately with intravenous megadose corticosteroids, acetazolamide and expeditious sequential optic nerve sheath fenestrations as described above. Adults are then referred for consideration of neurosurgical shunting procedures. Children with PTC rarely require neurosurgical shunts in spite of markedly elevated ICP. These optic nerves are very susceptible to decompensation, with permanent blindness sometimes occurring in spite of appropriate therapy.

A 23-year-old woman presented to a local emergency room (ER) complaining of headache. She was treated unsuccessfully with acetaminophen with codeine. She returned to the ER 3 days later, at which time the doctor looked at her fundus and noted papilledema. Imaging was normal. CSF pressure was > 550 mm CSF. She was

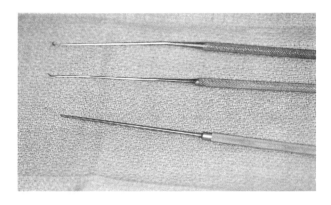

Figure 5.53 *A variety of modified neurosurgical nerve hooks help manipulate the overlying vessels and nerves, as well as elevate the incised optic nerve sheath.*

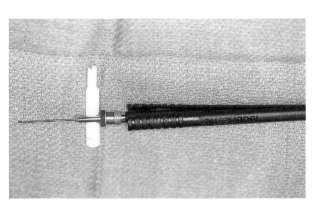

Figure 5.55 *Greishaber vitreoretinal scissors.*

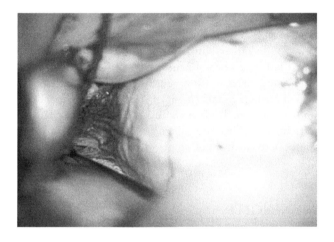

Figure 5.54 *Nerve hooks are utilized to elevate the incised optic nerve sheath from the underlying optic nerve.*

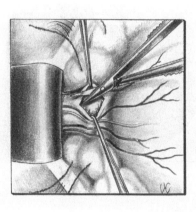

Figure 5.56 *Vitreoretinal scissors are used to extend the optic nerve sheath incision.*

treated with oral prednisone, acetazolamide and repeat lumbar punctures for 3 weeks. Her headache persisted and she was referred to a neurosurgeon for a shunting procedure. She complained to the neurosurgeon that she could not see and was referred to the present author that day. Her vision was 20/70 OU and visual fields were markedly constricted (Fig. 5.57). High-grade ischemic papilledema was present (Fig. 5.25). She was treated with intravenous methylprednisolone (250 mg every 6 hours) and acetazolamide 500 mg sequels twice daily, and underwent sequential optic nerve sheath fenestrations. Vision improved to 20/40 and the visual fields expanded. She was discharged from the hospital and her steroids were

tapered. One week later she returned, blind in one eye and hand motion in the other, complaining of headache. The orbits were explored and the fenestration sites in the optic nerve were open with freely flowing CSF evident. ICP was 350 mm CSF. A lumboperitoneal shunt was placed. Eventual visual function was light perception and 20/30 with a 5° visual field. Bilateral optic atrophy was present (Fig. 5.26).

Once ischemic papilledema is evident, optic nerves can decompensate with progressive visual loss in spite of treatment. Since treating this patient, the present author offers all similar patients neurosurgical shunting after treatment with intravenous steroids and optic nerve sheath fenestration.

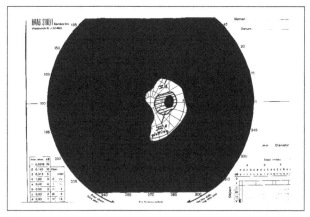

a

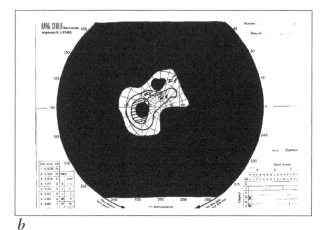

b

Figure 5.57 *Severely constricted visual fields in patient with ischemic papilledema.*

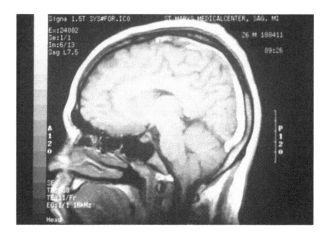

Figure 5.58 *MRI scan demonstrating sagittal sinus thrombosis.*

PSEUDO-PSEUDOTUMOR CEREBRI (PTC)

An occasional patient will present with PTC and have an atypical body habitus, i.e. they may be thin, male or a child. Pediatric PTC is different from adult PTC. It is self-limiting, patients are rarely morbidly obese and often have an underlying cause—minocycline ingestion, mastoiditis, inner ear infection or other causes. ICP may be exceptionally high, and papilledema and visual loss may be severe (Figs 5.38 and 5.39). These patients require prompt and aggressive treatment to prevent permanent visual loss from a usually self-limiting disease.

GLIOMATOSIS CEREBRI

This is an uncommon disorder that may present as typical PTC in either adults or children. Papilledema, elevated ICP and normal neuroimaging are the hallmarks. Eventually, deteriorating neurologic and mental status, and abnormal enhancement of the cerebral hemispheres and brain stem lead to the diagnosis. Several of these patients have died after diagnostic lumbar puncture and lumboperitoneal shunting prior to diagnosis.[14]

MENINGITIS

The diagnosis of PTC is predicated upon normal CSF cells and protein. Abnormal CSF contents are incompatible with the diagnosis of PTC and the clinician should consider meningitis due to Lyme disease or another etiology.

VASCULAR ABNORMALITIES

PTC, especially in males, may be the initial presentation of subclinical dural arteriole to cerebral venous sinus fistulas, which may elude diagnosis. These patients have a tendency to have progressive loss of vision in spite of treatment of their intracranial hypertension. Patients with sagittal sinus thrombosis (Fig. 5.58) or lateral venous sinus thrombosis may also present with clinical manifestations compatible with PTC.[15]

PSEUDOTUMOR CEREBRI (PTC) AND SYSTEMIC LUPUS ERYTHEMATOSUS (SLE)[16]

PTC may coexist with SLE. These patients do much better treated medically than surgically. Their elevated ICP and papilledema is more the result of lupus cerebritis than idiopathic PTC. The present author has learned the hard way that treatment of the underlying disease with systemic corticosteroids is more effective than treating the disc swelling with optic nerve sheath fenestration.

REFERENCES

1. Hayreh SS. Pathogenesis of optic disc edema. In: (Kennard C, Rose FC, eds) Physiologic Aspects of Clinical Neuro-ophthalmology. (Year Book: Chicago, 1988) 431–47.
2. Saunders M. The Bowman lecture. Papilledema: 'The pendulum of progress'. *Eye* 1997; **11**:267–94.
3. Brodsky MC, Glasier CM. Magnetic resonance visualization of the swollen optic disc in papilledema. *J Neuro-Ophthalmol* 1995; **15**:122–4.
4. Brodsky MC, Vaphiades M. Magnetic resonance imaging in pseudotumor cerebri. *Ophthalmology* 1998; **105**:1686–93.
5. Friedman DI, Forman S, Levi L et al. Unusual ocular motility disturbances with increased intracranial pressure. *Neurology* 1998; **50**:1893–6.
6. Round R, Keane JR. The minor symptoms of increased intracranial pressure: 101 patients with benign intracranial pressure. *Neurology* 1988; **38**:1461–4.
7. Wang SJ, Silberstein SD, Patterson S et al. Idiopathic intracranial hypertension without papilledema: a case-control study in a headache center. *Neurology* 1998; **51**:245–9.
8. Cinciripini GS, Donahue S, Borchert MS. Idiopathic intracranial hypertension in prepubertal pediatric patients: characteristics, treatment and outcome. *Am J Ophthalmol* 1999; **127**:178–82.
9. Scott IU, Siatkowski RM, Eneyni M et al. Idiopathic intracranial hypertension in children and adolescents. *Am J Ophthalmol* 1997; **124**:253–5.
10. Sugarman HJ, Felton WL, Salvant JB et al. Effects of surgically induced weight loss on idiopathic intracranial hypertension in morbid obesity. *Neurology* 1995; **45**:1655–9.
11. Beck RW, Greenberg HS. Post-decompression optic neuropathy. *J Neurosurg* 1985; **63**:196–9.
12. Liu GT, Volpe NJ, Galetta SL. Pseudotumor cerebri and its medical treatment. *Drugs Today* 1998; **34**:563–74.
13. Rizzuto PR, Spoor TC, Ramocki JM et al. Subtenon's local anesthesia for optic nerve sheath decompression. *Am J Ophthalmol* 1996; **102**:326–7.
14. Weston P, Lear J. Gliomatosis cerebri or benign intracranial hypertension? *Postgrad Med* 1995; **71**:380–1.
15. Lam BL, Schatz NJ, Glaser JS et al. Pseudotumor cerebri from cerebral venous obstruction. *Ophthalmology* 1992; **99**:706–12.
16. Li EK, Ho PCP. Pseudotumor cerebri in systemic lupus erythematosus. *J Rheumatol* 1989; **16**:113–16.

Chapter 6 Ischemic optic neuropathies

NON-ARTERITIC ANTERIOR ISCHEMIC OPTIC NEUROPATHY (NAION)

NAION is a potentially devastating infarction of the optic nerve head occurring in middle-aged to elderly patients. Patients are usually 50 years of age or over, most commonly in their sixth and seventh decades of life. The infarctions are often sectoral (Fig. 6.1) and the visual field defects are often easily correlated with the optic disc appearance (Fig. 6.2). Central visual acuity may be markedly or minimally disrupted.

Risk factors include hypertension, diabetes mellitus, atherosclerotic disease and smoking, and the disc at risk (Fig. 6.3)—a crowded optic disc with no cup is most common but NAION may occur less commonly in patients without discs at risk.[1,2]

Patients with NAION usually present with acute, painless, unilateral visual loss, often noted upon awakening. Hayreh et al[1] postulate that nocturnal hypotension in treated hypertensive patients may lead to hypoperfusion of a compromised optic nerve head circulation and subsequent infarction of the short ciliary artery circulation nourishing the prelaminar optic disc (Fig. 6.4).

Examination reveals a relative afferent pupillary defect (RAPD), sector optic disc swelling with peripapillary hemorrhages (Fig. 6.1), and optic-nerve-type visual field defects often correlating with the sector disc swelling. Visual loss ranges from minimal to devastating. Visual loss is usually static and stable, but progression may occur in some patients during the first 4–6 weeks (Fig. 6.5). The patient in Figs 6.4–6.6 presented with vague visual complaints, normal visual acuity, a relative central scotoma (Fig. 6.4) and subtle optic disc swelling (Fig. 6.5b). Five days later, he progressed to a dense inferior altitudinal defect (Fig. 6.6a) and marked optic disc swelling (Fig. 6.6b). Over the next week, visual field and acuity continued to deteriorate (Fig. 6.6c). Prodromal optic disc swelling may occur before there are any visual symptoms and may resolve spontaneously or progress to acute infarction.[2]

A 62-year-old lady had an episode of NAION with significant visual loss in her left eye 10 years ago. She had been followed yearly with no evidence of progression in the affected eye or occurrence in her sighted eye (Fig. 6.7). She was asymptomatic with a normal visual field in her sighted eye. The examiner thought that the optic disc appeared a bit fuller in her sighted eye but there was no

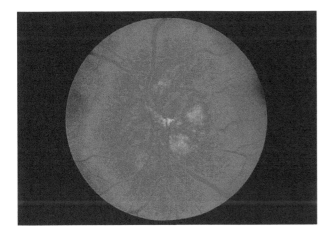

Figure 6.1 *Superior optic disc infarction in NAION.*

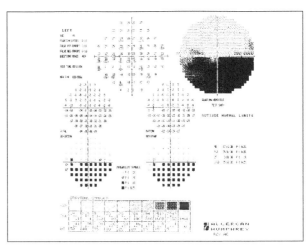

Figure 6.2 *Inferior visual field defect secondary to superior optic disc infarction.*

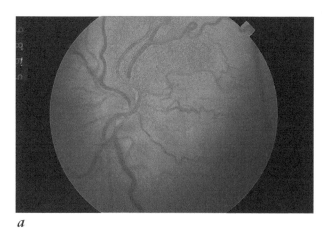

a

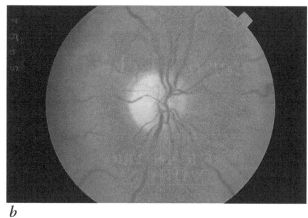

b

Figure 6.3 *The crowded disc at risk (a)—note that there is no cup-to-disc ratio—in a patient who had had a previous episode of NAION with resultant optic atrophy (b).*

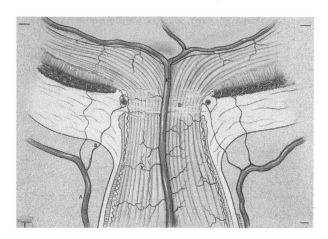

Figure 6.4 *Retinal and choroidal circulation to the optic nerve and retina. Note that the short ciliary vessels provide arterial blood supply to the lamina cribrosa and prelaminar optic nerve.*

visual dysfunction. She returned a few days later with vague visual complaints and no change in her examination except for some subtle, prodromal optic disc swelling (Fig. 6.8). She returned a week later with acute visual loss and infarction of her optic disc (Fig. 6.9). Visual function never recovered and optic atrophy ensued (Fig. 6.10). Thirty to 40% of patients with NAION will eventually have involvement of the second eye.

The diagnosis of typical NAION is usually straightforward if risk factors, the clinical setting, and the appearance of the optic disc and visual fields are all considered. Segmental optic disc swelling with peripapillary hemorrhages is typical (Fig. 6.11). Sector optic atrophy ensues (Fig. 6.12). Visual field changes may be diffuse but may correlate perfectly with the appearance of the optic disc (Figs 6.13 and 6.14). No further evaluation is necessary in these typical cases. Lifestyle modification—stopping

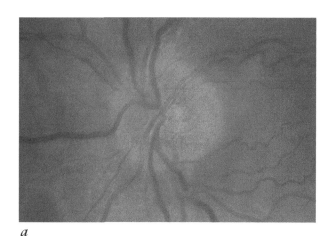

a

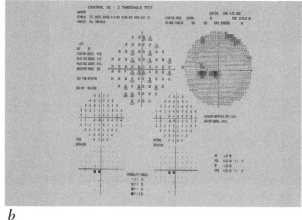

b

Figure 6.5 *A patient with NAION, normal visual acuity, subtle optic disc swelling (a) and a central scotoma (b).*

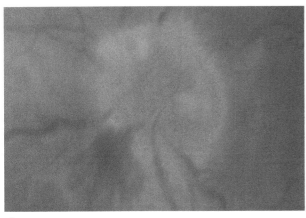

a

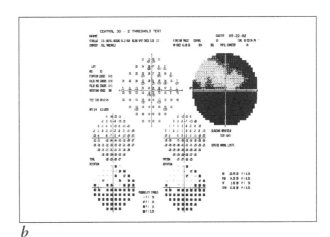

b

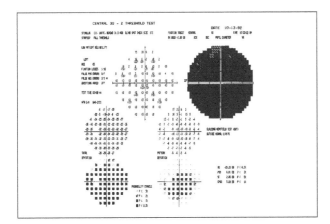

c

Figure 6.6 *The patient in Fig. 6.5 5 days later. Obvious NAION with optic disc swelling (a) and a dense inferior altitudinal defect (b). Visual field continued to deteriorate (c).*

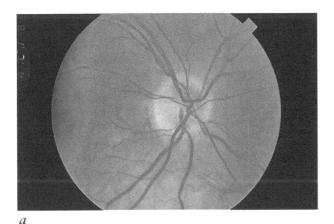

a

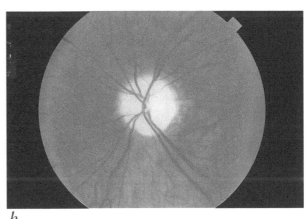

b

Figure 6.7 *A patient followed for 10 years after NAION with an atrophic optic disc right eye (OS) (a) and a disc at risk left eye (OD) (b).*

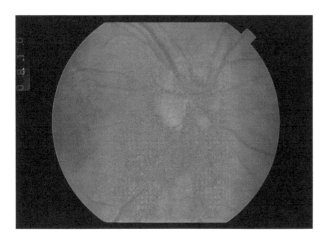

Figure 6.8 *Prodromal optic disc swelling.*

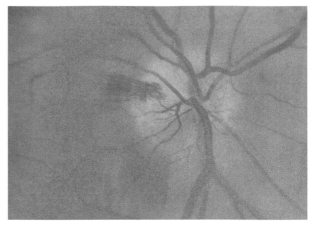

Figure 6.11 *Typical segmental optic disc swelling and peripapillary hemorrhage in patient with NAION.*

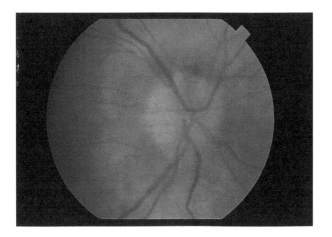

Figure 6.9 *Infarction of the optic disc.*

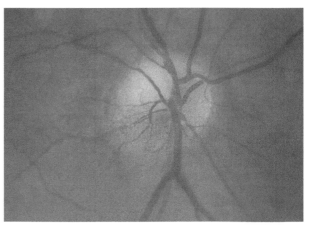

Figure 6.12 *The patient in Fig. 6.11 1 month later, sector optic atrophy ensues.*

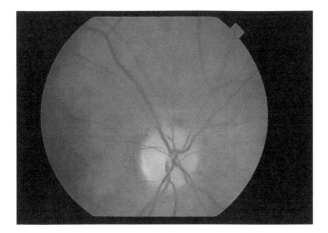

Figure 6.10 *Resultant optic atrophy.*

smoking, lowering cholesterol and controlling hypertension —is advisable. Neuroimaging is reserved for patients with an atypical-appearing optic disc swelling (Fig. 6.15) or involvement of the second eye and total optic disc swelling. Pseudo-Foster-Kennedy syndrome entails ipsilateral optic atrophy and contralateral optic disc swelling due to NAION (Fig. 6.16).

There is no effective treatment for NAION.[3,4] Various medical and surgical regimens have been advocated but none have been proven useful. Optic nerve sheath decompression surgery was reported to be effective by some[5,6] and ineffective by others[7,8] for progressive ischemic optic neuropathy. The Ischemic Optic Neuropathy Decompression Trial (IONDT) prospectively compared

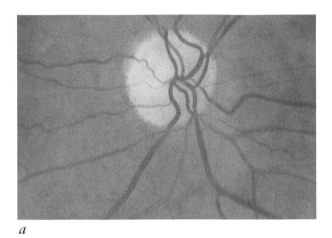
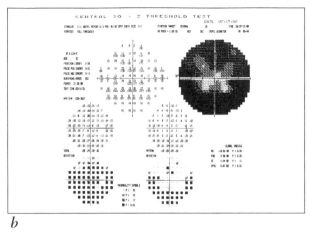

a

b

Figure 6.13 *A patient with bilateral NAION. The right optic disc has diffuse optic atrophy (a) with an accompanying diffuse, generalized visual field defect (b).*

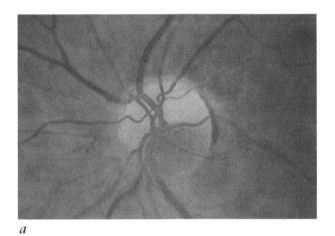
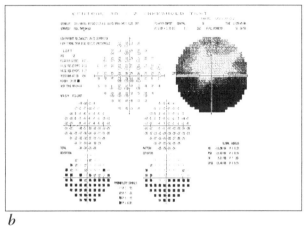

a

b

Figure 6.14 *The left optic disc demonstrates superior optic atrophy (a) and a corresponding inferior altitudinal visual field defect (b).*

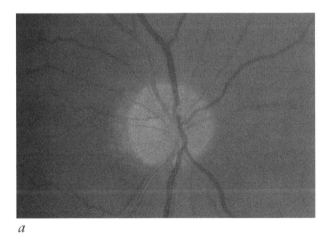
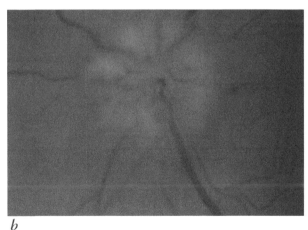

a

b

Figure 6.15 *Diffuse optic disc edema accompanying profound visual loss in the left eye. The right disc is crowded and at risk of NAION.*

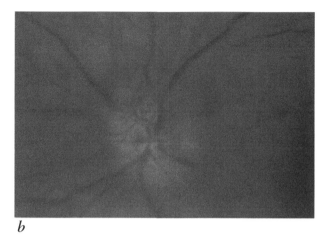

a   *b*

Figure 6.16 *Pseudo-Foster-Kennedy syndrome—optic atrophy OD and optic disc swelling OS.*

patients with NAION and visual acuity worse than 20/60 randomized to surgery or observation. Forty-three percent of the observed eyes improved three or more lines of visual acuity, while the surgical group had a lower rate of visual recovery and a higher rate of loss of three or more lines of visual acuity.[9] Some experienced optic nerve surgeons were appalled by the surgical technique utilized and the concept of operating on nonprogressive NAION, which was known to be ineffective.[5,6] The power of a prospective study, regardless of its merits or demerits, has effectively eliminated surgery as an option for patients with progressive NAION.[9]

DIAGNOSTIC PEARL

Be aware of the entity of amiodarone-induced optic neuropathy.[10] These patients usually have all the risk factors for NAION but present with bilateral visual loss and optic disc swelling. Discontinuing the medication may both resolve the optic disc swelling and restore visual function.

ARTERITIC ISCHEMIC OPTIC NEUROPATHY (AION)

Patients with AION secondary to giant cell arteritis (GCA) usually present with devastating visual loss and pallid optic disc edema (Fig. 6.17) caused by extensive infarction of the optic nerve head. However, visual loss

may not always be devastating. In a review of patients with biopsy-proven GCA, 30% had initial visual acuities between 20/20 and 20/100.[11] If undiagnosed, the second eye is often similarly involved days to weeks later. Many patients seen in a referral practice have both optic nerves infarcted, and are blind and untreatable. Simultaneous, bilateral visual loss is reported to occur in 20–62% of patients with GCA. Suspicion of the diagnosis and a timely sedimentation rate, C-reactive protein and superficial temporal artery (STA) biopsy are essential to prevent blindness in the second eye, and occasionally improve visual function in the involved eye.[12,13]

GCA is a disease of the elderly. The incidence is much greater in the 80-year-old Caucasian female than the 65-year-old black male, but it can occur in anyone over 60 years of age regardless of race. Systemic symptoms, often present, are often overlooked. Classic symptoms may include: headache, lethargy, weight loss, pain in and about the temples, pain while combing or brushing hair, polymyalgia, jaw and lingual claudication. Clinical signs include tender, ropy STA (Fig. 6.18), sector alopecia, and elevated sedimentation rate and C-reactive protein. A fluorescein angiogram may demonstrate markedly delayed filling of the peripapillary choroidal circulation prior to optic disc infarction or choroidal ischemia as the cause of the visual loss. Considering the possible devastating visual loss and the very real danger of unnecessarily treating elderly patients with high doses of corticosteroids, the present author and numerous others advocate an STA biopsy in any elderly patient with unexplained visual symptoms or systemic symptoms suggestive of giant cell arteritis.[12–16] An STA biopsy may often be done in the office with minimal morbidity, especially if the vessel is palpable and easily identified (Fig. 6.18).

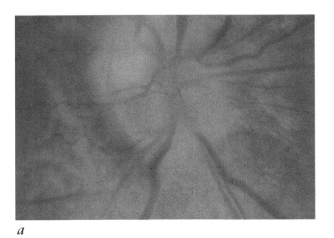
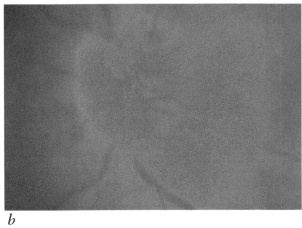

a   b

Figure 6.17   *Pallid optic disc edema in AAION (a) compared to the rather distinctive appearance of optic disc infarction of a patient with NAION (b).*

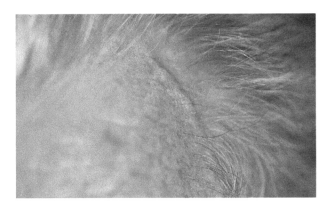
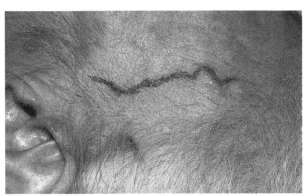

Figure 6.18   *Prominent, ropy STA in a patient with GCA.*

Figure 6.19   *Prominent STA marked prior to infiltration with local anesthetic. Note also the sector alopecia.*

TEMPORAL ARTERY BIOPSY TECHNIQUE

If the vessel is evident to inspection or palpation (Fig. 6.18), mark it with a marking pen before injecting the local anesthetic and obliterating your landmark (Fig. 6.19). Use a local anesthetic without epinephrine (adrenaline)—epinephrine will constrict the vessel and may make it very difficult to identify. If a vessel is not evident, a vertical incision may be made 1 cm anterior and superior to the ear (Fig. 6.20). An appropriate vessel may be located with Doppler ultrasound and marked prior to injecting anesthetic. This is not often necessary but is very helpful in patients with vessels that are difficult to locate or have had previous facial surgery (the forgotten face lift).

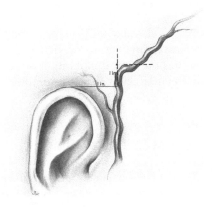

Figure 6.20   *If a prominent vessel is not evident, it can often be found by incising 1 cm anterior and superior to the top of the ear.*

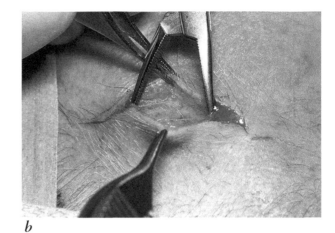

a   *b*

Figure 6.21 *Blunt dissection with a hemostat avoids trauma to the STA.*

An incision is made through the skin and superficial subcutaneous tissue. Both sides of the incision are grasped with forceps and elevated off the superficial temporal fascia (Fig. 6.21). The elevated subcutaneous tissue is incised with scissors. A hemostat is placed into the incision and spread to separate the tissue (Fig. 6.21). The incision is then opened along its entire length with scissors. The STA usually rests upon the superficial temporal fascia and is easy to identify (Fig. 6.22). Once identified, a hemostat is passed beneath the vessel to isolate it. A 4-0 silk tie is passed beneath the vessel and it is put on upward traction. Maintaining traction with the suture, the vessel is dissected free from the surrounding tissue for as long a distance as feasible. The vessel is clamped proximally and distally, and the specimen is excised (Figs 6.23 and 6.24). The proximal and distal segments of the vessel may be cauterized alone or cauterized and tied with a 4-0 silk suture if necessary. The subcutaneous tissue is closed with 5-0 Dexon suture and the skin approximated with suture or tissue glue. Pathology demonstrates the typical infiltration of giant cells (Fig. 6.25) and elastic stains demonstrate disruption of the interna elastica (Fig. 6.26).

MANAGEMENT ERRORS

The ultimate management error in treating patients with GCA is not thinking of the diagnosis until the second eye is involved. The patient in Fig. 6.27 was seen by her ophthalmologist and diagnosed with ischemic optic neuropathy. Two days later she returned with devastating visual loss in her other eye. The diagnosis was now obvious, but to no avail. There is a positive correlation between early diagnosis and treatment and some, albeit minimal, recovery of visual function.[15,16]

Systemic corticosteroids may not always protect the patient from further visual deterioration. Hayreh and Zimmerman[18] confirmed in a large series that early, high-dose steroids prevent visual deterioration in most patients whether administered orally or intravenously. A few patients continued to deteriorate in spite of adequate therapy.[17] It took at least 2 weeks of high-dose steroids to stabilize visual function.

Low-dose corticosteroids may not be protective of visual function. Most neuro-ophthalmologists have seen or heard of a patient with polymyalgia rheumatica being treated with low-dose prednisone suffering devastating visual loss due to AION. Kim et al[19] recently reported an

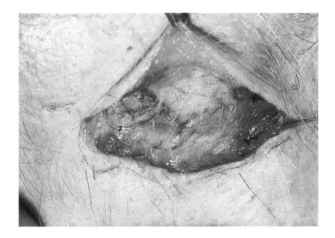

Figure 6.22 *STA lies on the superficial temporal fascia and is usually easy to identify.*

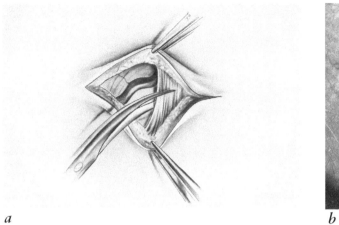

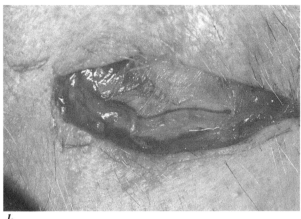

a

b

Figure 6.23   *The vessel is dissected free from the surrounding tissue (a) and isolated (b).*

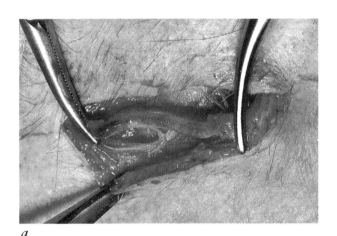

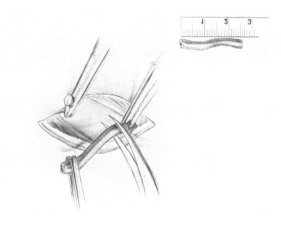

a

b

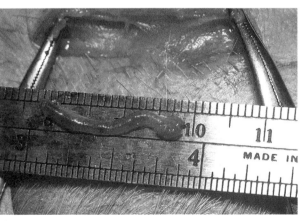

c

Figure 6.24   *Proximal and distal clamps are applied (a) and the specimen excised (b and c).*

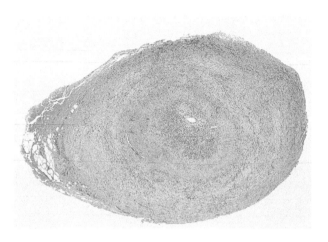

Figure 6.25 *Pathology demonstrates typical inflammation with giant cells (H&E stain).*

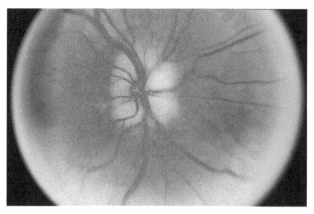

Figure 6.27 *Bilateral pallid optic disc edema in a patient with GCA.*

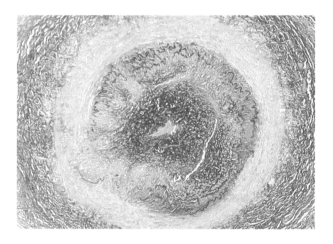

Figure 6.26 *Elastic stains demonstrate disruption of the interna elastica.*

asymptomatic patient with known GCA being treated with low-dose steroids in the face of a normalized erythrocyte sedimentation rate (ESR) and C-reactive protein having episodes of arteritic ischemic optic neuropathy 5 and 13 months after the original diagnosis of GCA. Temporal artery biopsy was very positive in spite of the prolonged treatment with corticosteroids. GCA is a devastating and humbling disease that may recur with a vengeance even many years after 'successful' treatment.

The patient in Fig. 6.28 was a 70-year-old black female presenting with visual loss and pallid disc edema.

Sedimentation rate was only mildly elevated but in view of the optic disc appearance, an STA biopsy was performed, which was negative. Steroids were discontinued. One month later she returned with devastating visual loss in her remaining eye and the appearance of pallid optic disc edema with peripapillary infarctions (Fig. 6.29). The diagnosis of GCA was again considered, steroids started and the contralateral side biopsied. It was again negative and steroids were discontinued. Bilateral temporal artery biopsies have their advocates, but actually the pathology on the second side is rarely different from the initial side. In one large series of bilateral biopsies, only six of 186 were different from the initial biopsy.[15]

Another error of omission is over-reliance on the ESR. Many elderly patients have unexplained elevated ESR, and 22% of patients with biopsy-proven GCA and visual symptoms have normal ESR. An elevated C-reactive protein and an elevated ESR are much more specific for GCA, but are not diagnostic. Clinical signs and symptoms may be helpful, but approximately 20% of patients with GCA and visual symptoms will have no systemic symptoms. Elderly patients with unexplained visual or systemic symptoms should have an STA biopsy to confirm the diagnosis of GCA. Starting treatment with systemic corticosteroids before biopsy is appropriate but the biopsy should be performed within 1 week, as steroid treatment > 1 week may obfuscate the histopathology. Treating elderly individuals for an extended period of time for GCA without a pathologic diagnosis is fraught with danger. Complications of steroid treatment are much more palatable to both physician and patient if the diagnosis is biopsy proven.

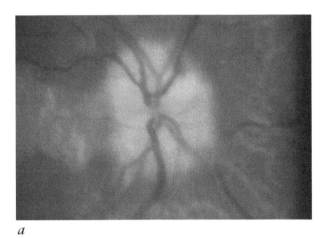
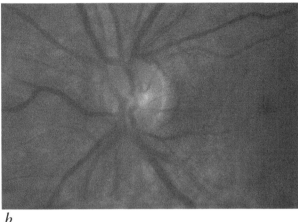

a   *b*

Figure 6.28   *Pallid disc edema right eye (a). The left optic disc is at risk for ischemic optic neuropathy (b).*

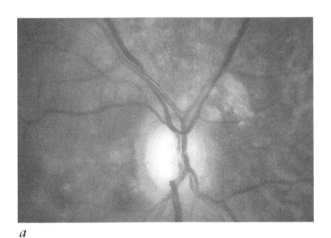
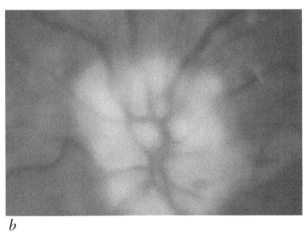

a   *b*

Figure 6.29   *One month later, optic atrophy OD and pallid optic disc swelling OS.*

DIAGNOSTIC PEARL

BILATERAL VISUAL LOSS AND PALLID DISC EDEMA

Patients presenting with bilateral visual loss and pallid optic disc edema in an ambulatory setting have GCA until proven otherwise (Figs 6.17a and 6.27). These patients should be treated immediately with high-dose intravenous corticosteroids and an expeditious temporal artery biopsy performed. Biopsy should be performed within 1 week of starting treatment with steroids to avoid false-negative results.

Patients awakening from major surgery with bilateral visual loss may have infarcted their optic nerves or have had a hypoperfusion infarction of their occipital lobes. Check the pupils. If the pupils are sluggish or there is an obvious afferent pupillary defect, the optic nerves have infarcted (Fig. 6.30). Pallid optic disc edema indicates massive infarction of the optic nerve head. If the optic discs appear normal and the pupils are dysfunctional, the posterior optic nerves have infarcted.

Posterior ischemic optic neuropathy (PION) may occur in the immediate perioperative period after major surgical procedures or may be a manifestation of non-arteritic or arteritic optic neuropathies.[20] Optic atrophy will ensue within 6–8 weeks, confirming the diagnosis. Patients with perioperative PION have a poor visual prognosis. If PION occurs spontaneously, evaluate the patient for systemic vascular disease, especially GCA. Patients with PION secondary to GCA have the same dismal visual prognosis as patients with AION. The present author has stated on several occasions that every time he has made the diagnosis of non-arteritic PION he has been mistaken. Sadda

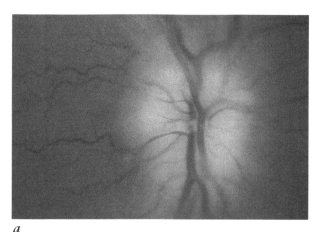
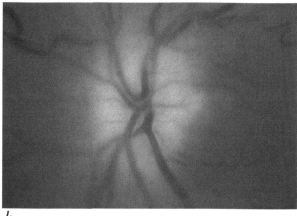

a   *b*

Figure 6.30 *Pallid infarction of the optic discs due to hypoperfusion anterior ischemic optic neuropathy.*

Circulation to Occipital Tip

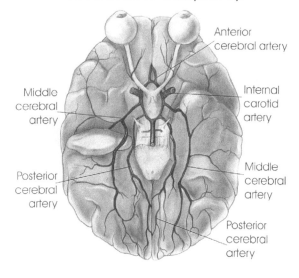

Figure 6.31 *The tip of the occipital lobe (central vision) has a dual blood supply from both posterior and middle cerebral circulations. Hypoperfusion causes an infarction at the watershed between the two circulations—the tip of the occipital lobes.*

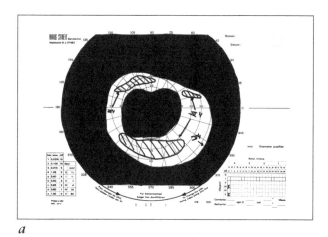
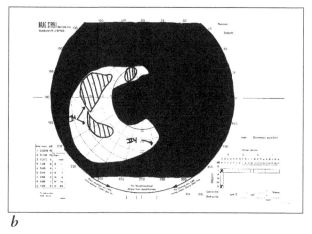

a   *b*

Figure 6.32 *Bilateral central visual field defects after watershed infarction of the occipital lobes due to hypoperfusion.*

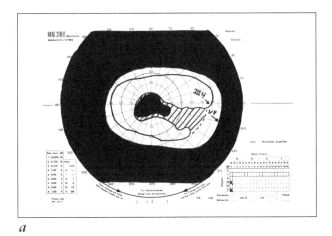 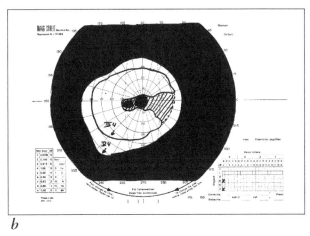

a   *b*

Figure 6.33   *Partial resolution of visual field defects in Fig. 6.25 with permanent, bilateral central scotomas.*

et al[20] describe about one half of their patients with PION resulting from non-arteritic PION. These patients had the same visual prognosis as patients with NAION: 34% improved, 28% stable and 38% had worsening visual function. For most of us dealing with real-time patient complaints, the diagnosis of PION should prompt an aggressive search for GCA and neuroimaging. The diagnosis of non-arteritic PION should remain a diagnosis of exclusion. If a patient awakens with visual loss after a major surgical procedure and the pupillary reactions are normal, the tip of the occipital lobe has infarcted due to hypoperfusion (Fig. 6.31). The blood supply to the occipital tip (macular vision) (Fig. 6.31) is derived from both the posterior and middle cerebral circulation. Hypoperfusion causes a watershed-type infarction affecting central vision in both eyes (Fig. 6.32). As edema subsides, this slowly resolves; but there is almost always a permanent bilateral visual field defect (Fig. 6.33).

REFERENCES

1. Hayreh SS, Joos KM, Podhajsky PA et al. Systemic diseases associated with nonarteritic anterior ischemic optic neuropathy. *Am J Ophthalmol* 1994; **118**:766–80.

2. Hayreh SS, Podhajsky PA, Zimmerman B. Non-arteritic anterior ischemic optic neuropathy: time of onset of visual loss. *Am J Ophthalmol* 1997; **124**:641–7.

3. Ischemic Optic Neuropathy Decompression Trial (IONDT) study group. Characteristics of patients with non-arteritic anterior ischemic optic neuropathy eligible for IONDT. *Arch Ophthalmol* 1996; **114**:1366–74.

4. Lessell S. Nonarteritic anterior ischemic optic neuropathy: enigma variations (editorial). *Arch Ophthalmol* 1999; **117**:386–8.

5. Sergott RC, Cohen MS, Bosley TM et al. Optic nerve sheath decompression may improve the progressive form of non-arteritic ischemic optic neuropathy. *Arch Ophthalmol* 1989; **107**:1743–54.

6. Spoor TC, McHenry JG, Lau-Sickon L. Progressive and static non-arteritic ischemic optic neuropathy treated by optic nerve sheath decompression. *Ophthalmology* 1993; **100**:306–11.

7. Glaser JS, Teimory M, Schatz NJ. Optic nerve sheath fenestration for progressive ischemic optic neuropathy. Results in second series consisting of 21 eyes. *Arch Ophthalmol* 1994; **112**:1047–50.

8. Yee RD, Selky AK, Purvin VA. Outcomes for optic nerve sheath decompression for non-arteritic ischemic optic neuropathy. *J Neuro-Ophthalmol* 1994; **14**:70–6.

9. Ischemic Optic Neuropathy Decompression Trial research group. Optic nerve decompression surgery for non-arteritic ischemic optic neuropathy (NAION) is not effective and may be harmful. *J Am Med Ass* 1995; **273**:625–32.

10. Nagra PH, Foroozan R, Savino PJ. Amiodarone induced optic neuropathy. *Br J Ophthalmol* 200; **34**:420–2.

11. Liu GT, Glaser JS, Schatz NJ et al. Visual morbidity in giant cell arteritis: clinical characteristics and prognosis for vision. *Ophthalmol* 1994; **101**:1779–85.

12. Weyland CM, Bartley GN. Giant cell arteritis: new concepts in pathogenesis and implications for management. *Am J Ophthalmol* 1997; **123**:392–5.

13. Ghanchi FD, Dutton GN. Current concepts in giant cell (temporal) arteritis. *Surv Ophthalmol* 1997; **42**:99–123.

14. Hayreh SS, Podhajsky PA, Zimmerman B. Ocular manifestations of giant cell arteritis. *Am J Ophthalmol* 1998; **124**:1611–14.

15. Hall JK, Volpe NJ, Galetta SL et al. The role of unilateral temporal artery biopsy. *Ophthalmology* 2003; **110**:539–42.

16. Hayreh SS, Zimmerman R, Kardon RL. Visual improvement with corticosteroid therapy in giant cell arteritis: report of a large study and review of the literature. *Acta Ophthalmol Scand* 2002; 80:353–4.

17. Foroozan R, Deramen VA, Buono LM et al. Visual recovery in patients with biopsy proven giant cell arteritis. *Ophthalmology* 2003; 110:539–42.

18. Hayreh SS, Zimmerman B. Visual deterioration in giant cell arteritis patients while on high dose corticosteroids. *Ophthalmology* 2003; **110**:1204–15.

19. Kim N, Trobe JD, Flint A et al. Reactivated giant cell arteritis. *J Neuro-ophthalmology* 2003; 23:113–16.

20. Sadda SR, Nee M, Miller NR et al. Clinical spectrum of posterior ischemic optic neuropathy. *Am J Ophthalmol* 2001; **132**;743–50.

Chapter 7 Traumatic optic neuropathies

Traumatic optic neuropathies may be obviously untreatable, obviously treatable, or treatment may be unproven and results of treatment equivocal. It is important to rapidly and decisively differentiate between these three options and make an intelligent and important management decision on behalf of your patient.

UNTREATABLE TRAUMATIC OPTIC NEUROPATHIES

Avulsion, transection and total infarction of the optic nerve is untreatable. There are no viable medical or surgical options for the optic neuropathies depicted in

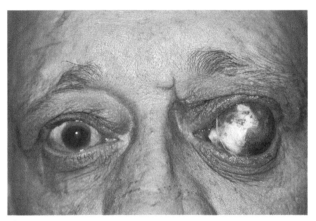

a

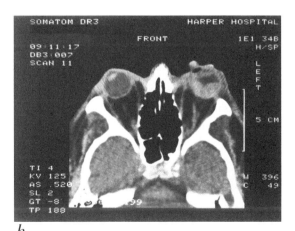

b

Figure 7.1 *Avulsion of the right eye by a finger injury (a). A CT scan demonstrating transection of the optic nerve as it exits the globe (b).*

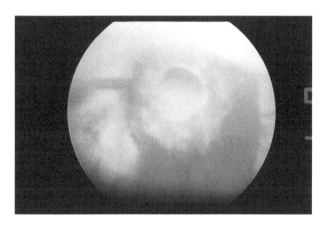

Figure 7.2 *Total avulsion of the optic nerve.*

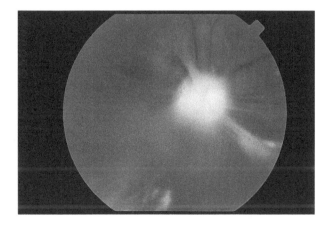

Figure 7.3 *Partial avulsion of the optic nerve.*

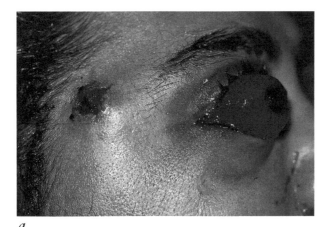

a

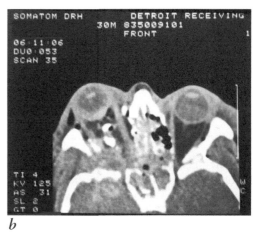

b

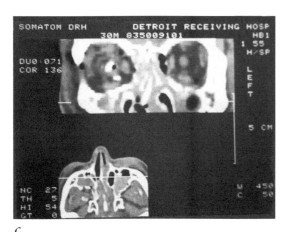

c

Figure 7.4 *Gunshot wound to the lateral orbit with resultant proptosis and blindness (a). CT scans (axial, b; coronal, c) demonstrating transection of the optic nerve by bullet fragment or bone.*

Figs 7.1–7.4. The patient in Fig. 7.1a had his eye avulsed from his optic nerve by a finger injury. The eye is without light perception. Fundus examination may reveal a total (Fig. 7.2) or partial (Fig. 7.3) avulsion of the optic nerve. The computerized tomography (CT) scan demonstrated what is clinically obvious—that the optic nerve has been severed from the back of the globe (Fig. 7.1b). The patient in Fig. 7.4a suffered a gunshot wound to his orbit. The CT scan demonstrates that the optic nerve has been completely transected and is irreparable (Fig. 7.4b).

TREATABLE TRAUMATIC OPTIC NEUROPATHY

Orbital hemorrhage is the most common treatable traumatic optic neuropathy. Although the diagnosis is often obvious (Fig. 7.5), it is rather incredible how often this potentially treatable disorder is untreated or inadequately treated. When confronted with an orbital hemorrhage, people have the tendency to equivocate, get imaging studies and wait for consultants. These delaying tactics are neither necessary nor appropriate. What is necessary is to take action, NOW. The patient with compromised vision from an obvious hemorrhage after trauma or periocular surgery needs to have the hemorrhage drained if it causing a compressive optic neuropathy. Open the wound and let the blood out. This is best done in the operating room but can be accomplished at the bedside or in the emergency department without difficulty. A patient with a traumatic orbital hemorrhage, decreased vision, elevated intraocular pressure (IOP) and a compressive optic neuropathy needs to be treated immediately. Do not wait, perform a canthotomy/cantholysis. This may be accomplished with local anesthesia. Clamp the lateral canthus and sever the inferior and superior crus of the lateral canthal tendons (Fig. 7.6). The appropriate end point is total disinsertion of the lateral upper

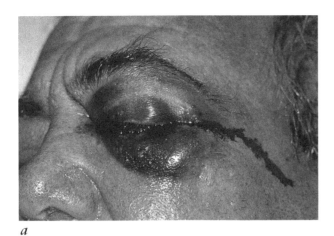

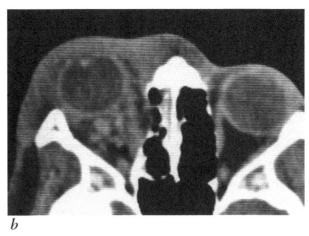

a *b*

Figure 7.5 *A patient with a visually threatening postoperative orbital hemorrhage (a). A CT scan demonstrates a significant orbital hemorrhage (b).*

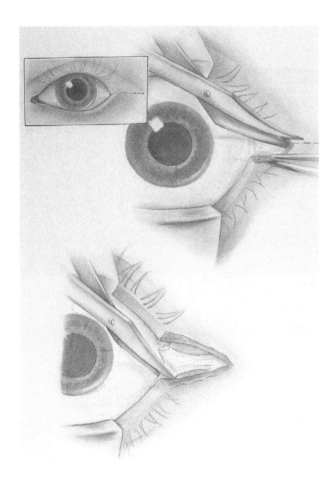

and lower eyelids (Fig. 7.7). This may be accomplished at the bedside, and you may obtain all the consultants and imaging studies you need after you have relieved the orbital pressure and restored visual function. There is a window of opportunity with these patients to restore vision. It varies with the patient's health, vascular system and risk factors; but suffice it to say that sooner is better than later. Waiting for imaging studies or a consensus of consultants is a recipe for a visual disaster.

The patient in Fig. 7.8 presented for a third opinion in reference to treatment of his traumatic optic neuropathy,

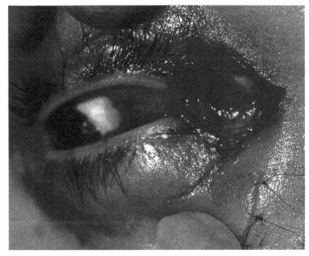

Figure 7.6 *Canthotomy/cantholysis. The lateral canthus is incised with scissors, and both the superior and inferior crus of the lateral canthal tendon are disinserted.*

Figure 7.7 *Total disinsertion of the lateral eyelids after an adequate canthotomy/cantholysis.*

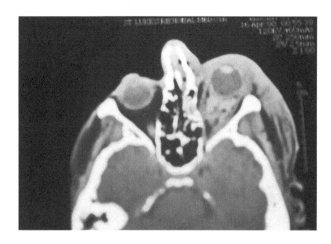

Figure 7.8 *A CT scan demonstrating a significant orbital and intraoptic nerve sheath hemorrhage.*

occurring when he was assaulted 1 month prior to examination. His vision in the involved eye was markedly decreased and his optic disc atrophic. On review of his original CT scans obtained at the time of his injury, there was evidence for a rather significant orbital hemorrhage and a questionable intraoptic nerve sheath hemorrhage (Fig. 7.8). One wonders whether this would have been a treatable optic neuropathy if treated appropriately. If the orbital pressure is elevated and visual function is compromised, relieve the pressure.

Another obvious, but sometimes overlooked, treatable optic neuropathy is the patient with decreased vision after surgery involving orbital implants and manipulation (orbital fracture repair). If there is a postoperative compressive optic neuropathy, take out the implanted material immediately. Do not wait for scans or consultants, it may be too late to restore visual function.

Optic nerve compression by a subperiosteal hemorrhage (Fig. 7.9a–c) is easily reversed by drainage of the hemorrhage. This can be accomplished without entering the orbit proper with minimal morbidity (Fig. 7.10).

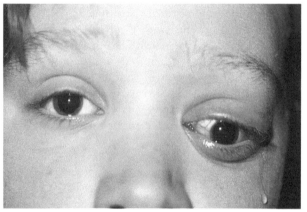

a

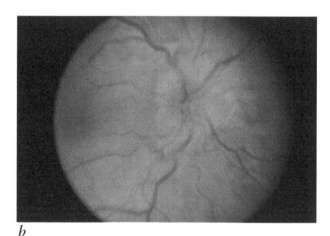

b

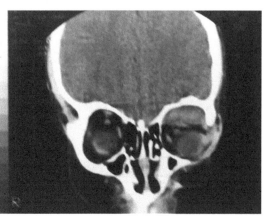

c

Figure 7.9 *A patient with proptosis (a), decreased vision due to optic nerve compression (b) and by a superior subperiosteal hemorrhage (c).*

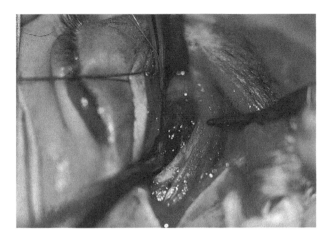

Figure 7.10 *Drainage of subperiosteal hemorrhage through a sub-brow incision.*

OPTIC NERVE SHEATH HEMORRHAGE

Hemorrhage into the optic nerve sheath may be an isolated event but is more commonly associated with a more diffuse orbital hemorrhage. Patients may have marked visual loss and a fundus picture of venous stasis (Fig. 7.11a and b). A CT scan will demonstrate significant blood in the optic nerve sheath (Fig. 7.11c). Optic nerve sheath decompression may be sight saving.

EQUIVOCALLY TREATABLE TRAUMATIC OPTIC NEUROPATHIES

In the present author's experience, approximately 25–30% of traumatic optic neuropathies are associated with obvious orbital hemorrhage or other craniofacial injuries that require treatment. The remainder are indirect

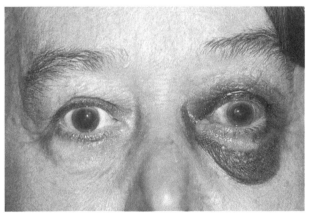

a

b

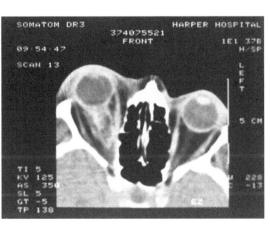

c

Figure 7.11 *A patient struck in left eye with immediate loss of vision (a). Venous stasis retinopathy (b). A CT scan demonstrating both orbital and intra-optic nerve sheath hemorrhages (c).*

injuries to the optic nerve as a result of blunt trauma to the cranium with resultant injury to the intracanalicular optic nerve. The course of the optic nerve from the back of the eye to the optic chiasm traverses the bony optic canal (Fig. 7.12). This is thought to be the site of indirect optic nerve injury. The mechanism is thought to be a combination of avulsion of the blood vessel nourishing the optic nerve in the bony optic canal (Fig. 7.13a) and increased pressure upon the intracanalicular optic nerve (Fig. 7.13b) with resultant swelling and compression of the intracanalicular optic nerve (Fig. 7.14). Obviously, avulsed blood vessels and the resultant dead nerve fibers are untreatable, but secondary damage to the optic nerve as it is compressed in the optic canal by swelling and edema may be treatable. This is the basis for treatment regimens ranging from intravenous megadose corticosteroids to surgical decompression of the bony optic canal.

The successful treatment of spinal cord injuries with intravenous megadose corticosteroids administered within 8 hours of injury rekindled interest in treatment of optic nerve injuries with megadose corticosteroids, in spite of the obvious differences between spinal cord and optic nerve.[1] There is no consensus as to the utility of megadose steroids or surgery for treating traumatic optic neuropathies.[2]

The data that show little beneficial effect from treatment with intravenous megadose corticosteroids seem flawed by the late onset of treatment. Traumatic blindness does not seem to carry the same degree of urgency as traumatic paraplegia, and it is rare for these patients to be diagnosed and treated within 8 hours of injury.

The diagnosis of indirect optic nerve injury is often delayed because the pupils are dilated prior to identifying an afferent pupillary defect (Fig. 7.15) and the fundus, especially the optic nerve, appears normal. The optic nerve will appear normal for 4–6 weeks, even if it is totally severed and the eye is amaurotic (Fig. 7.16a). Optic atrophy ensues as the ganglion cells die from retrograde degeneration (Fig. 7.16b).

Having treated a large number of patients with traumatic optic nerve injuries for over 20 years and publishing copiously about the experience,[3-8] the present author has learned that we do not have all the answers to this problem, and those who think they do either lack insight or experience. The old rules just do not apply. For example conventional wisdom states that total loss of vision to no light perception, especially when resulting from a penetrating injury, is totally untreatable. Let the following cases be instructive.

A 29-year-old man was stabbed with a stiletto up his right nostril during an altercation. He immediately lost all vision in his right eye and presented with an amaurotic eye

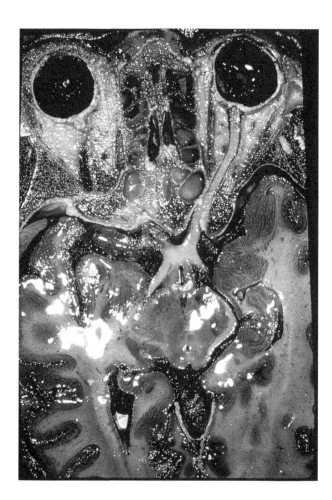

Figure 7.12 *Axial fresh cadaver section along the course of the optic nerve. Note how closely adherent the optic nerve is to the optic canal.*

and frozen globe (Fig. 7.17). A CT scan demonstrated pneumocephalus, confirming intracranial penetration. He was treated with intravenous methylprednisolone (250 mg every 6 hours) for 5 days and remained totally blind in his right eye. On day 6, he underwent an optic canal decompression through an external ethmoidectomy (Fig. 7.18). The following day vision improved to definite hand motion and 3 days later vision improved to 20/50 with a rather acceptable visual field (Fig. 7.19).[8]

Shortly afterwards, a 31-year-old man presented for a second opinion for a blind, immobile eye after a penetrating knife wound to the superior medial orbit (Fig. 7.20). He had been evaluated elsewhere and told that there was no treatment that would help restore his vision. After 5 days of megadose corticosteroids, visual acuity returned to 20/100 with a respectable visual field (Fig. 7.21), in spite of a significant degree of optic atrophy (Fig. 7.22).

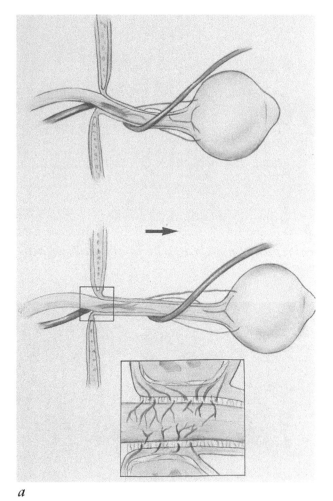

a

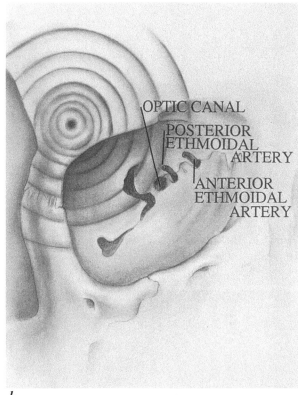

b

Figure 7.13 *Possible mechanisms for indirect injury to the optic nerve. Avulsion of the nutrient vessels in the optic canal (a) by an acceleration/deceleration injury and pressure waves transmitted from the supraorbital ridge to the optic canal (b).*

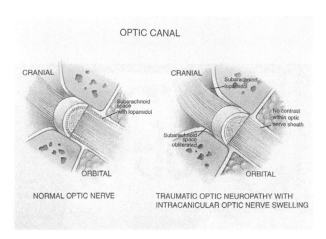

Figure 7.14 *Swelling and compression of the intracanalicular optic nerve. Normal anatomy allows the free flow of CSF from brain to orbit through the intracanalicular optic nerve. Axonal swelling due to injury compromises the still viable optic nerve fibers.*

These cases are not meant to be testimonials to miraculous cures but to reinforce the concept that we do not have all the answers to the problems of traumatic optic neuropathy. Many clinicians advocating therapeutic nihilism often lack the real-life experience with patients with isolated and complicated optic nerve injuries. How then should the clinician approach the patient with a traumatic optic nerve injury?

First, do not overlook obviously treatable causes of optic nerve dysfunction, i.e. orbital hemorrhage. Diagnose it and treat it expeditiously. Patients suffering indirect injury to their optic nerve, or from optic nerve injury associated with other facial injuries, may benefit from a course of high-dose intravenous corticosteroids. Modeled after the spinal cord treatment study, the present author prefers immediate treatment with intravenous methylprednisolone 30 mg/kg infused over 30 minutes, followed 2 hours later by 15 mg/kg infused in a similar fashion. The serum half-life of methylprednisolone is sufficiently short that these doses need to be given in

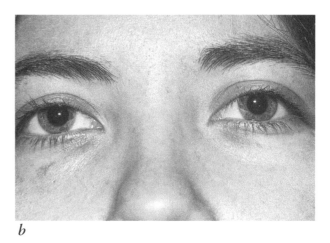

a   *b*

Figure 7.15 *Relative afferent pupillary defect. As light is directed into the sighted left eye, both pupils constrict equally (a). As the light is directed into the blind right eye, both pupils paradoxically dilate (b).*

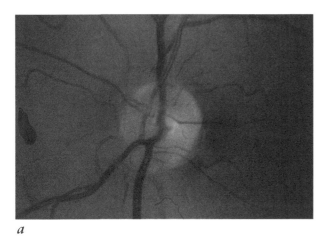

a   *b*

Figure 7.16 *Normal-appearing optic nerve in spite of total blindness immediately after injury (a). Optic atrophy ensues as ganglion cells die by retrograde degeneration (b).*

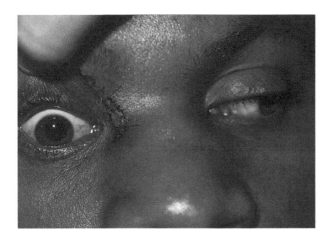

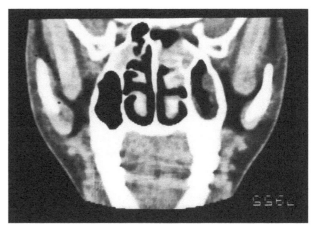

Figure 7.17 *Patient with total ophthalmoplegia and a blind eye after stiletto injury to the right orbit.*

Figure 7.18 *A CT scan after optic canal decompression demonstrating removal of the medial wall of the optic canal.*

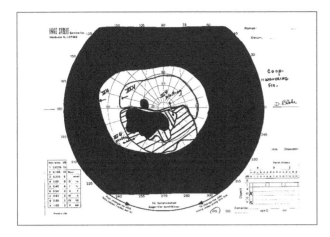

Figure 7.19 *Postoperative visual field.*

close proximity. Corticosteroids are then continued at 15 mg/kg every 6 hours for 24–48 hours.

In the present author's experience,[7] patients with initial visual acuity of 20/100 or better almost all improve on this regimen. Patients with initial visual acuity of 20/200 or worse may or may not improve. Those that improve are tapered from their steroids, usually by halving the daily dose for several days and then starting prednisone 80 mg/day and rapidly tapering by 20 mg every 3 days.

Patients who fail to improve with the intravenous steroid therapy or have recurrent visual loss as their steroids are being tapered are offered extracranial optic canal decompression via an external ethmoidectomy. The rare patient with documented, progressive visual

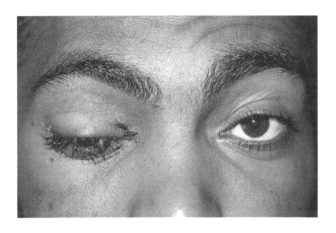

Figure 7.20 *Total ophthalmoplegia and amaurosis after knife injury to the superior medial orbit.*

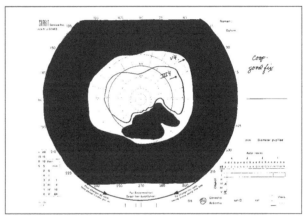

Figure 7.21 *Visual field after 5 days of megadose corticosteroid therapy.*

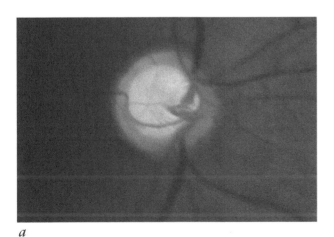
a

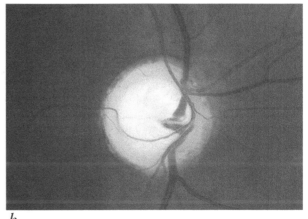
b

Figure 7.22 *Optic nerve appearance immediately after injury (a) and ensuing atrophy 6 weeks later (b).*

loss is especially encouraged to undergo surgery if medical therapy has failed to improve visual function.

Who benefits from aggressive medical and surgical treatment of traumatic optic nerve injuries? Experience indicates that 75% of patients treated by a combination of intravenous corticosteroids, with or without surgical intervention, improve two or more lines of vision, i.e. a doubling of their visual angle. Positive prognostic factors include early treatment (treatment with high-dose steroids initiated within 8 hours of injury) and a patient age of less than 40 years. Negative prognostic factors include initial visual acuity of no light perception, treatment onset after 8 hours and age greater than 40 years.[7]

The present author believes that early treatment with intravenous megadose steroids is the key to salvaging optimal vision for patients with traumatic optic nerve injuries. Our experience is unique in that the present author and his colleagues had control of the eye trauma service at a busy emergency department with a resident staff available 24 hours a day and attuned to optic nerve injuries. This does make a difference when comparing our visual results with those from other centers.[7]

Optic canal fractures were an original indication for bony decompression of the optic canal. The rationale was that the fragment of bone was impinging upon the optic nerve in the canal and causing a compressive optic neuropathy (Fig. 7.23). Most clinicians now agree that the presence of an optic canal fracture on a CT scan is a poor prognostic sign, usually indicating that the optic nerve has been transected or seriously injured. Patients without CT evidence for optic canal fractures appear to have a better visual prognosis than those who do.

EXTRACRANIAL OPTIC CANAL DECOMPRESSION[3,9]

The purpose of optic canal decompression is to remove the medial wall of the optic canal to relieve the pressure applied to the optic nerve by swollen axons confined by the bony optic canal (Fig. 7.14). The optic canal can be decompressed through a frontal craniotomy, transnasally with or without an endoscope or by an external ethmoidectomy with removal of the medial wall of the orbit and then the medial wall of the optic canal with direct, stereoscopic visualization. Many neurosurgeons are uncomfortable with performing a transcranial optic canal decompression in the setting of head injury in patients with a rather poor visual prognosis. Hence the popularity of taking an extracranial approach to the optic canal either endoscopically or under direct visualization (Fig. 7.24).

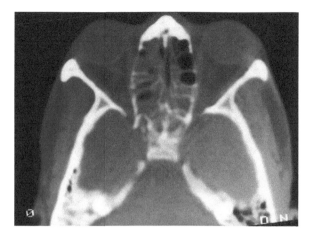

Figure 7.23 *A CT scan demonstrating medial optic canal fracture.*

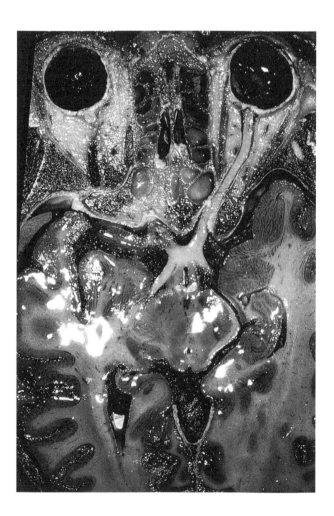

Figure 7.24 *Axial cadaver section demonstrating the accessibility of the intracanalicular optic nerve through the ethmoid sinus.*

TECHNIQUES

Extracranial optic canal decompression via external ethmoidectomy is performed under general anesthesia. After the patient is intubated, the area around the endotracheal tube is packed with gauze. Oxymethazoline 30 ml is poured into the nostril on the involved side. As it percolates through the nose and ethmoid sinuses, another 30–60 ml is instilled. Utilizing an Ascepto syringe in the involved nostril facilitates instillation. The surgical site is infiltrated with several milliliters of xylocaine with epinephrine (adrenaline) (1:200,000). This enhances hemostasis at the incision site. A gull-wing incision is outlined (Fig. 7.25) and made through skin and orbicularis muscle to the level of the periosteum with a 15-blade. The periosteum is incised with the same blade and dissected from the underlying bone. The medial canthal tendon, lacrimal sac and nasolacrimal duct are dissected from the bone subperiosteally. The medial orbital wall is infractured into the ethmoid sinus just posterior to the posterior lacrimal crest. The osteotomy is enlarged with Kerrison rongeurs (Fig. 7.26). The ethmoid sinus cells are removed from the sinus with a Takahashi forceps (Fig. 7.27). This effectively removes the ethmoid sinus and the medial wall of the orbit. The anterior and posterior ethmoidal neurovascular bundles are identified and bone removal is confined inferior to them (Fig. 7.26). Superior to these vessels is the anterior cranial fossa. Disorientation may result in a cerebrospinal fluid (CSF) leak or an inadvertent brain biopsy. It is important to maintain intact periorbita while removing the medial orbital wall. Incising the periorbita at this stage may make future dissection and removal of the optic canal much more difficult due to obliteration of the relevant anatomy by herniating orbital fat. After the

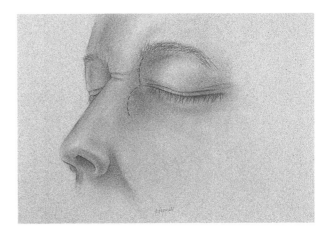

Figure 7.25 *A gull-wing incision is outlined between the bridge of the nose and the medial canthus.*

medial orbital wall is removed, hemostasis is obtained by packing the remains of the ethmoid sinus with neurosurgical cottonoids soaked with oxymethazoline. After excellent hemostasis is obtained, the operating microscope is brought into the field utilizing a 250–300 mm objective lens. In the operative field, the surgeon can visualize the confluence of periorbital fibers that mark the orbital apex (Fig. 7.28). With this as a landmark, the bony medial orbital wall and medial border of the optic canal is thinned with a diamond burr (Fig. 7.28). The surgical field is constantly irrigated and aspirated with normal saline solution instilled through the nose with an irrigating/aspirating cannula (Fig. 7.29). After the bone has been thinned, it may be removed from the underlying optic nerve with a curette, completing the optic canal decompression (Fig. 7.30). The optic nerve sheath may

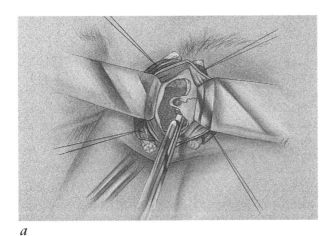

a

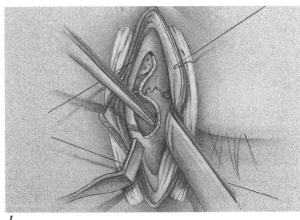

b

Figure 7.26 *Enlarging the osteotomy with Kerrison rongeurs. Note that the bone is removed inferior to the ethmoidal arteries.*

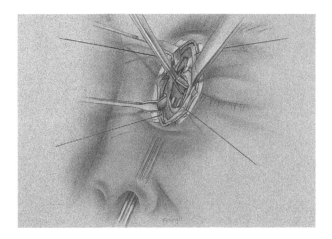

Figure 7.27 *Removal of the ethmoid cells and mucosa with Takahashi rongeurs.*

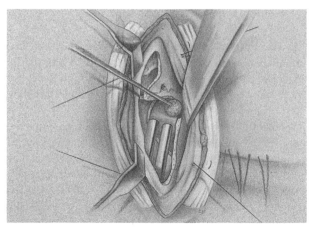

Figure 7.29 *Removal of the optic canal with a diamond burr. Constant irrigation and aspiration is accomplished through the nose.*

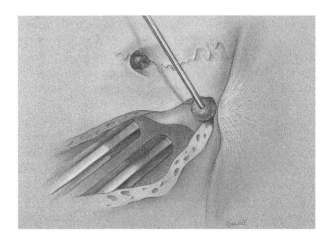

Figure 7.28 *Confluence of periorbital fibers at the orbital apex, inferior to the posterior ethmoidal artery.*

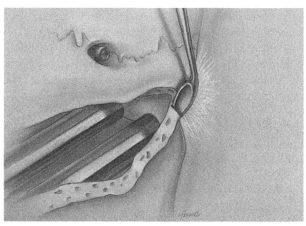

Figure 7.30 *Removal of the thinned optic canal with a curette.*

or may not be incised at the surgeon's discretion (Fig. 7.31). Adequate decompression of the optic canal may be verified by postoperative CT scans (Fig. 7.32).

This appears to be a very complicated surgical procedure. Actually it is rather straightforward if you utilize a few learning curves. First, practice on a few patients with dysthyroid optic neuropathy who require medial orbital decompressions for their compressive optic neuropathy (Fig. 7.33). The end point with their surgery is decompressing the medial orbit to the orbital apex: this is two-thirds of an optic canal decompression. Once you are comfortable with this procedure to obtain hemostasis, put the operating microscope into position and remove

the medial wall of the optic canal as described. There is always concern that you may injure the intracranial carotid artery. This has actually never been reported either in the literature or in small group discussions. It is theoretically possible, but if you remain superior to the optic nerve, it really should not happen and to the best of my knowledge has not.

No one can say with any degree of certainty which patients will improve with or without treatment for traumatic optic neuropathy. There are documented reports of patients improving both with and without treatment.[10-12] Some negative prognostic factors include: presence of blood in the posterior ethmoid sinus, age

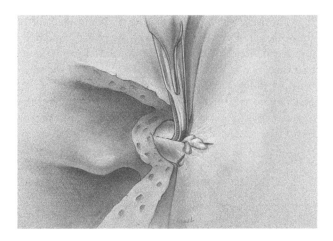

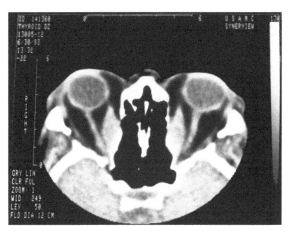

Figure 7.31 *Incision of the intracanalicular optic nerve sheath.*

Figure 7.33 *A CT scan demonstrating compression of the optic nerves by enlarged medial recti muscles.*

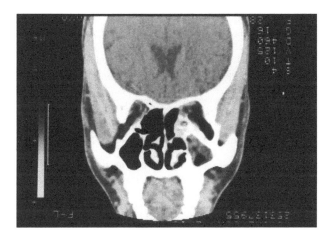

Figure 7.32 *A coronal CT scan demonstrates adequate decompression (removal) of the medial wall of the optic canal.*

greater than 40 years, loss of consciousness at the time of injury and no visual improvement after 48 hours of steroid therapy.[13] Two recent reviews demonstrate the lack of consensus as to the appropriate treatment of traumatic optic neuropathies. There are no absolute criteria for treatment with corticosteroids, surgery or observation. Clinical judgement must decide what, if any, treatment to offer individual patients.[13,14]

The consensus of this group's experience (well-known senior faculty members practicing neuro-ophthalmology, oculoplastic surgery and craniofacial surgery at a prestigious institution) is that patients with no light perception vision and orbital fractures have the worst visual prognosis. Most experienced clinicians agree. Patients

with blunt orbital injuries have a better visual prognosis than patients with penetrating injuries (19% versus 45% visual improvement). Eighty three percent of patients without orbital fractures had improved vision as opposed to 38% of patients with orbital fractures. Whether patients underwent surgical (optic canal decompression) or medical (corticosteroids) treatment made little difference in their ultimate visual outcome. Patient age and the timing of surgery had little bearing on the ultimate visual prognosis. Initial total blindness did not mitigate against some visual improvement—27% of patients with initial no light perception improved, while 100% of patients with light perception or better visual acuity improved.

Experienced surgeons also report significant improvements in visual function with medical and surgical treatment administered weeks to months after indirect optic nerve injury.[15] Twenty five patients were operated upon a median of 56 days after injury (range 16 days to 3 months). Patients without light perception for greater than 2 weeks had no positive response to surgery. Twenty of 25 patients with some residual vision had improved visual function after optic canal decompression. Again, the senior author of this series is a very experienced optic canal surgeon.

The present author's experience and prejudice opts for the aggressive treatment regimen outlined in this chapter, as well as offering treatment to all patients with traumatic optic nerve injuries. As the following case documents, you never know who will benefit from aggressive treatment of traumatic optic nerve injuries.

A 35-year-old lady struck her head and was rendered unconscious. Except for a blind right eye and an amaurotic pupil, her neuro-ophthalmic examination was normal. Her optic disc appeared a bit full and the nerve enlarged on CT scan. Ultrasound confirmed the presence of significant fluid in her optic nerve sheath, and optic nerve sheath fenestration was performed after vision failed to improve after 5 days of megadose corticosteroids. Visual acuity dramatically improved to 20/20 3 days after surgery. The basic lesson is never say never with visual loss.

It is almost always worthwhile to try some medical or surgical therapy rather than allow the patient to quietly and permanently lose vision. However, let me reiterate that there is no established standard of care for the treatment of indirect optic nerve injuries, and steroid treatment or no treatment would certainly be a much safer alternative than extracranial optic canal decompression by an inexperienced surgeon.

REFERENCES

1. Bracken MB, Collins WF, Freeman DF et al. A randomized controlled trial of methylprednisolone or naloxone in the treatment of acute spinal chord injury. *N Engl J* 1990; **322**:1405–11.
2. Levin LA, Beck RW, Joseph MP et al. The treatment of traumatic optic neuropathy. The international optic nerve trauma study. *Ophthalmology* 1999; **106**:1268–77.
3. Spoor TC, McHenry JG. Management of traumatic optic neuropathy. *J Cranio-Maxillofacial Trauma* 1996; **2**:14–26.
4. Spoor TC, Hartel WC, Lensink DB, Wilkinson MJ. Treatment of traumatic optic neuropathy with corticosteroids. *Am J Ophthalmol* 1990; **110**:665–9.
5. Spoor TC. Traumatic optic neuropathies. In: (Yanoff M, Duker JS, eds) Ophthalmology. (Mosby; London, 1999).
6. Spoor TC, McHenry JG, Bendel RE et al. Factors associated with the success of optic canal decompression and corticosteroids in traumatic optic neuropathy. Poster presentation, American Academy of Ophthalmology. San Francisco, CA, Nov 1994.
7. Spoor TC, Bendel RE, Ramocki JM, McHenry JG. Traumatic optic neuropathy and intravenous megadose corticosteroids. (Association for Research in Vision and Ophthalmology, Sarasota, FL, May 1993).
8. Spoor TC, Mathog RH. Restoration of vision after optic canal decompression following five days of total blindness and megadose corticosteroid therapy. *Arch Ophthalmol* 1986; **104**:804–6.
9. Joseph MP, Lessell S, Rizzo J et al. Extracranial optic nerve decompression for traumatic optic neuropathy. *Arch Ophthalmol* 1990; **108**:1091–2.
10. Lessell S. Indirect optic nerve trauma. *Arch Ophthalmol* 1989; **107**:382–6.
11. Li KK, Teknos TN, Lai A et al. Traumatic optic neuropathy: results in 45 consecutive surgically treated patients. *Otolaryngol Head Neck Surg* 1999; **120**:5–11.
12. Steinsapir KD, Goldberg RA. Traumatic optic neuropathy. *Surv Ophthalmol* 1994; **38**:487–518.
13. Carta A, Ferrigano L, Salvo M et al. Visual prognosis after indirect traumatic optic neuropathy. *J Neurol Neurosurg Psychiatry* 2003; **74**:246–8.
14. Wang BH, Robertson BC, Girotto JA et al. Traumatic optic neuropathy: a review of 61 patients. *Plast Reconstruc Surg* 2001; **107**:1655–64.
15. Thakar A, Mahaptra AK, Tandon DA. Delayed optic nerve decompression for indirect optic nerve injury. *Laryngoscope* 2003; **113**:112–19.

Chapter 8   Neuro-ophthalmic sequelae of closed head injury

Patients with neuro-ophthalmologic sequelae of cranio-cervical and closed head injuries are among the most challenging and gratifying patients encountered in a neuro-ophthalmology practice. They often arrive at the neuro-ophthalmologist's office unhappy and hostile, having seen an assortment of doctors who have been unable or unwilling to help them, or have tried to convince them that there is nothing wrong with them. The situation is muddied by lawyers trying to make money and insurance companies trying to save money. It is a fine balance of clinical judgement to determine which complaints are real, which are amplified and which are specious. It is best to examine these patients on several occasions with an open mind, treating their complaints as real unless they are proven contrived.

Neuro-ophthalmologic sequelae of cranio-cervical injury may be obvious or subtle. Whether the head strikes an immovable object or there is a sudden 'whiplash'-type injury, the skull stops and the brain keeps moving (Fig. 8.1). This may cause injury to the cerebral cortex (frontal and occipital lobes) or structures at the base of the brain (optic nerves, chiasm, cranial nerves and brain stem) (Fig. 8.2). To avoid errors of omission and missing a potentially

treatable entity, think of these neuro-ophthalmic sequelae as injuries to either the afferent or efferent visual systems. The former involves seeing, the latter involves the eyes working together to obtain binocular vision. Both systems may be involved. It is very important to remember that in a large series of patients examined at a university hospital, almost 60% of those patients with head injuries had an abnormal neuro-ophthalmic examination. Sixty percent of these patients were injured in motor vehicle accidents. There was no association between neuro-ophthalmologic findings and loss of consciousness. Loss of consciousness was not a significant indicator of either afferent or efferent neuro-ophthalmic function.[1]

AFFERENT VISUAL DEFECTS

Injuries to the afferent visual system may be obvious or subtle. A complete ophthalmic examination should detect any injuries to the eye causing media opacities or damage to the retina causing decreased vision.

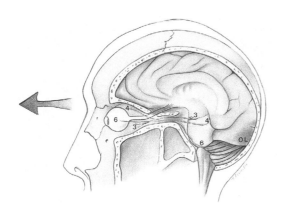

Figure 8.1 *The head strikes a solid object, the skull stops and the brain keeps moving. This may injure the occipital lobe, cranial nerves, optic nerves and chiasm.*

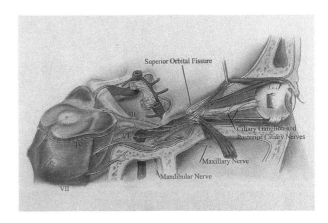

Figure 8.2 *Structures susceptible to traumatic injury along the base of the brain.*

Optic nerve injury may be more difficult to detect, especially if the patient has been dilated prior to examination, obscuring a relative afferent pupillary defect (RAPD) or light-near dissociation of the pupils caused by bilateral optic nerve or chiasmal injury. Optic nerve injury may be obvious with total loss of vision, amaurotic pupil and obvious injury to the optic nerve by computerized tomography (CT) scan (Fig. 8.3). It may also be quite subtle. The patient in Fig. 8.4 struck his occiput while loading his truck. He noted immediate visual loss to the extent that he was afraid to drive. Examination was 'normal', visual acuity was 20/20 in both eyes and he was labeled a malingerer. Subsequent neuro-ophthalmologic examination revealed subtle light-near dissociation of the pupils, bilateral superior altitudinal visual field defects and a hint of optic atrophy (Fig. 8.4a–d). Bilateral traumatic optic neuropathy was diagnosed and the patient underwent vocational rehabilitation since he could no longer safely drive a commercial vehicle.

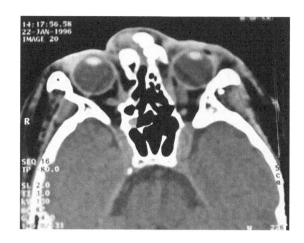

Figure 8.3 *A CT scan demonstrating transection of both optic nerves after cranial trauma.*

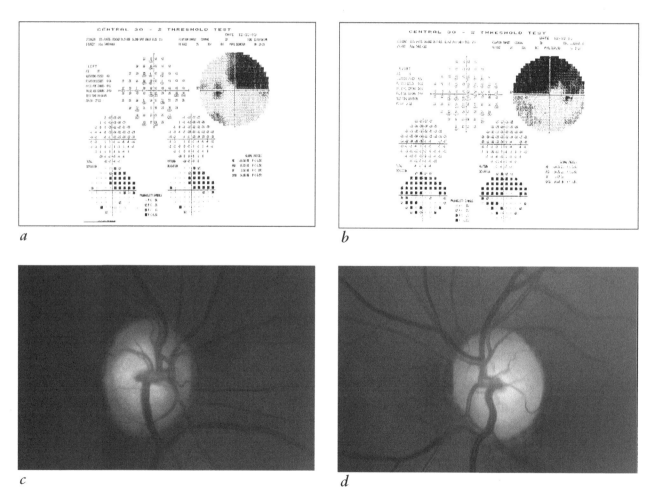

a

b

c

d

Figure 8.4 *Subtle traumatic optic neuropathy presenting with superior altitudinal visual field defects (a and b) and a corresponding degree of subtle optic atrophy (c and d).*

Chiasmal injuries are uncommon, usually caused by frontal trauma and manifest as a variation on the theme of bitemporal hemianopia. The patient in Fig. 8.5 awoke from sleeping under a roadway and struck his forehead on a metal beam. He immediately noticed decreased peripheral vision. The bitemporal nature of his field defect was confirmed by perimetry and, after negative neuroimaging, the diagnosis of traumatic chiasmal injury established.

Visual field examination is especially helpful in detecting subtle occipital lobe injuries. These patients may not complain of binocular visual loss but localize their complaints to one eye. Visual fields will invariably detect the bilateral, congruous defects diagnostic of occipital lobe lesion (Fig. 8.6), establishing the diagnosis in spite of the normal pupillary and ophthalmic examination. Imaging studies may well appear normal, especially if attention is not directed toward the occipital lobes. Retrochiasmal

visual field defects are very common in patients with head injuries accounting for > 50% of afferent visual defects in one large series.[1] Visual field defects may have significant financial and legal implications and should be sought in any patient suffering a head injury. This may be very difficult in those severely injured; however, as recovery progresses, visual field testing is facilitated.

Papilledema may result from closed head injury, causing thrombosis of the superior sagittal sinus, interfering with cerebrospinal fluid (CSF) reabsorption with resultant elevation of intracranial pressure (ICP) (Fig. 8.7). These patients may present with headache (elevated CSF pressure), diplopia (sixth-nerve paresis secondary to elevated CSF pressure) and evidence for superior sagittal sinus thrombosis on neuroimaging studies (Fig. 8.7c). In this setting, the diagnosis should be obvious. More challenging are those patients seen several months later, after the sagittal sinus has recanalized. Is their papilledema and

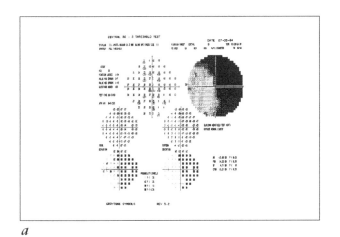

a

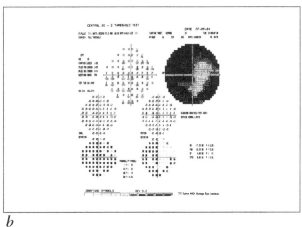

b

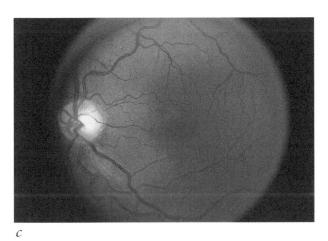

c

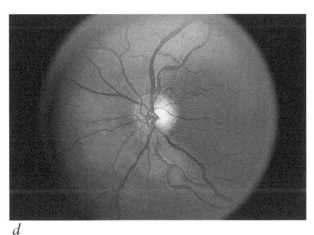

d

Figure 8.5 *Incomplete bitemporal hemianopia due to chiasmal injury after frontal trauma (a and b). Fundus photographs demonstrate bitemporal optic disc pallor (c and d).*

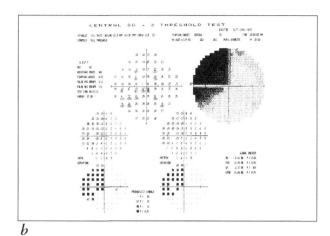

a   b

Figure 8.6   *Congruous visual field defects due to an occipital lobe injury.*

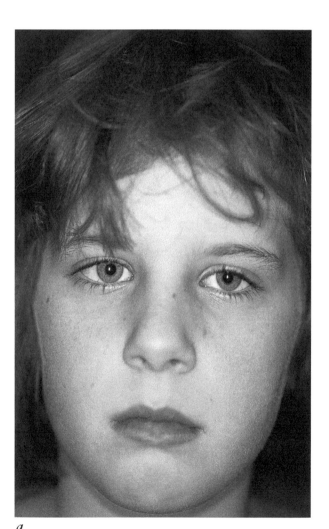

elevated ICP due to injury to the CSF reabsorption mechanism (villae) in the sagittal sinus (Fig. 8.8) or unrelated to their injury. This may be a perplexing medico-legal issue.

EFFERENT VISUAL DEFECTS

Efferent visual defects cause dysfunction in extraocular motility via injury to the brain stem or the third, fourth and sixth cranial nerves (Fig. 8.2). Patients present with a variation upon the theme of diplopia. Individual cranial nerve palsies are described in detail in other chapters, but they are often the result of cranial trauma. Efferent visual

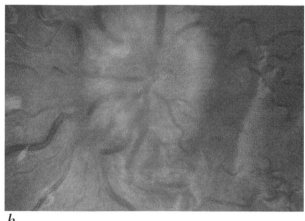

a   b

Figure 8.7   *A 12-year-old girl presenting with headache and diplopia secondary to a sixth-nerve paresis (a), papilledema (b and c) due to elevated ICP. An MRI scan demonstrates post-traumatic sagittal sinus thrombosis (d).*

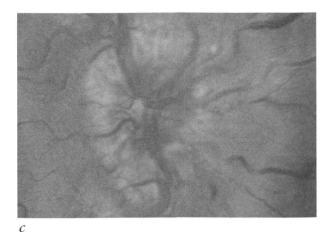

c

d

Figure 8.7 *(cont.)*

deficits account for almost 60% of neuro-ophthalmic manifestations of head trauma.[1]

After exiting the dorsal midbrain, the fourth nerve has a long tortuous course along the base of the brain through the cavernous sinus to innervate the superior

oblique muscle at the orbital apex (Fig. 8.9). A fourth nerve injury with a resultant superior oblique paresis is a common sequelae to head injury. Patients complain of vertical diplopia due to a hypertropia (Fig. 8.10a), adapt a compensatory head tilt to the opposite side (Fig. 8.10b) and often have a markedly overacting ipsilateral inferior oblique muscle (direct antagonist) (Fig. 8.11a and b). Patients with fourth-nerve palsies should be observed and reassured for at least 6 months prior to surgical intervention. Spontaneous resolution often occurs.

After the appropriate observation period, these patients invariably do well with a recession or myotomy of the overacting, ipsilateral inferior oblique muscle. The present author has rarely, if ever, operated upon the underacting, paretic superior oblique muscle. This is not inappropriate but, in my experience, it is rarely necessary in patients with fourth-nerve palsies. Inferior

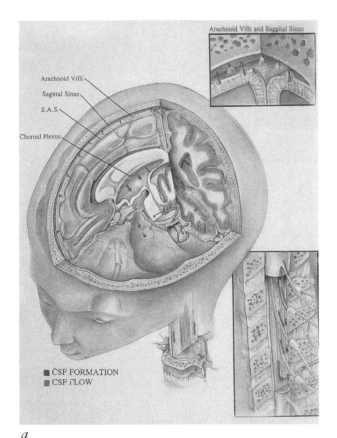

a

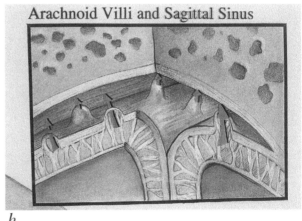

b

Figure 8.8 *CSF secretion in the choroidal plexi, circulation through the CNS and reabsorption by the arachnoid villae in the superior sagittal sinus (a); inset (b).*

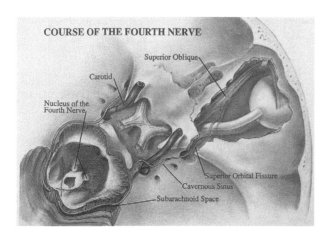

Figure 8.9 *Course of the fourth nerve from the brainstem to the orbit.*

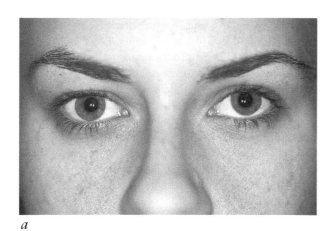

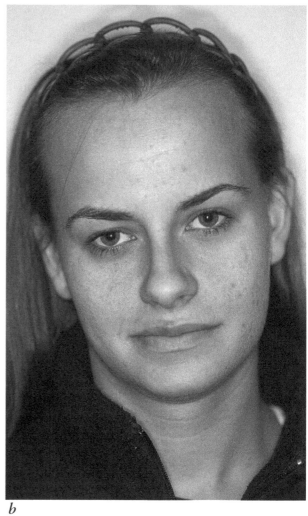

a   *b*

Figure 8.10 *Left hypertropia (a) due to superior oblique paresis with compensatory head tilt (b).*

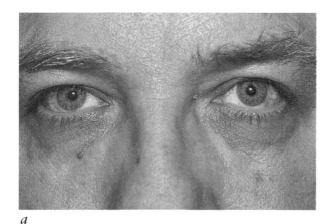

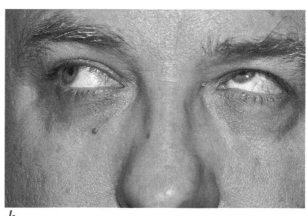

a   *b*

Figure 8.11 *A patient with a left hypertropia due to a superior oblique palsy (a) with a markedly overacting ipsilateral inferior oblique (b).*

oblique myectomy, recession or whatever weakening procedure is easy, effective and predictable should be used. The pundits of strabismology can debate ad nauseum the advantages or disadvantages of various weakening procedures but really whatever weakens the inferior oblique muscle is often an effective treatment for diplopia secondary to a superior oblique palsy.

The surgical procedure described below is effective, reproducible and has withstood the test of time. The bottom line is that whatever procedure is used to weaken the inferior oblique muscle, the muscle must be visualized directly in its entirety so that the whole muscle can be recessed, myotomized, transected or whatever. Under direct, complete visualization, probably any weakening procedure is effective.

INFERIOR OBLIQUE SURGERY

There is nothing esoteric about weakening the inferior oblique muscle except that it has to be done under direct visualization. Surgery is easily and effectively accomplished under local anesthesia with some supplemental intravenous sedation. Anesthetic solution is instilled beneath the conjunctiva in the inferior, temporal quadrant (Fig. 8.12). A Swan incision is made 8 mm from the limbus and enlarged superiorly and inferiorly. Anesthetic is instilled behind the globe with a blunt angiocatheter (Fig. 8.13). The inferior and lateral recti are isolated with muscle hooks (Fig. 8.14) and the conjunctiva is retracted with a Desmarres retractor (Fig. 8.15). This technique allows direct, total visualization

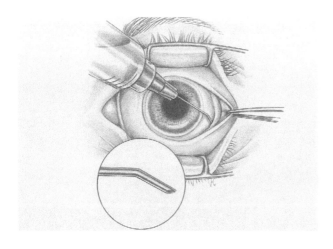

Figure 8.12 *Infiltrating anesthetic beneath the conjunctiva.*

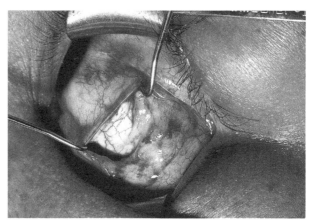

Figure 8.14 *Isolating the lateral and inferior recti with muscle hooks.*

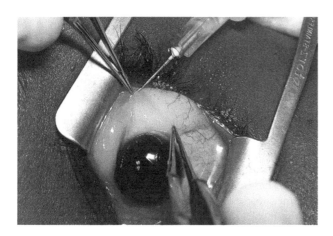

Figure 8.13 *Instilling anesthetic into the peribulbar space with a blunt cannula or angiocatheter.*

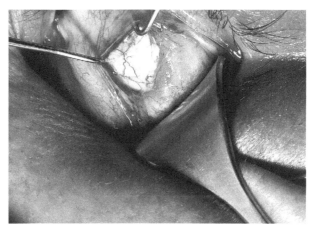

Figure 8.15 *Exposing the inferior oblique by retracting the temporal conjunctiva with a Desmarres retractor.*

of the inferior oblique muscle and prevents any inadvertent damage to the inferior and lateral recti. Once the muscle is visualized (Fig. 8.16), it can be isolated in its entirety (Fig. 8.17) and recessed, myotomized or weakened as the surgeon desires. Again, visualization is the key to appropriate treatment. The present author prefers to isolate the muscle, excise a portion of it (Fig. 8.18) and then suture the Tenon's capsule around it so that it will not migrate forward to its original insertion. Alternatively, the inferior oblique may be recessed and sutured to the globe 2 mm lateral and 3 mm posterior to the insertion of the inferior rectus. Either procedure is probably equally effective. The bottom line is to avoid violating the orbital fat pads and causing a fat-adherence syndrome. Make sure that the

entire inferior oblique is isolated under direct visualization and that it is weakened in an appropriate fashion, surgery will then be successful.

An occasional patient will continue to complain of diplopia in downgaze after apparently successful surgery. Look for a contralateral superior oblique paresis that may have been masked by the obvious paresis. This is relatively common and treatment entails weakening the overacting inferior oblique. Patients may also complain of torsional diplopia after 'successful' inferior oblique weakening. There may be no apparent ocular deviation but the patient complains that the vision is not right, especially at near. Occluding one eye obviates the complaint. Diagnosis is made by demonstrating torsion with Maddox prisms. Transposition of the anterior portion of the superior oblique tendon often relieves the torsional diplopia (Harada-Ito procedure).[2,3]

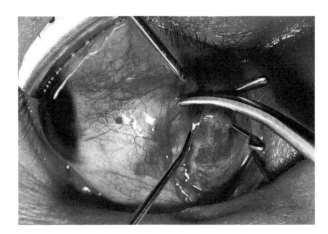

Figure 8.16 *The inferior oblique is isolated in its entirety.*

SIXTH-NERVE PARESIS

The sixth nerve is also commonly involved in patients with head injury. It exits the ventral pons and courses along the base of the brain through the cavernous sinus to innervate the lateral rectus muscle in the orbit (Fig. 8.19). These patients complain of horizontal diplopia, distance worse than near. There is decreased abduction of the involved eye. Sixth-nerve paresis may also result from elevated ICP (Fig. 8.7). The sixth nerve is stretched against the dura at Doral's canal as it enters the cavernous sinus. (Fig. 8.19) by the elevated CSF pressure pushing the brainstem caudally. Traumatic sixth-nerve

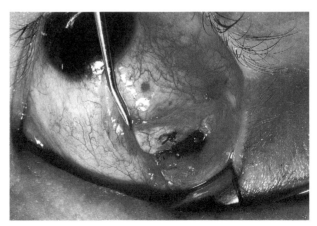

Figure 8.18 *The inferior oblique is sutured behind Tenon's fascia to prevent potential migration.*

Figure 8.17 *The inferior oblique is clamped and myotomized.*

palsies may resolve spontaneously and completely (Figs 8.20–8.22) or partially. Predictors of non-recovery include bilaterality, an inability to abduct the eye past the midline on initial presentation.[4]

Patients with partial resolution do very well with eye muscle surgery to correct their residual esotropia. These patients often resolve to an esotropia of 25-prism diopters. The image in the deviating eye lands on the optic nerve head, obviating the diplopia in spite of an obvious deviation. Patients with subtotal resolution of their lateral rectus palsy and symptomatic diplopia remaining in lateral gaze often have restriction by a contracted medial rectus muscle and may benefit from recession of the medial rectus.

If there is no resolution of lateral rectus function, the present author prefers a Hummelsheim transposition procedure, with or without a posterior fixation suture. The antagonistic medial rectus must first be recessed 5–6 mm (Fig. 8.23a). This may also be done pharmaco-

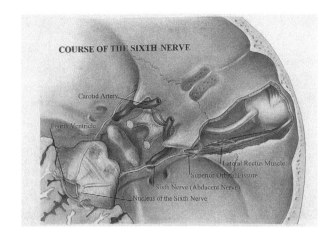

Figure 8.19 *Intracranial course of the sixth nerve exiting the ventral pons, traversing the base of the skull, and entering the cavernous sinus through Dorello's canal to innervate the lateral rectus muscle at the orbital apex.*

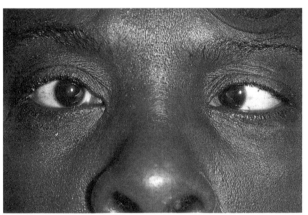

a

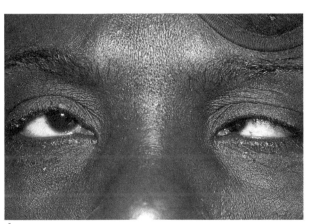

b

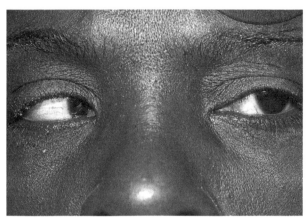

c

Figure 8.20 *Large-angle esotropia due to an asymmetric, bilateral sixth-nerve palsy (a) with absent abduction in right gaze (b) and partial abduction in left gaze (c).*

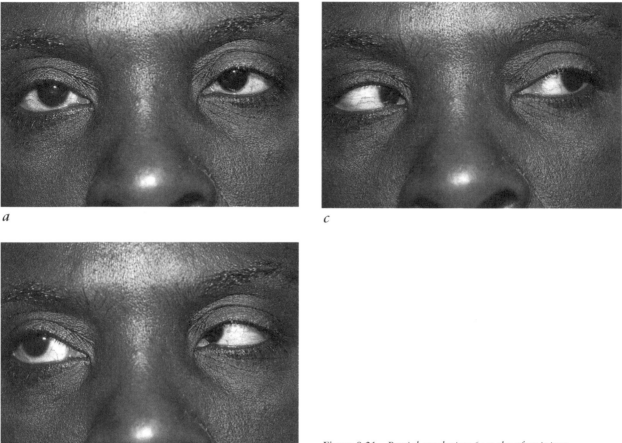

a

b

c

Figure 8.21 *Partial resolution 6 weeks after injury.*

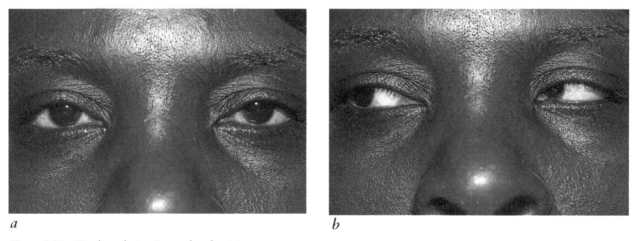

a

b

Figure 8.22 *Total resolution 3 months after injury.*

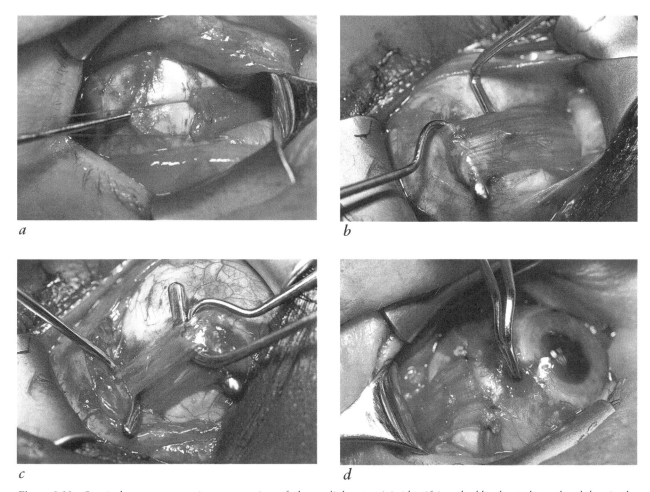

Figure 8.23 *Surgical sequence: maximum recession of the medial rectus (a); identifying the blood supply to the globe via the inferior and superior recti (b); splitting the vertical recti, sparing one of the blood vessels in each muscle to maintain the vascular supply to the eye (c); completed transposition of the lateral half of the superior and inferior rectus to the insertion of the lateral rectus (d). A posterior fixation suture strengthens the transposition.*

logically by injecting two units of botulinum-A toxin into the antagonistic muscle (medial rectus). The lateral rectus is then isolated, but not resected or disinserted, preserving its blood supply. The superior and inferior recti are identified and their blood supply examined. Each muscle is split with a tenotomy hook, leaving the medial vessels intact on each muscle (Fig. 8.23b). The lateral halves of the muscles are disinserted from the globe (Fig. 8.23c) and reinserted at the insertion of the lateral rectus (Fig. 8.23d). This procedure is not perfect but it does straighten the eyes and allows a bit of abduction (Figs 8.24 and 8.25). It may be strengthened considerably by a posterior fixation suture attaching each transposed muscle to the globe 8 mm posterior to the lateral rectus

insertion. In older individuals, anterior segment ischemia may occur if the vascular supply to the eye is sufficiently compromised. These patients develop corneal edema and iris atrophy secondary (Fig. 8.26) to their compromised anterior segment blood supply. Visual function usually normalizes after several months.

THIRD-NERVE PARESIS

The third nerve exits the ventral midbrain and passes along the base of the brain to enter the cavernous sinus and the orbit. In the orbit, it separates into an inferior and superior division. The superior division innervates the levator and superior rectus muscles. The inferior division innervates accommodation, the pupil, the inferior oblique, inferior rectus and medial rectus (Fig. 8.27). The third nerve may be partially or totally paretic (Fig. 8.28). Like the other cranial nerve pareses, they may resolve completely and spontaneously or not at all. Complete resolution requires no treatment, although aberrant regeneration may be a problem (Fig. 8.29).

Total third-nerve palsies (Fig. 8.28) with no resolution are best left alone. Raising the eyelid or straightening the eye often causes a significant keratopathy or symptomatic diplopia. If the involved eye needs to be straightened or is the only sighted eye, the lateral rectus may be disinserted from the globe and actually sutured to the

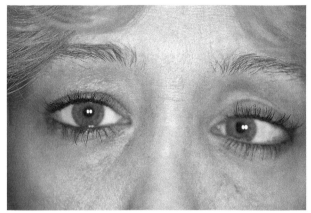

a

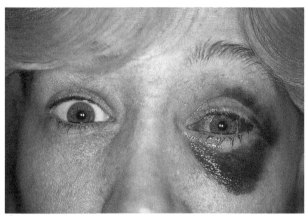

b

Figure 8.25   *A patient with a left sixth-nerve palsy before (a) and after (b) a Hummelsheim transposition.*

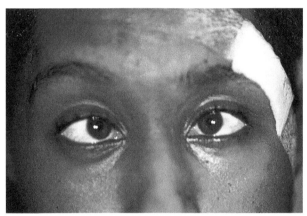

a

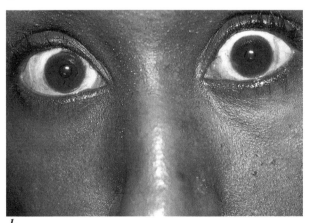

b

Figure 8.24   *A patient with bilateral sixth-nerve palsy before (a) and after (b) bilateral medial rectus recessions and Hummelsheim transposition procedures.*

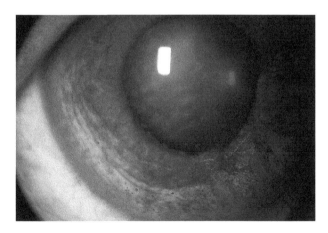

Figure 8.26   *Corneal edema and iris atrophy in a patient with resolving anterior segment necrosis.*

lateral periorbita. The eye may be fixed in primary gaze by transposing a piece of medial orbital periorbita to the medial rectus insertion. Alternatively, the superior oblique muscle may be transposed to the medial rectus insertion and resected. The denervated medial rectus may be resected, but it is rare that resecting a dead muscle is advantageous.[5–7]

Partial resolution allows the surgeon many options. As long as some muscles are functioning, something can be done and the patient's condition may be improved (Figs 8.30 and 8.31). If the vertical paretic component resolves, the eyes can be straightened horizontally. If the horizontal component resolves, the eyes can be straightened vertically (Figs 8.30 and 8.31). A reverse Hummelsheim procedure (moving the medial halves of the superior and inferior recti to the insertion of the medial rectus after maximally recessing or disinserting the lateral rectus 8 mm) may straighten an otherwise markedly exotropic eye. Some patients with complicated problems require very imaginative solutions.

Combined cranial nerve palsy may occur from base of the brain injury or injury to the cranial nerves in the cavernous sinus or orbital apex. Patients with base-of-skull fractures may have a combination of a sixth and seventh cranial nerve palsy and a hemotypanium (Fig. 8.32a–c). Patients with traumatic carotid–cavernous fistulas may initially present with an isolated sixth-nerve paresis rapidly progressing to multiple cranial nerve palsies and a frozen orbit (Figs 8.33, 8.34, 8.36 and 8.38). Cranial nerves III, IV, V1, V2 and VI and sympathetic nerve fibers pass through the cavernous sinus in close proximity to the carotid artery before entering the

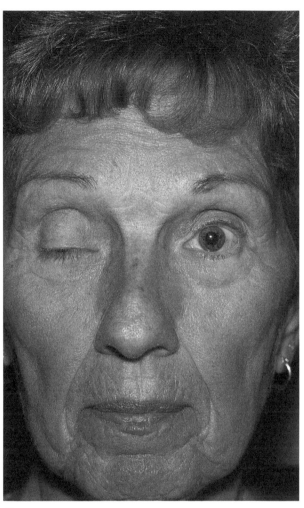

a

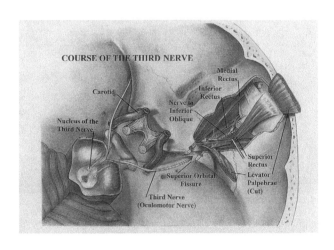

Figure 8.27 *Course of the third nerve from midbrain to orbit.*

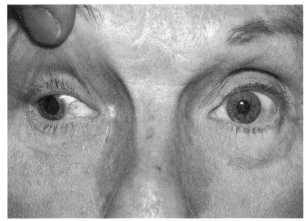

b

Figure 8.28 *Total third-nerve palsy: ptosis (a), a dilated pupil, exotropia (b), (continued overleaf)*

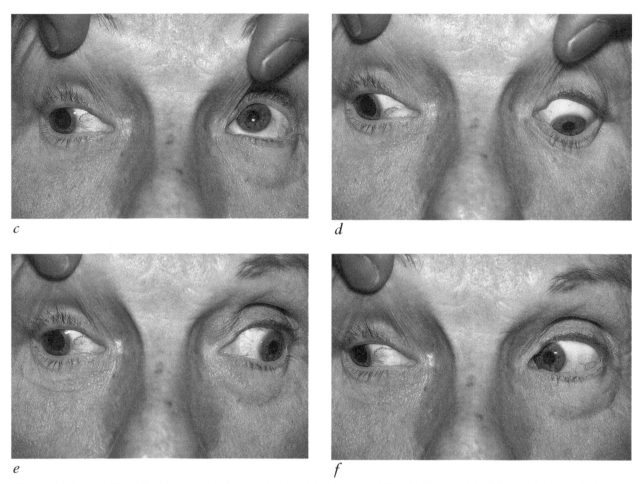

Figure 8.28 (cont.)   *Total third-nerve palsy: loss of elevation (c), depression (d) and adduction (e) of the involved eye. Only residual eye movements are abduction (f) and torsion with attempted adduction and depression.*

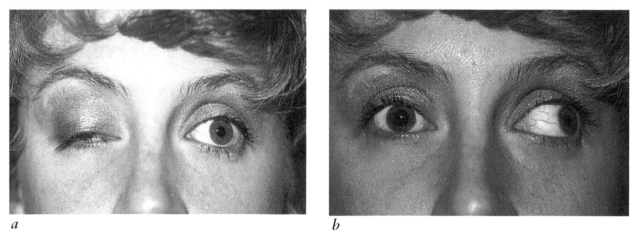

Figure 8.29   *Aberrant regeneration of a total third-nerve palsy. Complete ptosis (a) with resolution with attempted adduction of the right eye (b).*

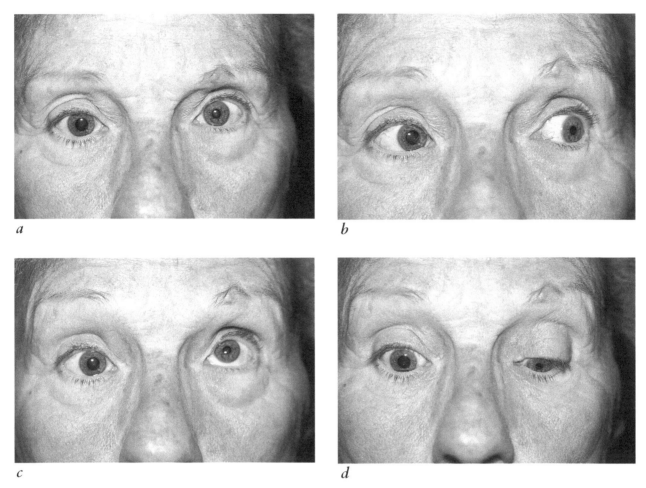

a   *b*

c   *d*

Figure 8.30 *Partial resolution of third-nerve palsy with residual, stable hypotropia (a), adduction has improved (b), elevation is absent in spite of ptosis resolution (c) and depression is decreased (d). Note the aberrant regeneration manifest as retraction of the upper eyelid with attempted downgaze (d).*

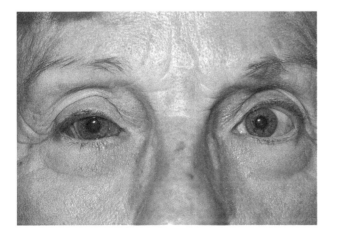

Figure 8.31 *Resolution of hypotropia after eye muscle surgery.*

orbit (Fig. 8.35). Injury to the intracavernous carotid artery causes high-pressure arterial blood to flow into the low-pressure cavernous sinus. The diagnosis is usually obvious (Figs 8.33, 8.34 and 8.36). The orbit is frozen, the conjunctival vessels are arterialized (Fig. 8.36b) and there is a very audible bruit. A dural arteriole may rupture into the cavernous sinus with more subtle manifestations (Fig. 8.38), presenting as a chronic red eye. Close examination reveals the arterialized conjunctival vessels and a CT scan demonstrates an enlarged superior ophthalmic vein (Fig. 8.39).

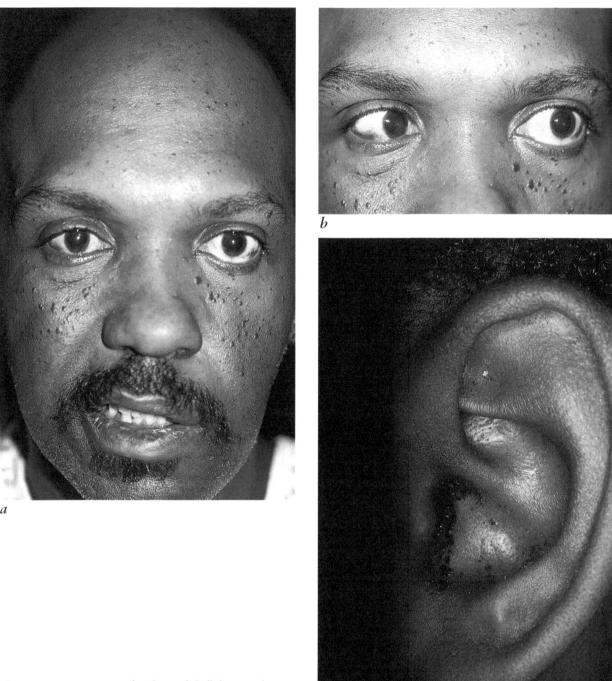

a

b

c

Figure 8.32 *A patient with a base-of-skull fracture demonstrating a subtle left facial weakness (a), lateral rectus paresis (b) and hemotypanium (c).*

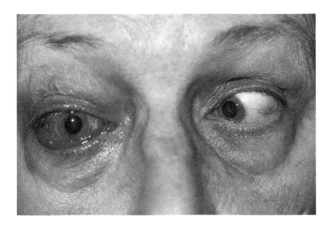

Figure 8.33 *Total sixth-nerve palsy as initial manifestation of carotid cavernous fistula.*

FACIAL NERVE

The facial nerve exits the brainstem at the ventral pons and travels along the base of the brain to exit the stylomastoid foramen. Along its course it is susceptible to injury, especially in patients with base-of-skull fractures. An ipsilateral sixth-nerve paresis and hemotypanium (Fig. 8.32) may accompany this, since the sixth nerve also has a long intracranial course along the base of the skull.

Patients with facial nerve paresis have difficulty closing their eyes (orbicularis oculi muscle), exposure keratopathy and often ectropion of the lower eyelid (Fig. 8.40). A dry eye may exacerbate the keratopathy since the parasympathetic fibers to the lacrimal gland are part of the facial nerve (Fig. 8.41). The use of psychotropic and antidepressant medications can also exacerbate dry eye and keratopathy.[8]

One of the most common causes of periorbital discomfort and photophobia is dry eye. Patients complain of gritty, aching, burning eyes often accompanied by blurring of vision due to corneal surface abnormalities and exposure of the sensory nerve endings secondary to corneal epithelial defects. Treatment with artificial tears and temporary punctal occlusion can be very effective.[9,10]

Many of these patients complain of transient blurring of vision. They notice that the quality of their vision is reduced and variable during the course of the day. More often than not these complaints are due to tear film abnormalities and dry eye exacerbated by the multiple medications that the patients are prescribed (psychotropics, antidepressants, pain relievers).[11]

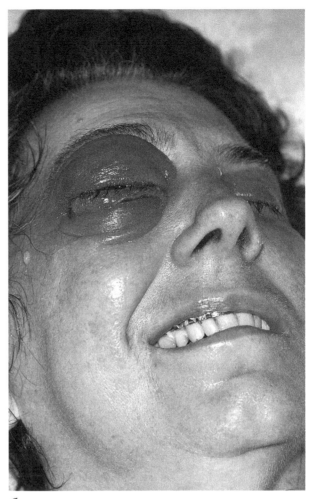

a

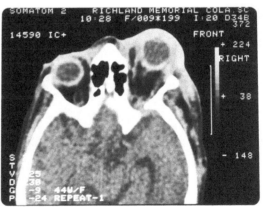

b

Figure 8.34 *Frozen orbit, swollen eyelids and intense pain due to a severe carotid cavernous fistula (a). Note the extensive proptosis evident on a CT scan (b).*

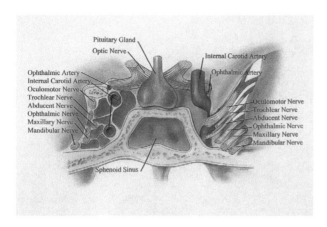

Figure 8.35 *Cross-section through the cavernous sinus demonstrating the relationships of the oculomotor nerves to the carotid artery, pituitary gland, sphenoid sinus and the optic chiasm.*

A patient with a recovered peripheral facial nerve injury may develop an apparent hemifacial spasm due to aberrant regeneration. The eyes may close upon attempted smiling or the mouth may contract with eyelid closure. This results from misdirected re-innervation between the orbicularis oculi and the orbicularis oris motor neurons. This may be differentiated from true hemifacial spasm (due to facial nerve hyperstimulation) by the latter's spontaneous occurrence. Aberrant regeneration of the facial nerve may also present as 'crocodile tears'. Parasympathetic nerves intended for the salivary glands are misdirected to the lacrimal gland. These patients complain of excessive tearing as they are preparing to eat or chew. Their doctors

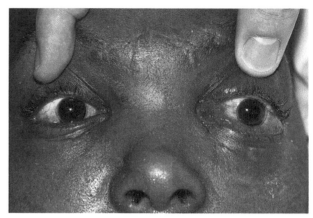

a

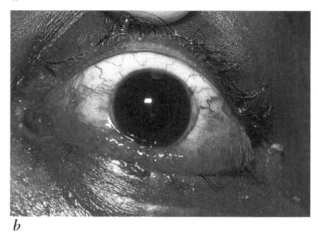

b

Figure 8.36 *Obvious carotid cavernous fistula (a) with arteriolized vessels (b), frozen orbit and a loud bruit.*

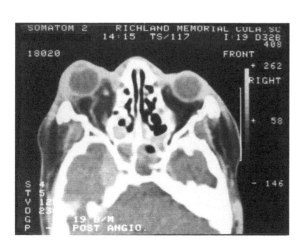

Figure 8.37 *A CT scan demonstrating enlargement of the orbit, superior ophthalmic vein and cavernous sinus.*

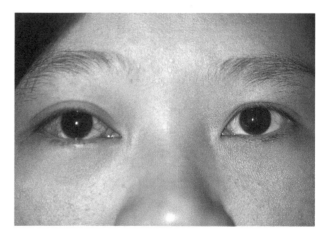

Figure 8.38 *Dural cavernous sinus fistula demonstrating arteriolized conjunctival vessels.*

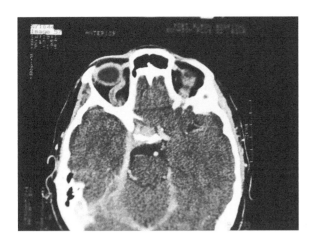

Figure 8.39 *A CT scan demonstrating obvious enlargement of the superior ophthalmic vein and subtle enlargement of the cavernous sinus.*

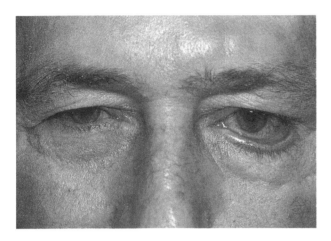

Figure 8.40 *Ectropion of the lower eyelid after a facial nerve injury, also note the ptotic left brow.*

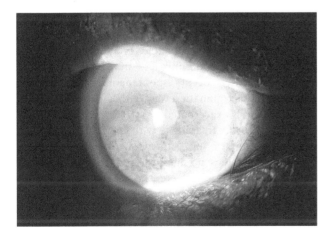

Figure 8.41 *Keratopathy due to severe dry eye.*

often think that they are crazy unless they ask them to chew or simulate chewing in the office and the diagnosis then becomes very obvious. Treatment with botulinum-A injections is very successful, but is often accompanied by significant, albeit transient, ptosis.

CONVERGENCE/ACCOMMODATIVE INSUFFICIENCY AND SPASM

In the present author's experience, almost all patients with closed head or cranio-cervical injuries have difficulties with either convergence or accommodation of their eyes. Other authors have found close to 15% of head injury patients seen in routine neuro-ophthalmologic consultation have significant accommodative convergence insufficiency.[1,12] The near reflex—convergence, accommodation and miosis of the pupil—is controlled by the rostral brainstem. This area seems to be very susceptible to injury in closed head or cranio-cervical trauma. One, two or all three mechanisms may be involved. The classic patient with accommodative convergence insufficiency recovers sufficiently from the injury to start trying to live a normal life. If normal life includes effort at near (reading, computer, writing, etc.), they become very symptomatic, complaining of blurred, double vision and headache after extended near effort. Young individuals may have 'instant presbyopia,' accommodating like someone aged 50. They are immediately relieved with a +1.50 sphere at near.

Convergence insufficiency may be more difficult to diagnose and treat. Awareness is the key to diagnosis. Historically, patients complain of blurring and doubling of vision after near effort, often accompanied by headache. Measuring the convergence amplitudes with a light and a prism bar not only establishes the diagnosis, but allows treatment to proceed. Treatment may be accomplished with minus lenses, prisms on the glasses or base-out prism exercises. Occasionally, eye muscle surgery may be required. Once the diagnosis is made, these patients are very treatable. Patients with severe convergence insufficiency may be exotropic at near greater than distance (Figs 8.42 and 8.43). Eye muscle surgery may be necessary to restore function at near.

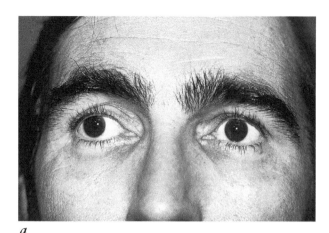

a

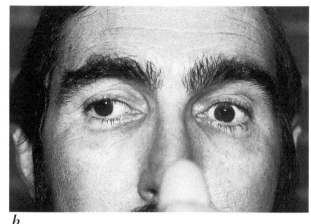

b

Figure 8.42 *Patient with severe convergence insufficiency exotropia (a) and total lack of convergence (b) due to head injury.*

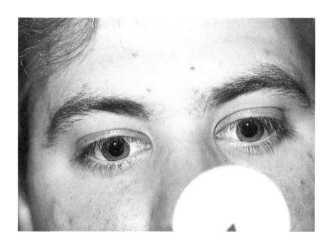

Figure 8.43 *Total loss of near reflex: note absent miosis with attempted convergence accompanied by loss of accommodation.*

SPASM OF ACCOMMODATION AND CONVERGENCE [13,14]

Unlike convergence/accommodative insufficiency, spasm of the near reflex—convergence, accommodation and miosis—is extraordinarily difficult to treat effectively. These patients present with headache and blurred vision (excess accommodation), and diplopia (excess convergence) with a pseudo-sixth-nerve paresis (Fig. 8.44). The keys to diagnosis are consideration and noting that the patient has blurred vision caused by myopia induced by excessive accommodation. This is an abduction defect that does not make sense in that it does not appear to be a typical sixth-nerve paresis, and the pupil constricts with attempted abduction of the eye. Treatment is very difficult. Cycloplegia is sometimes helpful but often fails.

The patient in Fig. 8.44 had severe accommodative convergence spasm. She was treated with the ultimate cycloplegia (atropine drops) with no real resolution of her symptoms except for a marked decrease in her accommodative myopia. Her eyes still crossed and her headache remained (Fig. 8.45). Differentiation of accommodative/convergence spasm from a sixth-nerve paresis is especially important in young individuals where a sixth-nerve paresis may connote dire neurologic consequences (see Chapter 10).

BLEPHAROSPASM

Blepharospasm—uncontrollable bilateral contractions of the orbicularis oculi muscles—may be subtle or very obvious. It often occurs spontaneously but is often preceded by a traumatic event, either psychological or physical, and is exacerbated by stress.[15]

If diagnosed, treatment with periodic botulinum injections is gratifying. Patients with benign essential blepharospasm have no significant underlying neurologic problems. They rarely, if ever, need neuroimaging—just an informed physician to make the often obvious diagnosis and administer the toxin. Treatment is by injection of botulinum-A toxin into the involved orbicularis muscles. Injection of 2 units of botulinum-A toxin per site at 10 sites on each side of the face is very effective.

Botulinum toxin is the single most effective treatment for blepharospasm. Maiming treatments like orbicularis oculi muscle extirpation and section of the facial nerve may be devastating and are rarely effective. Some variation upon the theme of botulinum injection is the treatment of choice. Orbicularis extirpation procedures may have their advocates[16] but the vast majority of patients respond to botulinum toxin.[17]

If it is believed that the patient has developed immunity to botulinum-A, try botulinum-B toxin (Myobloc) in those patients unresponsive or no longer responsive to botulinum-A toxin. Chemomyectomy with doxyrubicin also has its advocates in refractory cases.[18]

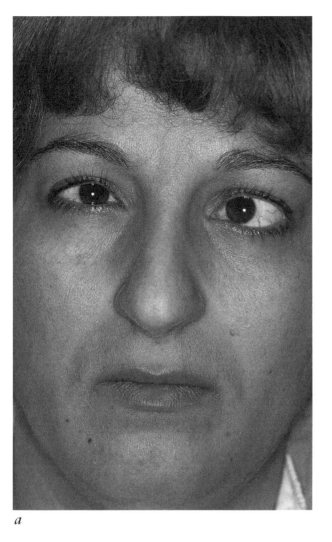

a

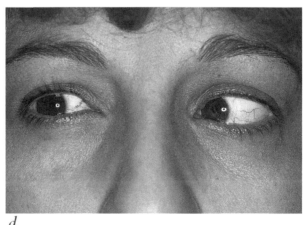

b

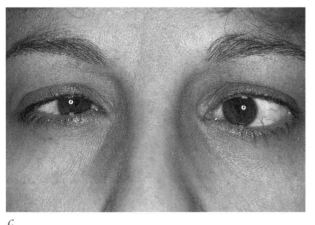

c

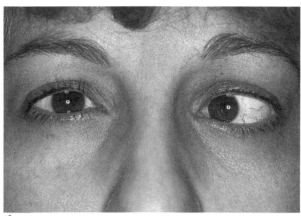

d

Figure 8.44 *Accommodative/convergence spasm: vision is blurred due to excessive accommodation, eyes are esotropic (a and b) due to excessive convergence, abduction is limited bilaterally (c and d).*

POST-TRAUMATIC HEAD AND NECK PAIN

In the present author's experience, patients with post-traumatic head injuries and cranio-cervical injury develop a distinctive pattern of head and neck pain. The common complaint is pain wrapping around the head and radiating either to the neck and upper back or from the neck and upper back to wrap around the head. Muscle spasm is often palpable in the upper back and neck. The pain is often refractory to multiple medications and adjunctive therapies. The present author and others have treated these often-refractory patients with injections of botulinum-A or -B toxin into the intrinsic muscles of the forehead, the trapezius muscles and the strap muscles of the neck from the base of the neck to the splenius capitis muscle with a success rate > 80%.[19-23]

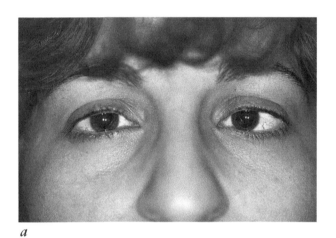

a

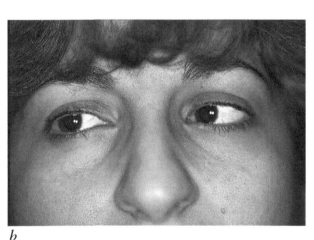

b

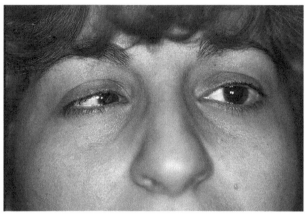

c

Figure 8.45 *Ocular abduction defect remains even after cycloplegia with atropine. Note the dilated pupils (a–c).*

REFERENCES

1. Van Stavern GP, Bioousse V, Lynn MJ et al. Neuro-ophthalmic manifestations of head trauma. *J Neuro-ophthalmol* 2001; 21:112–17.
2. Simons BD, Saunders TG, Siatkowski RM et al. Outcome of surgical management of superior oblique palsy: a study of 123 cases. *Binoc Vis Strabis Q* 1998; 13:273–82.
3. Helveston EM, Mora JS, Lipsky SN et al. Surgical treatment of superior oblique palsy. *Trans Am Ophthalmol Soc* 1996; 94:315–28.
4. Holmes JM, Beck RW, Kip KE et al. Predictors of non-recovery in acute traumatic sixth nerve palsy and paresis. *Ophthalmology* 2001; 108:1457–60.

5. Kose S, Uretman O, Pamukcu K. An approach to surgical management of total oculomotor palsy. *Strabismus* 2001; 9:1–8.

6. Simons BD. Surgical management of ocular motor cranial nerve palsies. *Semin Ophthalmol* 1999; 14:81–94.

7. Lee V, Bentley CR, Lee JP. Strabismus surgery in congenital third nerve palsy. *Strabismus* 2001; 9:91–9.

8. Calonge M. Treatment of dry eye. *Surv Ophthalmol* 2001; 45 (Suppl 2):S222–S239.

9. Goto E, Yagi Y, Kaido M et al. Improved functional visual acuity after punctal occlusion in dry eye patients. *Am J Ophthalmol* 2003; 135:704–5.

10. Nava-Castanda A, Tevilla-Canales JL, Rodriguez L et al. Effects of lacrimal occlusion with collagen and silicon plugs in patients with conjunctivitis associated with dry eye. *Cornea* 2003; 22:10–14.

11. Volpe NJ, Liu GT, Galetta SL. Transient visual loss. *Curr Concepts Ophthalmol* 1998; 6:55–9.

12. Lepore FE. Disorders of ocular motility following head trauma. *Arch Neurol* 1995; 52:924–6.

13. Goldstein JH, Schneekloth BB. Spasm of the near reflex: a spectrum of anomalies. *Surv Ophthalmol* 1996; 40:268–78.

14. Chan RV, Trobe JD. Spasm of accommodation associated with closed head trauma. *J Neuro-ophthalmol* 2002; 22:15–17.

15. Diamond EL, Trobe JD, Belar CD. Psychologic aspects of essential blepharospasm. *J Nerv Ment Dis* 1984; 172:749–56.

16. Anderson RL, Patel BCV, Holds JB. Blepharospasm: past, present and future. *Ophthal Plast Reconstr Surg* 1998; 14:305–17.

17. Mauriello JA, Dhillon S, Leone T et al. Treatment selections of 239 patients with blepharospasm and Meige syndrome over 11 years. *Br J Ophthalmol* 1996; 80:1073–6.

18. Wirtschafter JD, McLoon LK. Long term efficacy of doxyrubicin chemomyectomy in patients with blepharospasm and hemifacial spasm. *Ophthalmology* 1998; 105:342–6.

19. Rollnik JD, Tannenberger O, Schubert M et al. Treatment of tension-type headache with botulinum-A toxin: a double blind placebo controlled study. *Headache* 2000, 40:300–3.

20. Schmitt WJ, Slowey E, Fravi N et al. Effect of botulinum-A injections in the treatment of chronic tension type headache: a double-blind placebo controlled study. *Headache* 2001; 41:658–64.

21. Freund BJ, Schwartz M. Treatment of whiplash associated neck pain with botulinum-A toxin. *J Rheumatol* 2000; 27:481–4.

22. Spoor TC, Spoor DK. Treatment of head and neck pain with botulium-A toxin in 200 patients poster presentation. North American Neuro-ophthalmologic SOG. Snowbird, Utah. Feb 10, 2003.

23. Blumenfeld A. Botulinum type A as an effective prophylactic treatment in primary headache disorders. *Headache* 2003; 43:853–60.

Chapter 9　Ptosis: differential diagnosis and treatment

The ptotic eyelid is overdiagnosed by the neurologist and neurosurgeon, and underdiagnosed by the ophthalmologist and oculoplastic surgeon. The former often embark on major diagnostic endeavors for patients with an 'obvious' dehiscence of the levator aponeurosis, while the latter may overlook some significant associated neurologic signs and symptoms. After accurate diagnosis and treatment, ptosis may be repaired by a levator advancement procedure if the levator muscle has any function, or a slinging procedure (preferably open sky) if there is no levator function.[1] Good eyelid function with excellent cosmesis is the desired result of ptosis surgery.

DIFFERENTIAL DIAGNOSIS

Accurate diagnosis is essential prior to treatment. Inaccurate diagnosis may lead to inappropriate treatment as in the following case. A 40-year-old lady presented to her physician with slowly progressive ptosis. She was diagnosed as having myasthenia gravis (without benefit of a Tensilon test) and treated with Mestinon to the verge of urinary incontinence. Referred with obvious ptosis (Fig. 9.1) and excellent levator function (Fig. 9.2a and b), the Mestinon was discontinued and a subsequent Tensilon test was negative. Her incontinence resolved and her ptosis was treated by levator advancement.

A 12-year-old girl presented to an optometrist with acute onset ptosis and an inflamed eyelid (Fig. 9.3). She was referred to a plastic surgeon for repair. He told her to wait 6 months for the condition to stabilize prior to eyelid surgery. She then saw a neurologist and a neurosurgeon, and underwent a computerized tomography (CT) scan that was read as negative. A four-vessel angiogram was normal (no aneurysm). She was referred to an ENT surgeon who diagnosed orbital cellulitis (sinus were normal and she was afebrile) and was treated with a 7-day course of intravenous antibiotics without improvement. While in the hospital, she was seen in consult by the neuro-ophthalmology service. The CT scan

was repeated with coronal reconstructions revealing an enlarged levator/superior rectus complex (Fig. 9.4). The diagnosis of orbital myositis was made and she was treated with systemic prednisone. Her symptoms resolved in 48 hours.

Caveat: Ptosis can result from a variety of causes—neurologic, myogenic, or involvement of the orbit or the eyelid itself.

NEUROGENIC ANATOMY

Both levator muscles are innervated by a single central caudal nucleus in the midbrain. Injury to the central caudal nucleus must result in bilateral ptosis with absent levator function. Except for bilateral third-nerve palsies (Fig. 9.5), it is the only neurogenic cause of bilateral ptosis. As with any unexplained extraocular motility dysfunction, myasthenia gravis must be considered in the differential diagnosis.

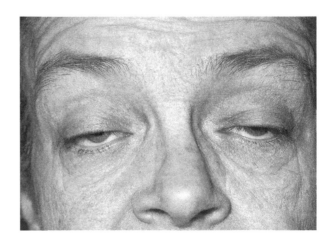

Figure 9.1 *Ptosis of the upper eyelids.*

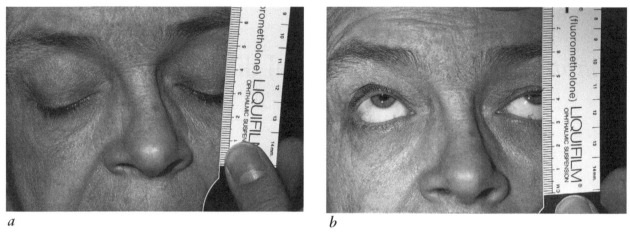

Figure 9.2   *Levator function is measured from extreme downgaze (a) to upgaze (b). Excellent function is > 15 mm excursion.*

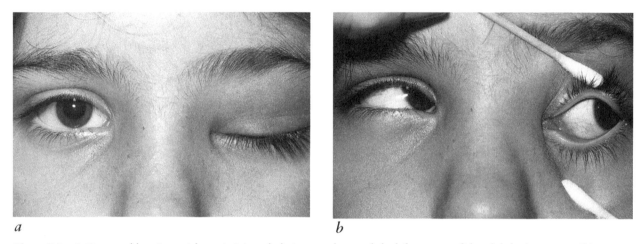

Figure 9.3   *A 12-year-old patient with ptosis (a), and obvious erythema of the left upper eyelid and defective upgaze (b).*

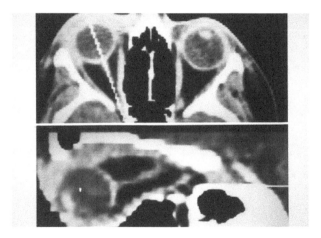

Figure 9.4   *A CT scan demonstrating enlargement of the levator superior rectus complex due to orbital myositis.*

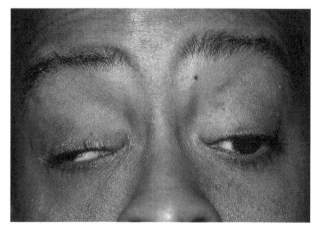

Figure 9.5   *Traumatic bilateral third-nerve palsies—bilateral ptosis, exotropia and dilated pupils.*

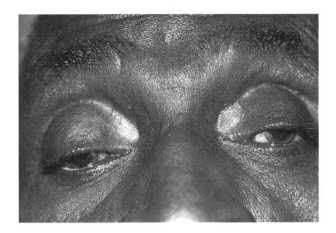

Figure 9.6 *Bilateral ptosis with no levator function.*

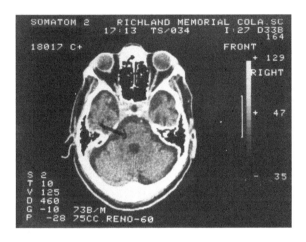

Figure 9.7 *A CT scan demonstrating lacunar infarct in the vicinity of the central caudal nucleus of the midbrain.*

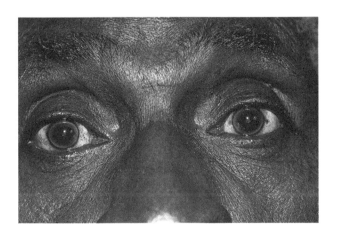

Figure 9.8 *The same patient as in Fig. 9.7 2 weeks later, showing normal eyelid position and levator function.*

CASE STUDY 1

A 60-year-old man was referred from his neurologist with acute onset, bilateral ptosis and no levator function (Fig. 9.6). A Tensilon test was performed that was negative; the test was repeated and it remained negative. A CT scan demonstrated a lacunar infarction of the midbrain in the vicinity of the central caudal nucleus (Fig. 9.7). Two weeks later ptosis completely resolved and levator function was normal (Fig. 9.8). Similar cases have been described by others.[2]

The levator muscle is innervated by the superior branch of the oculomotor nerve (see Chapter 10) after it enters the orbit. Since the superior division of the oculomotor nerve also innervates the superior rectus muscle, involvement results in ptosis combined with superior rectus muscle dysfunction (Fig. 9.9). Isolated ptosis, i.e. no associated pupillary or extraocular motility deficits, almost never has a neurogenic cause. A myogenic cause or myasthenia gravis must be considered.

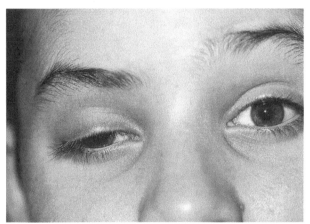

a

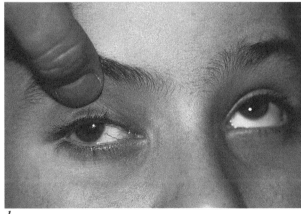

b

Figure 9.9 *Ptosis (a) and upgaze palsy (b) secondary to superior division third-nerve paresis.*

CASE STUDY 2

A 15-year-old boy was noted to have increased ptosis after football practice. Examination in the morning was normal but in the late afternoon isolated ptosis of the right upper eyelid was very evident (Fig. 9.10a). The ptosis was rapidly resolved (Fig. 9.10b) after administration of intravenous edrophonium (Tensilon), confirming the clinical suspicion of myasthenia gravis (MG). In a recent series of 24 patients with childhood MG, 96% had ptosis, 88% strabismus (usually an exotropia with a vertical component) and 21% amblyopia.[3]

A patient with ptosis, oculomotor motility deficits and pupillary enlargement represents a neuro-ophthalmologic/neurosurgical emergency (Fig. 9.11a–c). Although these presentations are usually obvious, internal carotid artery/posterior communicating artery (ICA/PCA) aneurysms may also present in a much more subtle fashion.

A 16-year-old girl complained of ptosis and diplopia (Fig. 9.12 a and b). Two to 3 mm of ptosis, decreased levator function, limited upgaze and a mildly dilated pupil (Fig. 9.12 c and d) alerted the examiner to the diagnosis of aneurysm, which was confirmed by cerebral angiography.

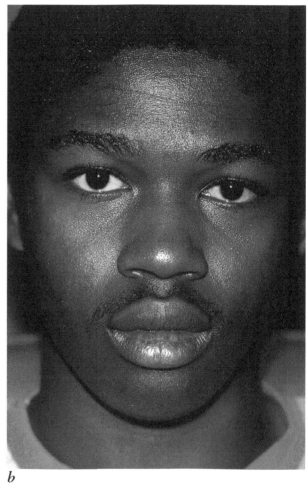

b

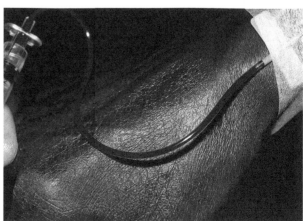

a   *c*

Figure 9.10 *Ptosis of the right upper eyelid (a). Resolution of ptosis (b) after administration of 10 mg intravenous edrophonium (c).*

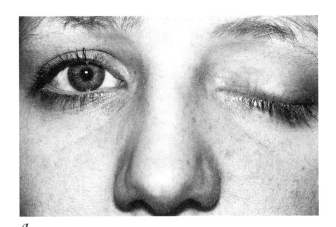

a

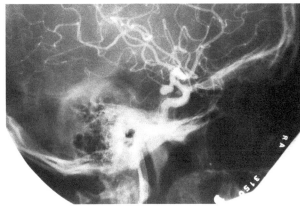

c

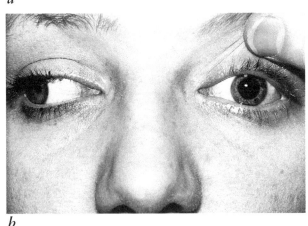

b

Figure 9.11 *A patient presented with ptosis (a), a dilated pupil and total third-nerve palsy (b). Cerebral angiography confirmed the presence of an ICA/PCA aneurysm (c).*

To reiterate, isolated ptosis with good levator muscle function is rarely, if ever, of neurological significance. If levator function is poor, think of MG (see Chapters 10, 11). If other muscles innervated by the oculomotor nerve are involved, refer to the differential diagnosis of oculomotor nerve palsies (see Chapter 10). If the pupil is dilated, even in the presence of minimal extraocular motility dysfunction, rule out an intracranial compressive lesion or an aneurysm. If other oculomotor nerves are involved, carefully image the cavernous sinus region for tumor or carotid aneurysm.

A 46-year-old man was referred for evaluation of a ptotic right upper eyelid (Fig. 9.13a). Examination revealed a partial third-nerve paresis with pupillary involvement and an associated sixth-nerve paresis (Fig. 9.13a–c). Neuroimaging revealed a mass in the cavernous sinus (Fig. 9.14) that proved to be an undifferentiated carcinoma. The associated sixth-nerve paresis keyed the clinician to evaluate the cavernous sinus rather than pursue angiography to rule out an aneurysm.

Aberrant regeneration of the oculomotor nerve may result in a patient with significant ptosis (Fig. 9.15a) that improves completely with adduction of the eye. This results from a synkinesis between the superior and inferior division of the third nerve resulting in elevation of the eyelid with adduction (Fig. 9.15b).[4]

OPHTHALMOPLEGIC MIGRAINE

Ophthalmoplegic migraine usually occurs in children, has an uncertain etiology and is repetitive (Figs 9.16 and 9.17), totally resolving several weeks after occurrence. This is a diagnosis of exclusion, predicated upon normal neuroimaging and neurologic examination. After multiple similar episodes, clinicians may be comfortable with the diagnosis of ophthalmoplegic migraine in a known migraineur; but if any doubt exists, magnetic resonance imaging (MRI) and MR angiography imaging should be obtained. With a negative history, cerebral angiography should be performed.[5,6]

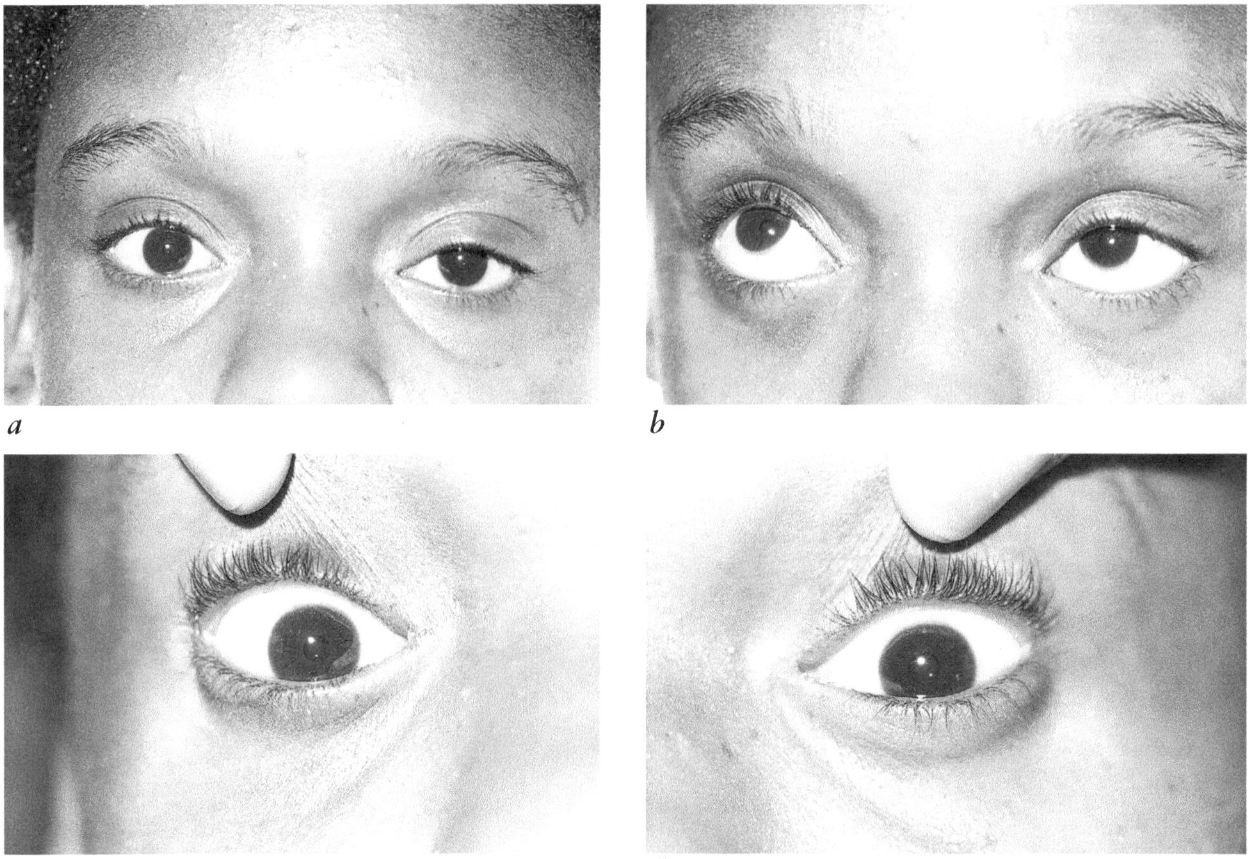

Figure 9.12 *A patient with a more subtle, partial third-nerve paresis, manifest by ptosis and upgaze paresis (a and b). Mild pupillary dilatation (c and d) cinched the diagnosis of third-nerve compression by aneurysm.*

CYCLIC OCULOMOTOR PALSY

Patients with cyclic oculomotor paresis present with episodic ptosis, mydriasis and decreased accommodation occurring approximately every 2 minutes. The pupil then constricts, the lid elevates and the eye adducts. This is unilateral and usually occurs in infancy. Over time, lid motion may decrease but the pupillary mydriasis remains. This should also be considered in the differential diagnosis of episodic pupillary mydriasis.

SYMPATHETIC DYSFUNCTION

The upper eyelid is elevated not only by the levator muscle but also by the sympathetically derived Mueller's muscle (Fig. 9.18) (see Chapter 1). Sympathetic denervation of Mueller's muscle results in 1–2 mm of ptosis. Since the sympathetic nerves also innervate the iris dilator muscle, the involved pupil is miotic. The combination of ptosis and miosis is Horner's syndrome, resulting from sympathetic denervation (Fig. 9.19). This may also be accompanied by anhydrosis, but it is not often of clinical significance in a busy ophthalmic practice. It is important to remember that 20% of the elderly population has some degree of anisocoria and levator dehiscence is also quite common in these patients. A miotic pupil due to sympathetic denervation (true Horner's syndrome) does not dilate to 4–10% cocaine drops (Fig. 9.20). A miotic pupil due to physiologic anisocoria dilates quite readily to cocaine testing. Also, ptosis due to Horner's syndrome is always minimal (1–2 mm). If a greater degree of ptosis is present, it is most likely caused by dehiscence of the levator aponeurosis (Fig. 9.21 a and b).

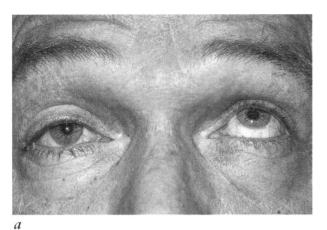

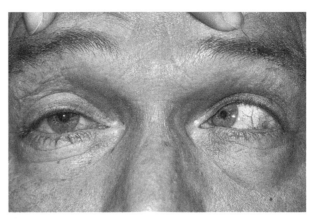

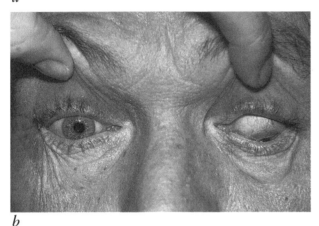

Figure 9.13 *Patient with partial third-nerve paresis (a and b) accompanied by an obvious sixth-nerve palsy (c) implicating the cavernous sinus.*

MYOGENIC PTOSIS

The hallmark of congenital ptosis is ptosis and decreased levator function (Fig. 9.22). The levator muscle is abnormal and dysfunctional. Contraction and relaxation of the muscle are abnormal with subsequent ptosis and lagophthalmos. At surgery the levator muscle is often fibrotic and infiltrated with fat. Children with congenital ptosis may develop either occlusion, anisometropic or strabismic amblyopia. Occlusion amblyopia should be obvious; the ptotic eyelid blocks the visual axis. Children often try to compensate for this by adapting a chin-elevated head position in an attempt to clear their visual axis. Anisometropic amblyopia (resulting from disparate refractive errors) is not as obvious. Forty to 50 percent of children with congenital ptosis may have associated anisometropia or strabismus.[6] A careful motility examination and cycloplegic refraction is essential in evaluating children with congenital ptosis. These amblyogenic factors should be diagnosed and treated prior to ptosis repair unless occlusion is the obvious cause of the amblyopia.

Figure 9.14 *A CT scan demonstrating an enhancing mass proven to be a metastatic undifferentiated carcinoma.*

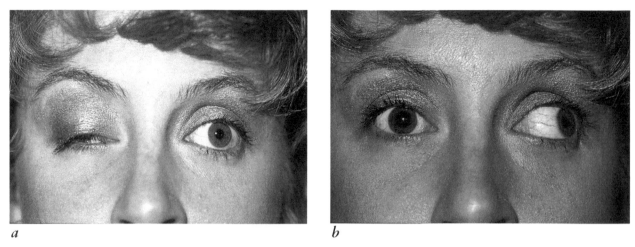

Figure 9.15   *Aberrant regeneration of a traumatic third-nerve palsy. Complete ptosis with absent levator function (a) completely resolves with adduction of the involved eye (b).*

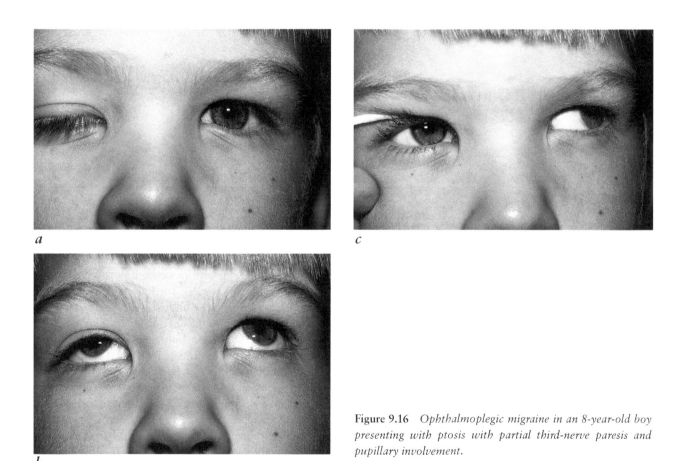

Figure 9.16   *Ophthalmoplegic migraine in an 8-year-old boy presenting with ptosis with partial third-nerve paresis and pupillary involvement.*

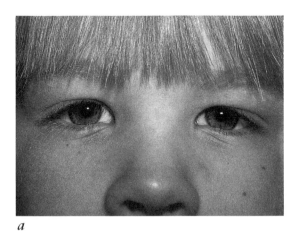

a

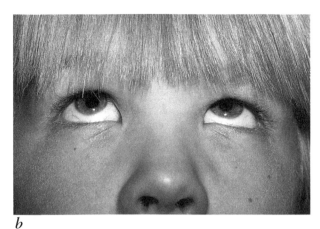

b

Figure 9.17   *The same child as in Fig 9.16 2 months later with total resolution of the third-nerve paresis.*

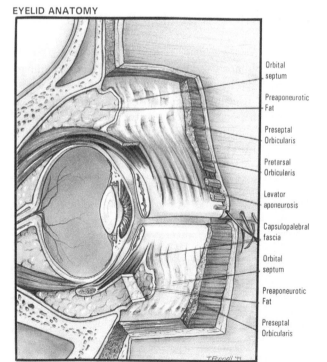

c

EYELID ANATOMY

Orbital septum
Preaponeurotic Fat
Preseptal Orbicularis
Pretarsal Orbicularis
Levator aponeurosis
Capsulopalebral fascia
Orbital septum
Preaponeurotic Fat
Preseptal Orbicularis

Figure 9.18   *Anatomy of the upper eyelid demonstrating the relationship between the levator and the underlying Mueller's muscle.*

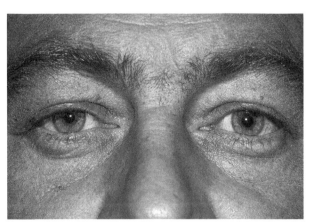

Figure 9.19   *Horner's syndrome with minimal ptosis and miosis due to sympathetic denervation.*

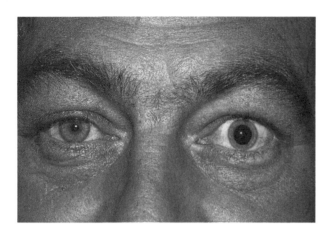

Figure 9.20   *Failure of the sympathetically denervated pupil to dilate after instillation of 4% cocaine.*

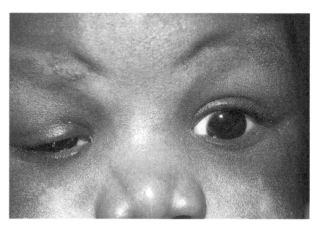

Figure 9.22   *Congenital ptosis with obstruction of the pupillary axis.*

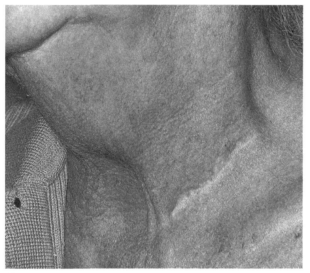

a

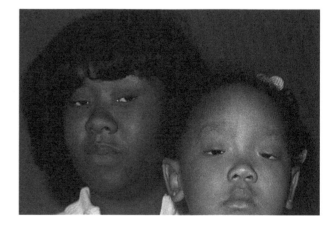

b

Figure 9.21   *Horner's ptosis from previous neck surgery (a) exacerbated by a levator dehiscence (b).*

Be careful when evaluating adults with recent-onset ptosis, retracting upper eyelid in downgaze and poor to fair levator function. This may be a sign of an orbital malignancy infiltrating superior orbital structures.[7] These orbits should be imaged prior to any treatment.

BLEPHAROPHIMOSIS SYNDROME

Blepharophimosis syndrome is an autosomally dominant inherited syndrome (Fig. 9.23) that includes blepharophimosis, telecanthus, epicanthus inversus and severe ptosis with poor to absent levator function (Fig. 9.24). Ectropion and hypoplasia of the superior orbital rims and nasal bridge may also be present.

Figure 9.23   *Mother and daughter with autosomal dominant blepharophimiosis syndrome.*

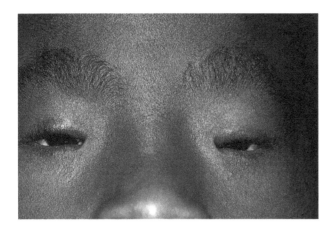

Figure 9.24 *Blepharophimosis syndrome consisting of ptosis with poor levator function, telecanthus and ectropion of the lower eyelids.*

MARCUS GUNN JAW-WINKING SYNDROME

Jaw winking results from a synkinesis between the third and the fifth cranial nerves. There is an abnormal connection between the motor division of the trigeminal nerve (innervates the masseter muscle) and the superior division of the oculomotor nerve (innervates the levator and superior rectus muscles). As the ptotic individual chews or sucks, their eyelid elevates, obviating the ptosis, which may actually retract the upper eyelid (Fig. 9.25 a and b). Since the superior division of the oculomotor nerve is involved, there may also be an associated double elevator palsy and superior rectus dysfunction. As with congenital ptosis there may be associated superior rectus weakness, double elevator palsy, anisometropia and amblyopia.[8]

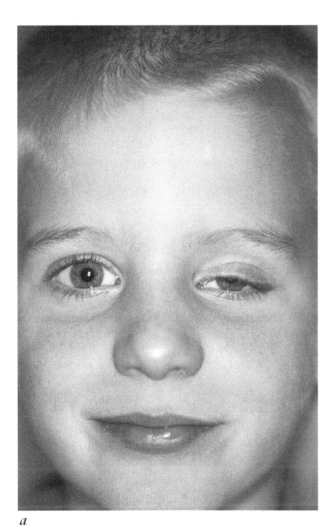

a

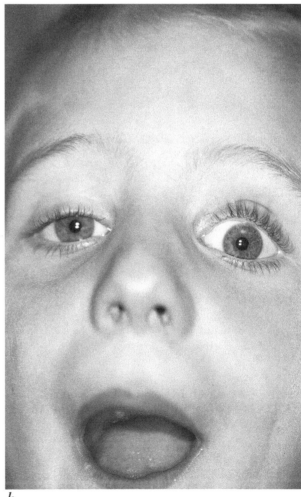

b

Figure 9.25 *Jaw-winking ptosis (a); the upper eyelid retracts with chewing (b).*

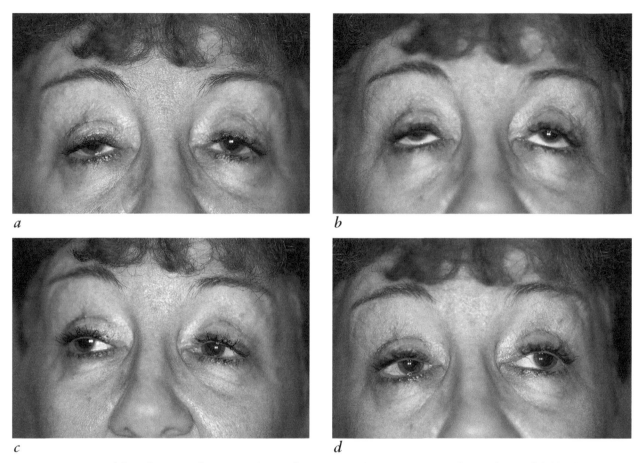

a

b

c

d

Figure 9.26   *CPEO: bilateral ptosis with poor to no levator function (a) and decreased extraocular motility in all fields of gaze (b–d).*

ACQUIRED MYOGENIC PTOSIS

Localized or diffuse muscular diseases may cause an acquired myogenic ptosis. These include chronic progressive ophthalmoplegia, oculopharyngeal dystrophy or myotonic dystrophy.

CHRONIC PROGRESSIVE EXTERNAL OPHTHALMOPLEGIA (CPEO)

Ptosis is a prominent component of CPEO. Patients present in adulthood with slowly progressive ptosis and ophthalmoplegia. Ptosis is usually severe with poor levator function (Fig. 9.26). Extraocular motility dysfunction is often severe and symmetrical, but asymmetric presentations may occur. As opposed to MG, there is no diurnal variation or exacerbation with fatigue of either the ptosis or extraocular motility dysfunction. A remarkably positive Tensilon test was performed on the patient in Fig. 9.27. The patient had been followed elsewhere for several years with the diagnosis of CPEO. The present author performs Tensilon testing pro forma on all patients with presumed CPEO, especially if there is an asymmetric presentation. A peripheral pigmentary retinopathy and heart block (Kearns-Sayre variant) may accompany CPEO.

OCULOPHARYNGEAL DYSTROPHY

Patients with oculopharyngeal dystrophy usually present later in life than do those with CPEO. These patients present with ptosis and dysphagia. Inheritance is autosomal dominant and often found in patients with French-Canadian ancestry.

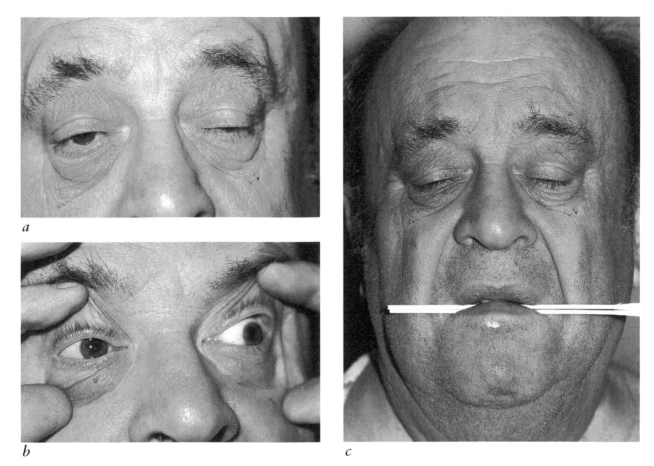

Figure 9.27   *A patient followed for many years with ptosis (a), gaze paresis (b) and the diagnosis of CPEO. Generalized weakness and masseter weakness (c) alerted the present author to an alternate diagnosis. The patient's markedly positive Tensilon test confirmed the diagnosis of MG.*

MYOTONIC DYSTROPHY

Patients with myotonic dystrophy present in late childhood with ptosis, generalized myotonia, hatchet facies (Fig. 9.28) and wasting of the hand muscles. Males also manifest frontal balding and testicular atrophy. Extraocular motility involvement is usually minimal. In addition to prominent ptosis and mild to negligible ophthalmoplegia, ocular findings may include Christmas tree cataracts, hypotony, corneal changes and chorioretinitis. Inheritance is autosomal dominant.

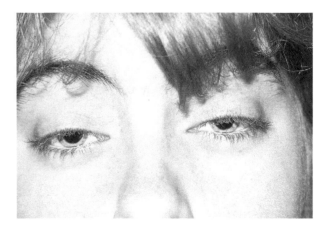

Figure 9.28   *Myotonic dystrophy.*

LEVATOR DEHISCENCE

Patients with disinsertion, dehiscence or attenuation of their levator aponeurosis present with constant, stable ptosis, excellent levator function, elevation of their upper eyelid crease and thinning of the upper eyelid (Fig. 9.29). If these criteria are not present, the patient should be further evaluated for another cause of ptosis (i.e. Horner's syndrome or MG). Ptosis caused by levator dehiscence is very common in the aging population, may be masked by dermatochalasis, compensated for by using the frontalis muscles to elevate the eyelids and does not require an extensive neurologic or neuro-radiologic evaluation. Levator dehiscence may result from trauma, swelling of the eyelid (Fig. 9.30), contact lens wear, previous ocular surgery or aging. Ptosis

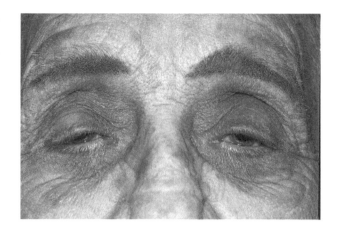

Figure 9.29 *Extreme ptosis with excellent levator function due to levator dehiscence.*

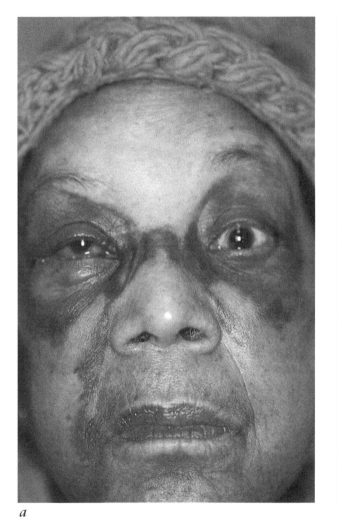

a

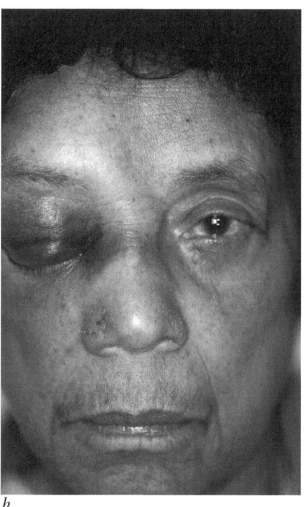

b

Figure 9.30 *Ptosis due to levator dehiscence (a) after blunt trauma to the eye and orbit (b).*

after ocular surgery may be transient or permanent (levator dehiscence), resulting from eyelid edema, hematoma, an eyelid speculum, myotoxicity from the anesthetic or a superior rectus bridle suture.[9] Treatment, when necessary, entails identifying and advancing the levator aponeurosis until the desired eyelid height is obtained. This is best done under local anesthesia, adjusting the eyelid height at the time of surgery (Fig. 9.31a–e).

PSEUDOPTOSIS

PROTECTION

Patients may appear ptotic due to other causes. The eyelid may be closed in an attempt to protect the eye from pain due to ocular irritation or a foreign body under the eyelid. Eversion of the upper eyelid should be a part of the initial evaluation of any ptotic patient.

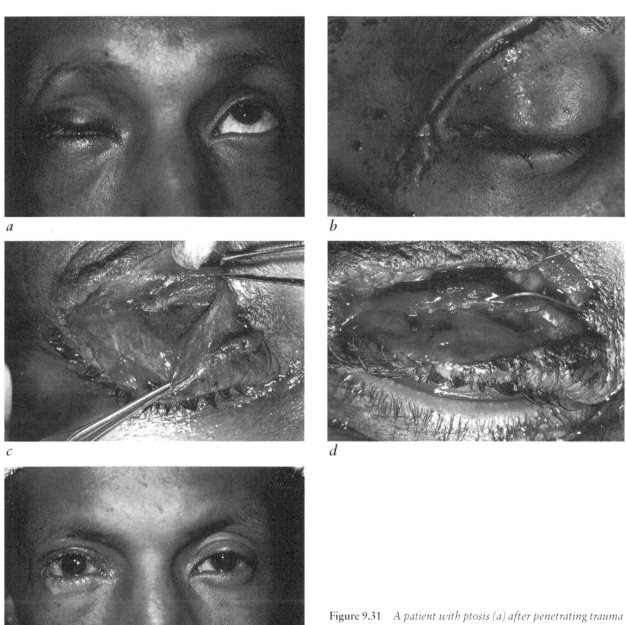

a

b

c

d

e

Figure 9.31 *A patient with ptosis (a) after penetrating trauma to the orbit and eyelid (b). Exploration of the upper eyelid revealed a total transection and dehiscence of the levator aponeurosis (c). Surgical repair (d) resolved the ptosis (e).*

ENOPHTHALMOS

Enophthalmos may result from antecedent trauma to the orbit (orbital fracture), scirrhous carcinoma metastatic to the orbit (Fig. 9.32), atrophy of orbital fat or chronic maxillary sinusitis (the shrinking sinus syndrome; Fig. 9.33).[10] Patients with enophthalmos have a superior sulcus deformity that may mimic the elevated eyelid crease evident in patients with dehiscence of the levator aponeurosis.

VERTICAL STRABISMUS

If the eye is hypertrophic, the upper eyelid may appear ptotic (Fig. 9.34). A cover test with the patient fixating on an accommodative target reveals the vertical deviation and the proper diagnosis.

CONTRALATERAL PROPTOSIS OR EYELID RETRACTION

When confronted with a patient with either unilateral ptosis or proptosis (Fig. 9.35), the clinician must question which side is abnormal, i.e. the ptotic side or the proptotic side. This simple question and its answers will save time, expense and potential embarrassment. Dysthyroid patients in particular may be proptotic with upper eyelid retraction on one side and appear ptotic on the contralateral side by Hering's law (Fig. 9.36). Evaluation and treatment of the proptosis and eyelid

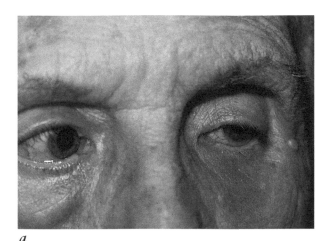

a

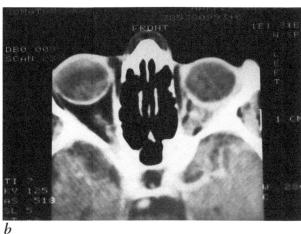

b

Figure 9.32 *Pseudoptosis caused by enophthalmos due to scirrhous gastric carcinoma metastatic to the orbit.*

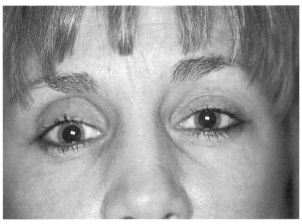

a

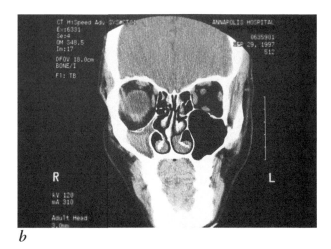

b

Figure 9.33 *Pseudoptosis (a) caused by chronic maxillary sinusitis; (b) the shrinking sinus syndrome evident on coronal CT scan.*

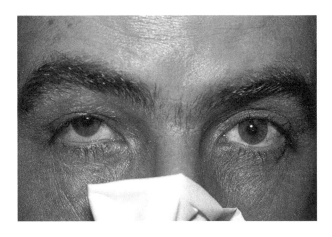

Figure 9.34 *Pseudoptosis due to hypertropia. Cover testing reveals the obvious diagnosis.*

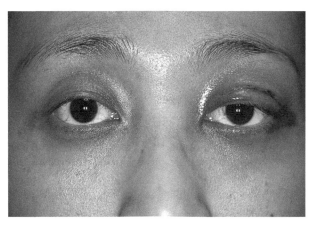

Figure 9.36 *Ptosis resolved after recession of the contralateral levator muscle.*

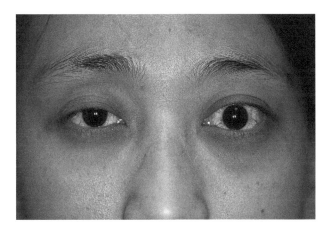

Figure 9.35 *Pseudoptosis due to contralateral proptosis and upper eyelid retraction.*

retraction would be more appropriate than elevating the seemingly ptotic upper eyelid.

BLEPHAROSPASM AND HEMIFACIAL SPASM

Patients with blepharospasm may appear to have bilateral ptosis from squeezing of the eyelids due to excessive orbicularis contraction. Patients with hemifacial spasm may similarly appear to have unilateral ptosis. Observation of the patient usually reveals the correct diagnosis. Patients with blepharospasm (Fig. 9.37) have

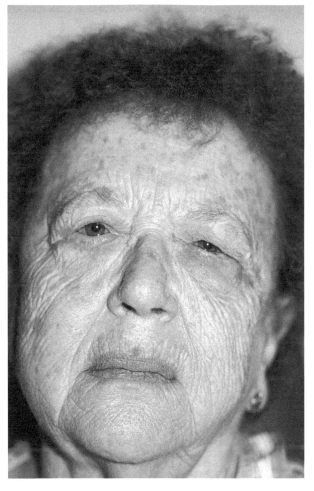

Figure 9.37 *Ptosis due to benign essential blepharospasm causing dehiscence of the levator aponeurosis.*

characteristic bilateral, involuntary contracture of their orbicularis oculi muscles. Other facial muscles may also be involved but they are always bilateral. Early in the clinical course, these twitches may not be very obvious, but as the disease progresses they become much more forceful and may result in functional blindness. Blepharospasm is absent during sleep and originates in the central nervous system. It is best treated with periodic injections of botulinum-A toxin (Botox, Allergan), although surgical extirpation of the orbicularis oculi has been advocated for refractory cases.[11]

Blepharospasm should be differentiated from hemifacial spasm. Hemifacial spasm is always unilateral and manifests synchronous contracture of one side of the entire face (Fig. 9.38). Hemifacial spasm occurs

during sleep and is often due to vascular compression of the facial nerve at the brainstem. Hemifacial spasm may also be treated by Oculinum injections or by neurosurgical decompression of the facial nerve. Patients with both blepharospasm and hemifacial spasm may develop true ptosis due to dehiscence of the levator aponeurosis by the constantly contracting orbicularis muscles.

MALINGERING

For a variety of reasons, patients may feign ptosis. This is usually quite obvious, and normal levator function and eyelid height is usually evident while testing extraocular motility (Fig. 9.39a–d).

ORBITAL DISORDERS

Superior orbital masses may cause an apparent ptosis of the upper eyelid. This is usually accompanied by depression of the globe (hypo-ophthalmia; Fig. 9.40a and b), but depression may be subtle and missed if not considered. The lacrimal gland is divided into its palpebral and orbital portion by the levator aponeurosis (Fig. 9.41). Lacrimal fossa masses often depress the temporal portion of the upper eyelid causing a distinctive S-shaped ptosis (Fig. 9.42). Frontal sinus infections may drain into the upper eyelid causing recurrent eyelid infections and ptosis, refractory to inappropriate treatment (Fig. 9.43).

An occasional child (Fig. 9.44) may present with sudden onset ptosis, minimal to no levator function, 'normal' imaging studies and negative Tensilon testing on several occasions. The orbit should be carefully imaged with special attention to the superior rectus/levator complex to detect enlargement that may be caused by a rhabdomyosarcoma (Fig. 9.44). Remember to look for the 'downgaze "hangup" sign' and poor levator function, and consider the possibility of a subtle malignancy.[7]

LOCAL ETIOLOGIES

Hemorrhage, infection, inflammation and eyelid tumors may be misdiagnosed as ptosis. Patients with a history of significant eyelid swelling may develop ptosis secondary to levator dehiscence after resolution of the edema and hemorrhage (Fig. 9.31). Eyelid infections (Fig. 9.45) should be obvious and differentiated from pre- or post-septal orbital cellulitis (Fig. 9.46). Orbital

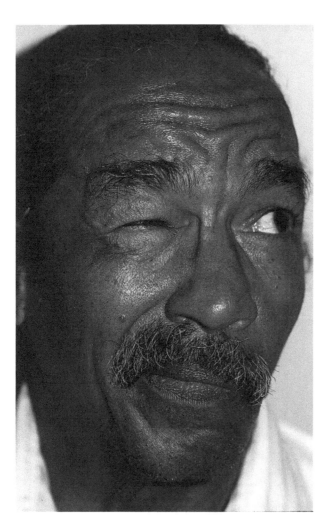

Figure 9.38 *Hemifacial spasm—unilateral rhythmic contraction of the facial musculature.*

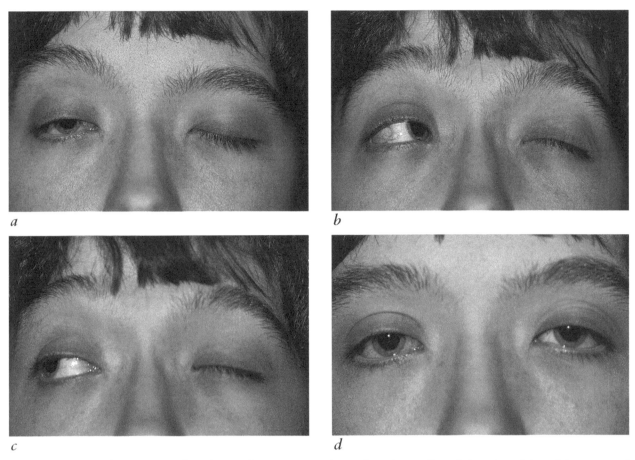

Figure 9.39 *Feigned ptosis (a) with no levator function, improving on lateral gazes (b and c), and resolving with upgaze and distraction (d).*

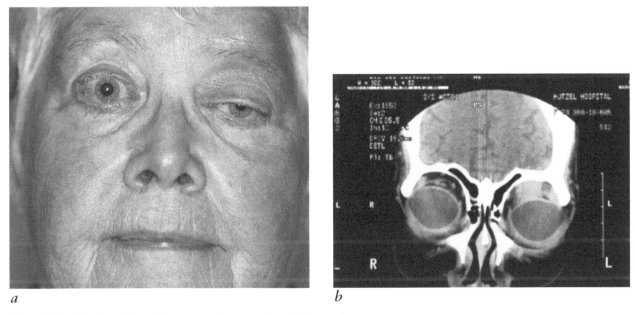

Figure 9.40 *Ptosis and hypoglobus caused by superior orbital neoplasm.*

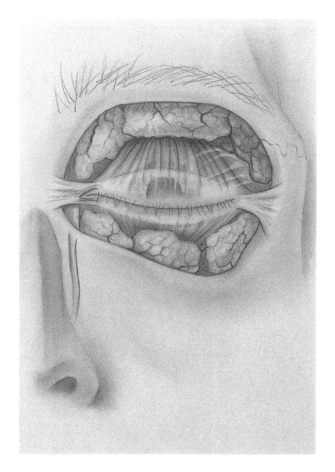

Figure 9.41 *The levator aponeurosis splits the lacrimal gland into an orbital and palpebral lobe. Also note the relationship of the preaponeurotic fat pads to the underlying levator aponeurosis.*

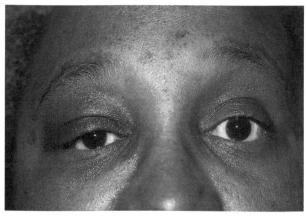

a

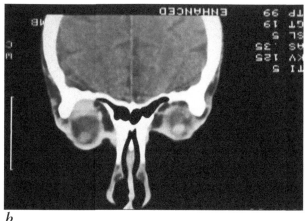

b

Figure 9.42 *S-shaped ptosis (a) due to enlargement of the lacrimal gland due to chronic dacryoadenitis (b).*

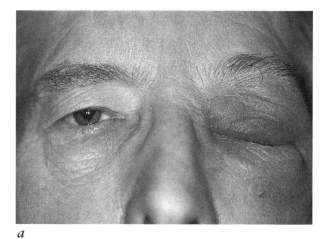

a

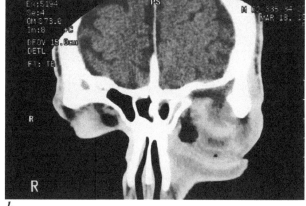

b

Figure 9.43 *Ptosis (a) secondary to chronic frontal sinusitis draining into the upper eyelid (b).*

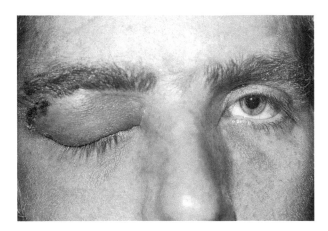

Figure 9.44 *Child presenting with isolated ptosis and absent levator and normal imaging studies.*

Figure 9.45 *Ptosis from eyelid infection due to a foreign body.*

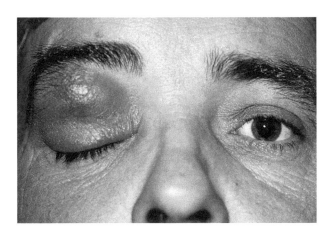

Figure 9.46 *Preseptal cellulitis causing eyelid swelling and ptosis.*

inflammation may be confined to the levator/superior rectus complex (myositis; Fig. 9.47), or from the lacrimal gland (dacryoadenitis), the latter cause a distinctive S-shaped ptosis (Fig. 9.42). Eyelid tumors may be obvious (Fig. 9.48) or evident only upon eversion of the upper eyelid (Fig. 9.49). Eversion of the eyelid should be part of every ptosis evaluation. Giant papillary conjunctivitis, large conjunctival follicles or foreign bodies may also cause ptosis.

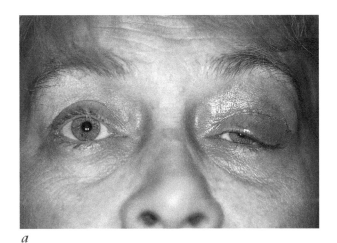

a

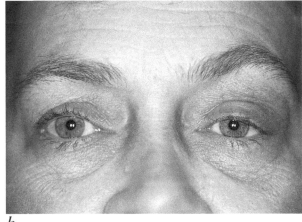

b

Figure 9.47 *Orbital myositis involving the levator and superior rectus muscle (a). Resolution after systemic corticosteroids (b). Note the resultant ptosis due to levator dehiscence.*

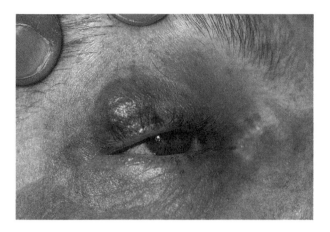 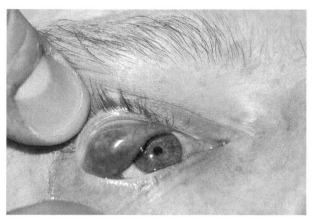

Figure 9.48 *Ptosis resulting from a cavernous hemangioma of the eyelid.*

Figure 9.49 *Eversion of the eyelid reveals a subconjunctival mass causing ptosis.*

REFERENCES

1. Spoor TC, Kwitko GM. Blepharoptosis repair by fascia lata suspension with direct tarsal and frontalis fixation. *Am J Ophthalmol* 1990; **109**:314–17.

2. Martin TJ, Corbett JJ, Babikian PV et al. Bilateral ptosis due to mesencephalic lesions with relative sparing of ocular motility. *J Neuro-ophthalmol* 1996; **16**:258–63.

3. Kim JH, Hwang JM, Hwang YS et al. Childhood myasthenia gravis. *Ophthalmology* 2003; **110**:1458–62.

4. Sibony PA, Lessell S, Gittinger JW Jr. Acquired oculomotor synkinesis. *Surv Ophthalmol* 1984; **28**:382–90.

5. Spoor TC, Troost BT, Slamovits T, Kennerdell JS. Recurrent, isolated oculomotor paresis. *J Headache* 1981; **21**:58–62.

6. Troost BT. Ophthalmoplegic migraine. *Biomed Pharmacother* 1996; **50**:49–51.

7. Uddin JM, Rose GE. Downgaze 'hangup' of the upper eyelid in patients with adult onset ptosis: an important sign of possible orbital malignancy. *Ophthalmology* 2003; **110**:1433–6.

8. Doucet TW, Crawford JS. The quantification, natural course and surgical results in 57 eyes with Marcus Gunn (jaw winking) syndrome. *Am J Ophthalmol* 1981; **92**:702–7.

9. Bernadino CR, Rubin PA. Ptosis after cataract surgery. *Semin Ophthalmol* 2002; **17**:144–8.

10. VanderMeer JB, Harris G, Toohill RJ. The silent sinus syndrome. *Laryngoscope* 2001; **111**:975–8.

11. Anderson RL, Patel BC, Holds JB. Blepharospasm past, present and future. *Ophthal Plast Reconstruc Surg* 1998; **14**:305–17.

Chapter 10 Horizontal gaze disorders

Patients with horizontal gaze dysfunction complain of horizontal diplopia. When asked to describe their double vision they respond that it is side by side. Volitional horizontal saccadic gaze is controlled in the frontal lobe. Horizontal pursuit gaze is controlled in the occipital lobe (Fig. 10.1). Saccadic gaze goes from fovea to fovea (20/20 to 20/20) with blur in between. Pursuit gaze maintains the fovea on the object of regard, following it with 20/20 acuity. An apt analogy would be a dove hunter walking through a field. He spots a dove and raises his shotgun and sights the dove—that's the saccade. Following the dove (keeping it on his fovea) prior to shooting is the pursuit movement. Seeing the dove fall (or escape) requires another saccade.

Area 9 of the right frontal lobe controls saccadic gaze to the left. The message leaves the frontal lobe via the fronto-mesencephalic tract, crosses the midline in the upper midbrain and synapses at the left parapontine reticular formation (PPRF) (Fig. 10.1). A frontal lobe lesion will cause a transient gaze palsy. If the right frontal gaze center is damaged, no cortical message gets to the left PPRF; therefore, left horizontal conjugate gaze is defective. The eyes deviate to the right. Hence, with a destructive cortical gaze palsy, the eyes deviate to the side of the lesion. An irritative lesion in the right frontal gaze center would stimulate the left PPRF and cause the eyes to deviate to the left. With an irritative frontal lesion the eyes deviate away from the lesion.

Supranuclear control of pursuit movements arise in area 18 of the occipital lobe, pass uncrossed (or double crossed) via the occipito-mesencephalic tract to the ipsilateral PPRF, i.e. left occipital lobe goes to left PPRF for

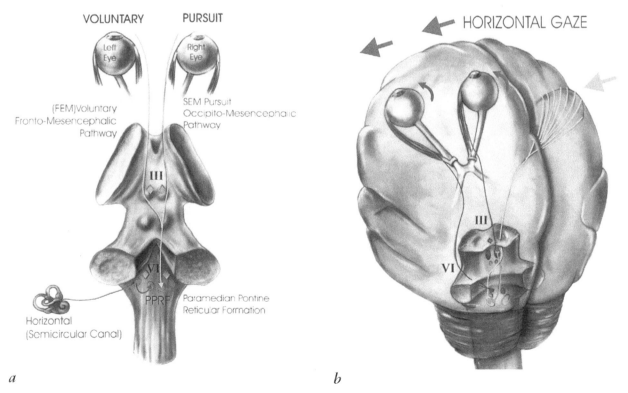

a *b*

Figure 10.1 *Pathway for supranuclear control of horizontal eye movements. Pursuit movements arise from the occipital lobe via uncrossed fibers in the occipito-mesencephalic tract to synapse in the PPRF (a and b). Saccadic movements arise in the frontal lobe and pass crossed to the PPRF via the fronto-mesencephalic tract (b).*

left gaze. The PPRF is the final common pathway for horizontal gaze. It is intimately related to the sixth-nerve nucleus. There is no isolated nuclear sixth-nerve palsy. A lesion in either the PPRF or the sixth-nerve nucleus causes paresis of ipsilateral horizontal gaze (Figs 10.2 and 10.3).

In order to initiate conjugate gaze to the left, the left lateral rectus must contract and the right medial rectus must contract simultaneously. The left PPRF/sixth-nerve nucleus (horizontal gaze center) stimulates the left lateral rectus to contract via the sixth nerve (Fig. 10.2). The gaze center must simultaneously send a message across the pons and up the brainstem to the contralateral (right) medial rectus subnucleus in the midbrain. This is accomplished through the median longitudinal fasciculus (MLF) (Fig. 10.2). The right medial rectus is stimulated to contract via a third-nerve subnucleus. This explanation is a gross simplification of a very complicated and not well-understood phenomenon, but it serves well to understand the clinical neuro-anatomy of common brainstem syndromes.

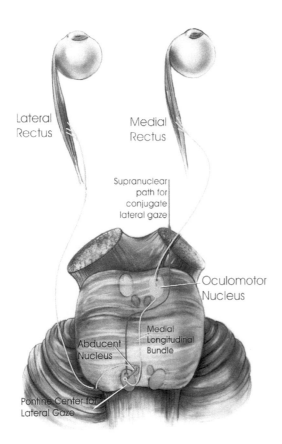

Figure 10.2 *Horizontal gaze palsy and PPRF diagram.*

How do you distinguish between a supranuclear (cortical) gaze palsy and an infranuclear (pontine) gaze palsy (Fig. 10.4)? Stimulate the pons directly with the doll's-head maneuver or caloric testing. The vestibulo-ocular reflexes stabilize the retinal image during head movement. These are tested by either the oculocephalic maneuver (doll's-head reflex) or directly tested with cold caloric testing. Turn the head; the eyes should deviate in the opposite direction. This represents an intact doll's-head maneuver. Failure of the eyes to move conjugately may reveal a sixth-nerve paresis, internuclear ophthalmoplegia or a pontine gaze palsy. This maneuver may also differentiate between frontal and pontine gaze palsies. Oculocephalic movements are intact with frontal gaze palsies and absent in patients with pontine gaze palsies. Do not perform the oculocephalic maneuver on patients with suspected cervical spine injuries!

Cold caloric testing provides a stronger stimulus to elicit brainstem motility dysfunction. After elevating the head to 30°, so the horizontal semicircular canals are perpendicular to the floor, 30–60 ml of ice-water is instilled into the ear. The cold water inhibits the ipsilateral vestibular system, allowing the contralateral system to be unopposed. Therefore, the eyes slowly and conjugately move toward the tested ear due to the uninhibited vestibulo-ocular connections from the contralateral ear. The eyes then rapidly return to their starting position and the cycle then repeats itself. The fast phase is a saccadic movement mediated by the frontal eye fields.

Warm-water calorics do just the opposite. The warm water stimulates the vestibulo-ocular system on the tested side causing tonic, conjugate deviation of the eyes away from the stimulation and the rapid saccade back towards the stimulated side. This rapid eye movement has been remembered by several generations of physicians by the pneumonic COWS—cold opposite, warm same. If the brainstem is dysfunctional, neither cold nor warm water will elicit eye movements. If the brainstem is intact and there is diffuse bilateral hemispheric dysfunction, caloric stimulation will only produce the tonic, slow eye movements. The saccadic recovery movement will be lost.

Irrigating both ears with either warm or cold water can test vertical gaze. Bilateral cold-water stimulation causes a slow, tonic downward deviation of the eyes. Bilateral warm-water stimulation results in an upward deviation of both eyes. Theoretically, by using a combination of unilateral and bilateral calorics one can differentiate upper and lower brainstem dysfunction, since vertical gaze is controlled at a higher level in the brainstem (midbrain) than horizontal gaze is (pons). Fig. 10.2 represents the pons at the level of the PPRF. A lesion in the PPRF, be it a

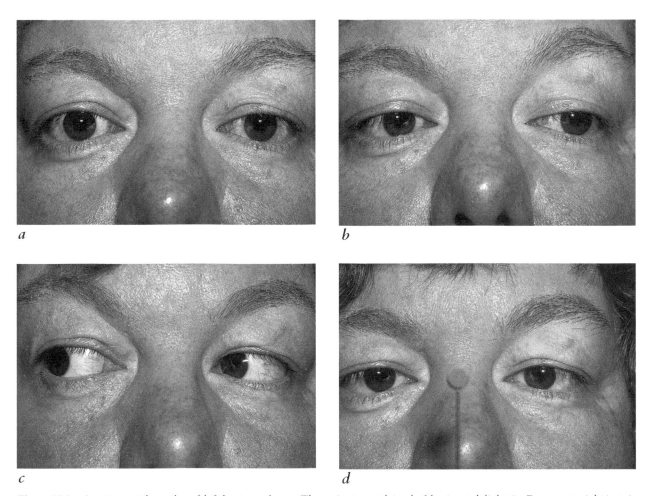

Figure 10.3 *A patient with a palsy of left horizontal gaze. The patient complained of horizontal diplopia. Eyes are straight in primary gaze (a), left gaze is absent (b), right gaze is intact (c) and convergence is intact (d).*

lacunar infarction, demyelination or tumor, will cause a paresis of ipsilateral horizontal gaze (Fig. 10.3a and b). Horizontal gaze in the opposite direction remains intact (Fig. 10.3c), as does convergence.

Refer to Fig. 10.2 and place the lesion in the contralateral MLF. The patient in Fig. 10.5a has a lacunar infarction in the right MLF. Since the PPRF is intact the right eye abducts normally. The MLF lesion blocks the message for horizontal gaze to the right medial rectus. The right eye fails to adduct as the left eye abducts (Fig. 10.5b). There is often excessive end-point nystagmus of the abducting eye. The resultant motility dysfunction is an internuclear ophthalmoplegia (INO). An INO is usually an obvious clinical diagnosis. It is named according to the side of the dysfunctioning medial rectus muscle. The example above is a right INO since the right medial rectus is dysfunctional.

Patients with INO may present complaining of horizontal diplopia and no obvious ocular adduction defect is evident on examination. A subtle underaction of the adducting eye may be missed, but the accompanying nystagmus of the contralateral abducting eye may be obvious. This exacerbated end-point nystagmus results from overshooting of the normal abducting eye. This phenomenon of overshooting of the unaffected eye and undershooting of the affected eye may also be evident as ocular dysmetria. Ask the patient to look from one object to the other. The normal abducting eye will overshoot the target then make a quick saccade back to the target. The undershooting eye (subtle INO) will undershoot the target and then make a quick saccade to fixate the target. Looking for ocular dysmetria in a patient complaining of horizontal diplopia and manifesting no obvious motility deficits may help diagnose a subtle INO.

If the MLF is dysfunctional on both sides, neither eye can adduct. Both the right and the left PPRF are intact, therefore both eyes abduct normally and the patient

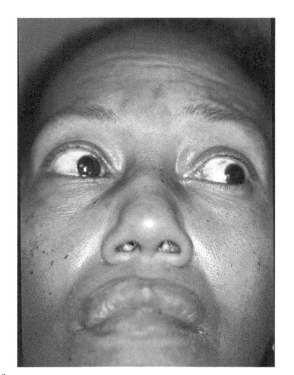

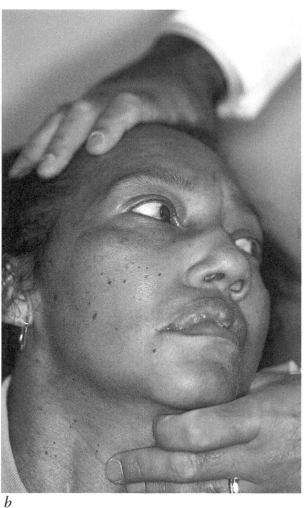

a

Figure 10.4 *Doll's-head maneuver to differentiate frontal from pontine gaze palsies. The patient has a right gaze palsy (a). Eyes fail to move right when rotating head to the left (b), confirming that the lesion is in the pons. If the patient had a frontal gaze palsy, the eyes would move to the right with the doll's-head maneuver.*

b

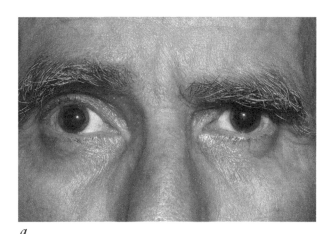

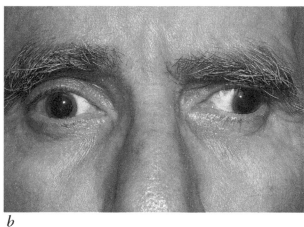

a

b

Figure 10.5 *A patient with a right INO. He is exotropic in primary gaze (a). Horizontal gaze to the right is intact. On attempted left gaze, the right eye fails to abduct past the midline (b).*

appears exotropic (Fig. 10.6a–c). This is known as wall-eyed bilateral internuclear ophthalmoplegia (WEBINO). If the offending lesion is at the pontine level, convergence will be intact. A more rostral lesion, in the midbrain, may cause an INO and, since the convergence centers are at that level, convergence will be dysfunctional.

Fig. 10.7 depicts a lesion involving the left PPRF and the ipsilateral MLF. What would be the resultant motility deficit? Since the left PPRF is involved, there is no horizontal conjugate gaze to the left. The right PPRF is spared, but the left MLF is involved. On attempted right gaze, the right eye abducts normally, but the message to the left eye to adduct does not pass through the damaged MLF so the left eye fails to adduct. The only functional horizontal eye motion is abduction of the right eye (Fig. 10.8b). This is known as the one-and-one-half syndrome (Fig. 10.8). Since the lesion is at the pontine level, convergence remains intact, i.e. the medial recti can converge the eyes but cannot move them in horizontal conjugate gaze. Since the lesion is at the pontine level the doll's-head and caloric reflexes are dysfunctional.

OCULAR ABDUCTION DEFECTS

ABDUCENS NERVE PALSIES

As mentioned above, the sixth-nerve nucleus is intimately related to the PPRF. A nuclear sixth-nerve palsy does not exist. A lesion in the sixth-nerve nucleus causes a horizontal gaze palsy. The sixth nerve can however be involved in the pons, often in conjunction with adjacent structures, resulting in well described ventral and dorsal pontine syndromes that have been obfuscated with eponyms for years.

Fig. 10.9 represents a cross-section through the pons at the level of the sixth-nerve nucleus. The corticospinal tract lies in the ventral portion of the pons. The corticospinal tract carries motor innervation to the contralateral arm and leg. The sixth-nerve fascicle passes adjacent to the corticospinal tract as it exits the ventral pons to innervate the lateral rectus muscle. The facial nerve lies lateral to the sixth nerve as it exits the pons to innervate the face. Lesions in the ventral pons may be

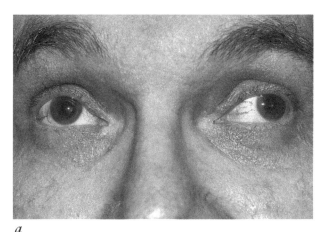

a

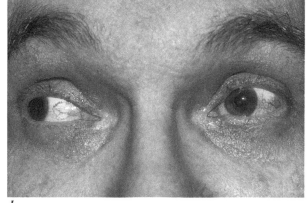

b

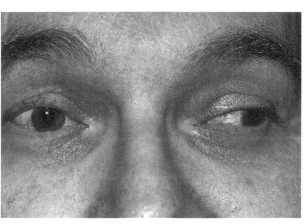

c

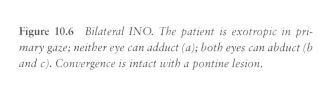

Figure 10.6 *Bilateral INO. The patient is exotropic in primary gaze; neither eye can adduct (a); both eyes can abduct (b and c). Convergence is intact with a pontine lesion.*

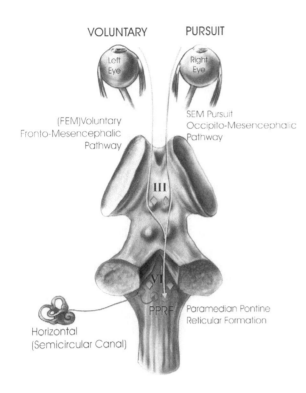

Figure 10.7　*Anatomy of the one-and-one-half syndrome.*

very localizing and involve any or all of these structures. A patient with a ventral pontine lesion involving the sixth nerve and corticospinal tract (Fig. 10.9) presents with horizontal diplopia accompanied by contralateral hemiparesis (Fig. 10.10) (Raymond's syndrome). This may be subtle and missed if not actively sought. If the lesion extends a bit more dorsal and lateral to involve the

seventh nerve, the patient will have an ipsilateral abduction defect, peripheral seventh-nerve paresis and contralateral hemiparesis (Millard-Gubler syndrome) (Fig. 10.11).

Patients with more dorsal pontine lesions are rarely seen in an ambulatory practice. More centrally located dorsal pontine lesions involve the sixth and seventh nerves near their nuclei. Hence the medial nuclei, as well as the median longitudinal fasciculi, and the parapontine reticular formation (PPRF). Sensory nuclei of the trigeminal nerve and descending sympathetic pathways may be involved. These patients with dorsal pontine pathology may manifest any combination of the previously mentioned brainstem motility dysfunctions.[1]

ISOLATED ABDUCENS PARESES

As the sixth nerve exits the ventral pons (Fig. 10.12), it traverses the base of the brain, along the clivus, passing through Dorello's canal, into the cavernous sinus and enters the orbit (Fig. 10.12). Isolated sixth-nerve paresis may be vasculopathic and totally benign, as in an elderly diabetic (Fig. 10.13), or be the harbinger of significant neurologic dysfunction (Fig. 10.14). As a general rule, isolated sixth-nerve paresis in an elderly adult is most often vasculopathic and has a benign course with spontaneous recovery occurring within 60–90 days. An extensive neuroradiologic evaluation is not necessary in these patients with isolated sixth-nerve paresis and vasculopathic risk factors (hypertension, diabetes and atherosclerotic disease). If, however, they do not recover function in 90 days a full neuro-ophthalmologic and neuroradiologic evaluation is necessary. Evaluation

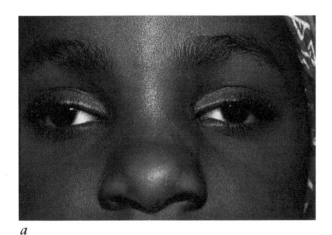

a

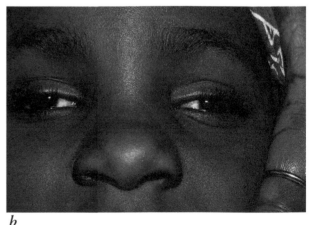

b

Figure 10.8　*A patient with the one-and-one-half syndrome has dysfunctional right horizontal gaze (a) due to MLF involvement, inability to adduct the adduct the right eye (b). The only horizontal eye movement is abduction of the left eye (b).*

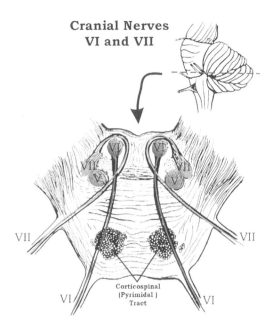

Cranial Nerves VI and VII

Figure 10.9 *Cross-section of the pons at the level of the sixth-nerve nucleus.*

should include magnetic resonance imaging (MRI) of the brain with attention to the brainstem and cavernous sinus. If imaging is negative, a Tensilon test may be diagnostic of myasthenia gravis (MG). Neuro-ophthalmic examination should be repeated to be certain that the sixth-nerve paresis is indeed isolated and there are no subtle findings for associated cranial nerve palsies (Fig. 10.15). Other causes for defective ocular abduction should be considered (see below).

In a younger adult (aged 20–45), the causes of an isolated sixth-nerve paresis are often more sinister. Vasculopathic neuropathies are decidedly uncommon in this age group and other causes need to be considered. Demyelination, aneurysm and neoplasm are all very real possibilities in these patients (Fig. 10.16). An individual in this age group must have appropriate neuroimaging studies. If imaging studies are negative, a Tensilon test and a careful follow-up neuro-ophthalmic examination are necessary.[2,3]

A child who becomes esotropic may have a sixth-nerve paresis or his family may have just noted the onset of an accommodative or congenital esotropia. Does the eye

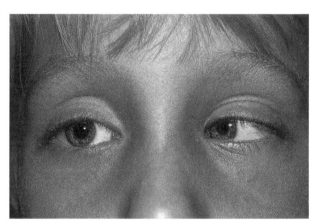

a

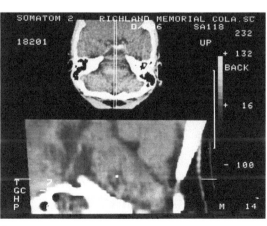

c

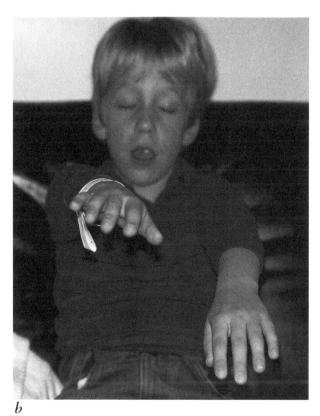

b

Figure 10.10 *A patient presents with esotropia, decreased abduction of the right eye and a left hemiparesis (a and b). A CT scan demonstrates a cystic pontine glioma (c).*

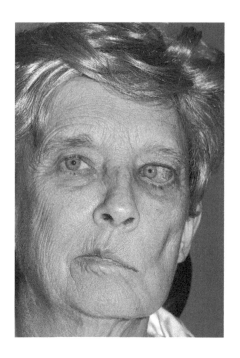

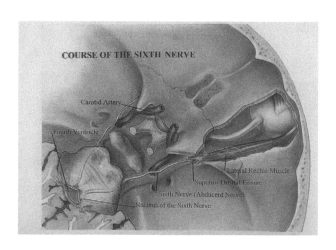

Figure 10.12   *The course of the sixth nerve from the pons to the orbit.*

Figure 10.11   *A patient with a more dorsal pontine lesion also has involvement of the ipsilateral facial nerve.*

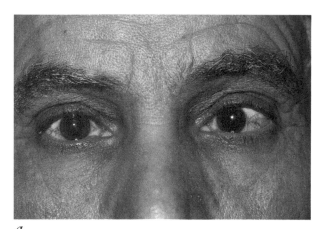

a

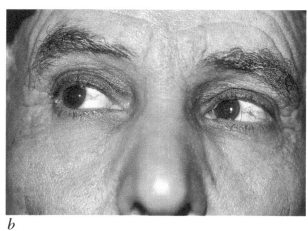

b

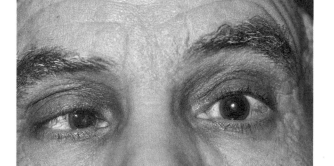

c

Figure 10.13   *Vasculopathic sixth-nerve paresis in an elderly diabetic patient: this will resolve spontaneously and further evaluation is rarely necessary.*

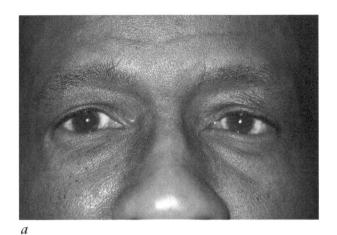

a

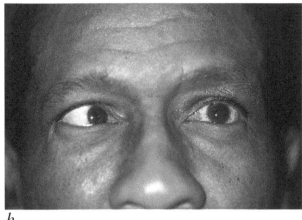

b

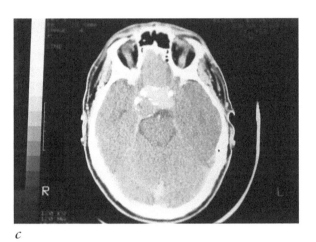

c

Figure 10.14 *A sixth-nerve paresis in a younger patient (a and b) needs further evaluation. A CT scan demonstrates a large parasellar mass (c).*

fully abduct? Play with the child. Try to get him/her to abduct the esotropic eye. Keys, toys, little things that make a noise may get the child's attention for long enough to abduct the involved eye towards the object of regard. Once you see the eye fully abduct, that is the moment of truth. The deviation is an esotropia and the baby needs a strabismus evaluation not a neuro-ophthalmologic evaluation. What if you cannot make the child abduct the eye? Patch the opposite eye and see if he/she will abduct the involved eye after the other eye is patched. Why not just get an MRI? A MRI in an infant requires varying degrees of sedation with its inherent risks. Is the deviation comitant (the same in all fields of gaze)? Formal measurements are impossible in an infant, but in an older child the esotropia may be measured in primary, left and right gaze. If an esotropia is laterally comitant, a sixth-nerve paresis is unlikely. An isolated sixth-nerve paresis may be a benign sequel to a viral infection in a young child. Again, this prognosis is predicated upon an otherwise normal neuro-ophthalmologic examination. You must actively seek an associated neuro-ophthalmic sign like an ipsilateral facial weakness or a contralateral hemiparesis (Fig. 10.14) and view the fundus to rule out papilledema (Fig. 10.17). A sixth-nerve paresis may be a sequelae to elevated intracranial pressure (ICP). Elevated ICP, either due to a mass lesion or pseudotumor cerebri, pushes the brainstem caudally, tethering the sixth nerve or nerves on the dura as they enter the cavernous sinus (Dorello's canal; Fig. 10.12). This causes a sixth-nerve paresis that is totally reversible after ICP is normalized. A similar mechanism causes a sixth-nerve paresis that is a benign, reversible sequelae, occasionally seen after lumbar puncture and myelograms. These findings may be subtle. Suspect a sixth-nerve paresis in any patient with an esotropia or phoria greater at distance than near.

The sixth nerve is also very susceptible to trauma as it traverses the base of the brain, and may be injured in conjunction with the facial nerve by basilar skull trauma. This may be accompanied by a hemotypanium (see Chapter 7). There are only two areas where a single

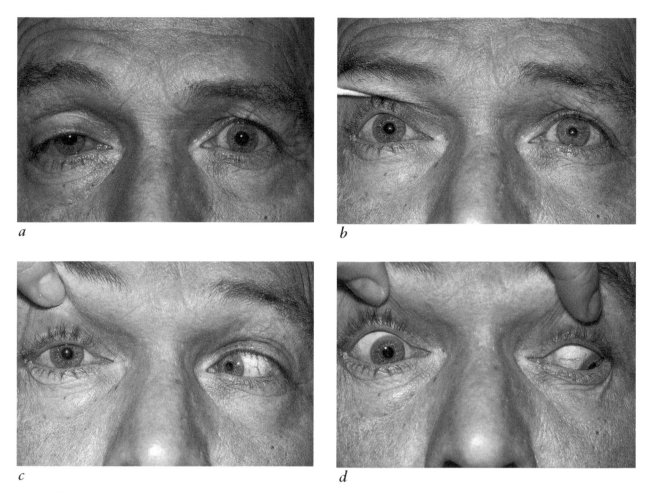

Figure 10.15 *A patient developing a partial third-nerve paresis in addition to his initial sixth-nerve paresis. Note the mild anisocoria (b), absent ocular abduction (c) and decreased ocular adduction (d).*

lesion may cause a sixth- and seventh-nerve paresis—the pons (Fig. 10.9) and the base of the brain. Trauma may also cause an isolated unilateral or bilateral (Figs 10.18 and 10.19) sixth-nerve paresis. These patients have diplopia and are uncomfortable; they want something done now. Do not offer them surgery too soon. Wait a full 6 months for partial or total improvement.[4] If sixth-nerve function partially recovers, patients are left with an esotropia, often on their blindspot, that responds very well to eye muscle surgery. If no resolution of sixth-nerve function occurs, a medial rectus recession and a Hummelsheim transposition of half the inferior and superior recti to the insertion of the lateral rectus will straighten the eye. Posterior fixation sutures applied to the transposed vertical recti will strengthen the procedure but abduction will never be good. It is worth waiting for partial recovery. Some authors advocate injection of Oculinum toxin (Botox, Allergan) into the medial

recti very soon after lateral recti paresis. Although there have been some vocal advocates,[5] the results have not been proven better than observation and surgery as necessary[6] (see also Chapter 7).

Prior to entering the cavernous sinus, the sixth nerve lies adjacent to the inner ear and the semilunar ganglion (trigeminal sensory). Inner ear infection or tumor involving the base of the brain may affect both the sixth nerve and semilunar ganglion causing a syndrome of facial pain and sixth-nerve paresis (Gradenigo's syndrome). Facial pain and ophthalmoplegia may also result from perineural metastasis of facial, sinus or base of tongue squamous cell carcinomas to the semilunar ganglion and affect the adjacent sixth nerve. The cancer travels along the sensory nerve to the semilunar ganglion. Other cranial nerves are often affected and this rarely involves an isolated sixth-nerve paresis. Nasopharyngeal carcinoma may behave in a similar fashion. The nasopharynx is

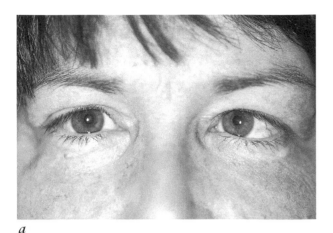

a

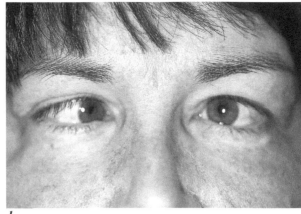

b

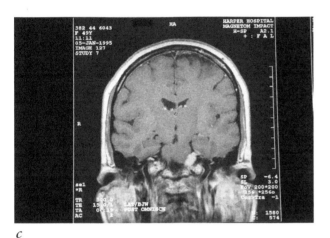

c

Figure 10.16 *Sixth-nerve palsy (a and b) secondary to a base of brain meningioma evident on an MRI scan (c).*

separated from the base of the brain by just a few millimeters of bone (Fig. 10.20) and an isolated unilateral or bilateral sixth-nerve paresis may be the initial manifestation of nasopharyngeal carcinoma (Fig. 10.21). As with squamous cell carcinomas, other cranial nerves are often rapidly involved as the carcinoma spreads along the clivus potentially affecting many cranial nerves.[6]

CAVERNOUS SINUS

The sixth nerve lies in the middle of the cavernous sinus and seems more vulnerable than the other cranial nerves in the cavernous sinus (Fig. 10.20). Cavernous sinus inflammation, aneurysms and tumors, both meningiomas and metastasis, may initially present with a sixth-nerve paresis (Fig. 10.22). Aneurysms of the infraclinoidal carotid artery may present initially as an isolated sixth-nerve paresis with or without an ipsilateral Horner's syndrome, since the sympathetic nerves are wrapped around the carotid artery in the cavernous sinus.

PSEUDO-SIXTH-NERVE SYNDROMES

SPASM OF THE NEAR REFLEX

Accommodative/convergence spasm may present as an apparent defect of horizontal gaze or as a sixth-nerve paresis. These patients complain of diplopia, blurred vision and headache. Motility findings are inconsistent (Fig. 10.23). The pupil remains miotic with attempted lateral gaze.

This is classically the key to making this diagnosis, but practically this may be rather hard to see. Blurred vision in the distance (induced myopia due to accommodative spasm), normal acuity at near and normalization of distance visual acuity after cycloplegia cinch the diagnosis. No further evaluation or neuroimaging is really necessary. Treatment with cycloplegic agents may be frustrating for both patient and physician. Some patients respond extraordinarily well to cycloplegia, whereas others maintain their spasm even when fully atropinized (see Chapter 7).

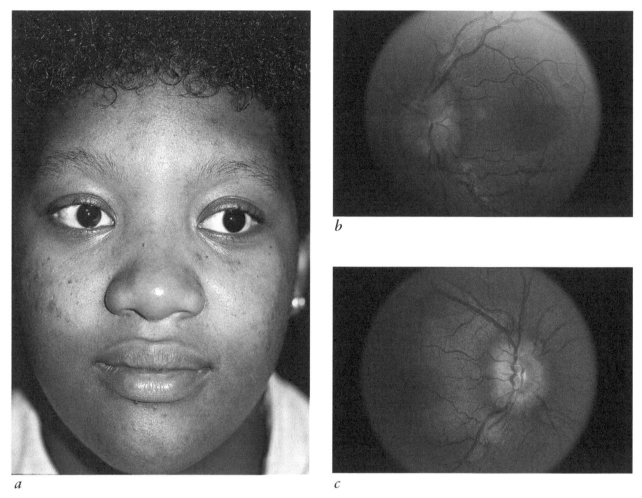

Figure 10.17   *A child with sixth-nerve paresis secondary to elevated ICP from pseudo-tumor cerebri (a). Fundus examination demonstrates high-grade papilledema (b and c).*

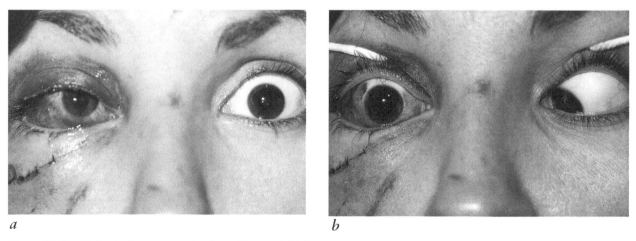

Figure 10.18   *Right sixth-nerve paresis after orbito-cranial injury.*

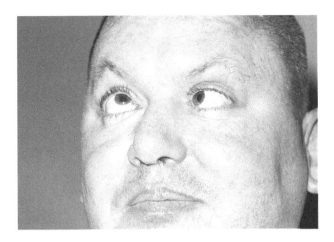

Figure 10.19 *Bilateral sixth-nerve paresis after closed-head injury.*

Figure 10.20 *Cross-section through the cavernous sinus.*

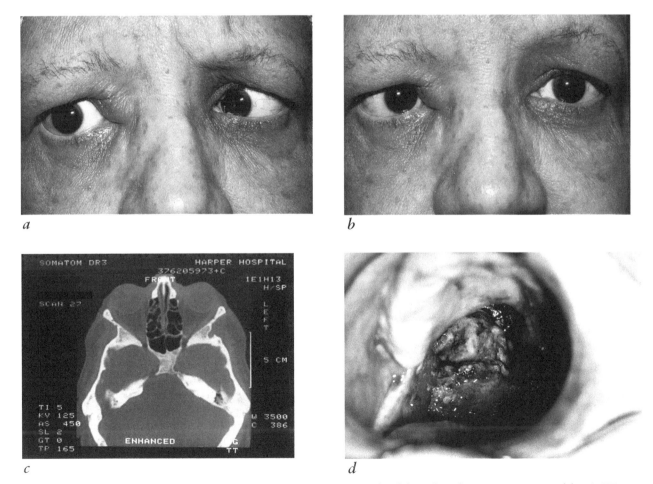

Figure 10.21 *A patient with nasopharyngeal carcinoma presenting with a bilateral sixth-nerve paresis (a and b). A CT scan demonstrates erosion of the clinoids (c); fungating mass viewed intranasally (d).*

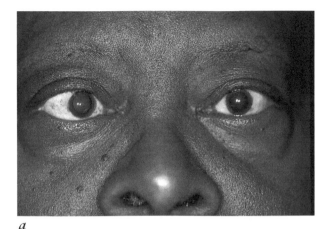

a

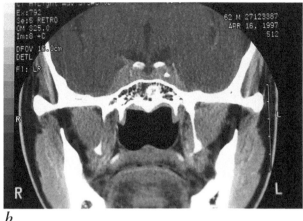

b

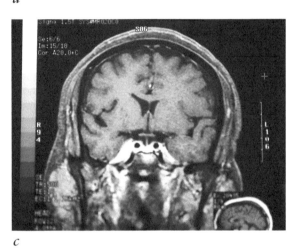

c

Figure 10.22 *A patient with a cavernous sinus inflammation (a) presenting with a sixth-nerve paresis. Contrast-enhanced CT scan (b) and MRI (c) demonstrate enlargement of the right cavernous sinus.*

DYSTHYROID ORBITOPATHY

Dysthyroid orbitopathy is often an obvious clinical diagnosis (Fig. 10.24) confirmed by typical muscle enlargement on a computerized tomography (CT) scan and markedly positive forced ductions. The abduction defects may be obvious (Fig. 10.25) and accompanied by massive enlargement of the medial recti (Fig. 10.25b), or be much more subtle (Fig. 10.26) and accompanied by subtle enlargement of the medial recti (Fig. 10.27) on a CT scan. The neuroradiologist unfamiliar with the patient's clinical signs and symptoms may miss these subtle findings. If dysthyroid orbitopathy is suspected as the etiology of the patient's horizontal diplopia, review the CT scans; make sure that both axial and coronal sections are available. Subtle extraocular muscle enlargement may only be evidenced by a slight convexity, instead of concavity, of the extraocular muscle viewed in coronal section (Fig. 10.28). Medial rectus enlargement may be extreme (Fig. 10.29) and cause an associated compressive optic neuropathy

which needs treatment prior to the motility defect (see below). If there is no evidence for a compressive optic neuropathy, a 5 mm medial rectus recession usually improves extraocular motility significantly. If the posterior medial recti are significantly enlarged, recession may cause a compressive optic neuropathy (Fig. 10.30).

If a patient's dysthyroid motility problem does not make sense or is atypical, consider concomitant MG. MG is evident in 5% of patients with dysthyroid orbitopathy and a Tensilon test may be very revealing. The patient in Fig. 10.31 had known Graves' orbitopathy and presented with diplopia; an enlarged medial rectus was evident on a CT scan (Fig. 10.32). What is wrong with this figure? Patients with dysthyroid involvement of their medial recti have limited abduction of the involved eye (Figs 10.24–10.26). If there is an adduction deficit or an exotropia be careful of diagnosing dysthyroid orbitopathy as the etiology for the motility dysfunction. It is much more likely to be MG (Fig. 10.31) or orbital myositis (Fig. 10.33).

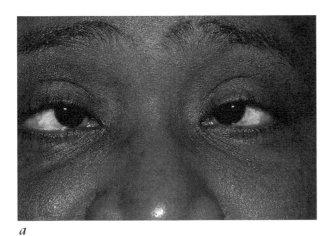

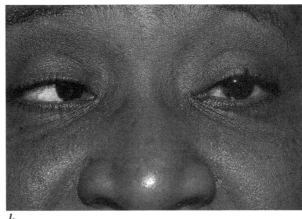

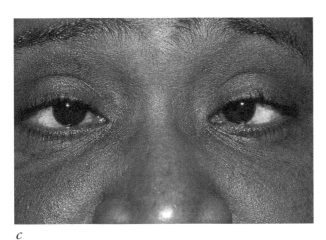

Figure 10.23 *Accommodative convergence spasm: note the inability to abduct either eye (a and b) and the miotic pupils with attempts at abduction (c).*

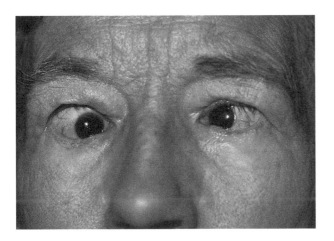

Figure 10.24 *Obvious dysthyroid orbitopathy with restrictive horizontal strabismus accompanied by upper eyelid retraction.*

ORBITAL MYOSITIS

Patients with orbital myositis involving the medial or lateral recti may present with horizontal diplopia secondary to defective ocular abduction. Acute orbital myositis is usually obvious (Fig. 10.33) the patient has pain, an inflamed orbit, defective abduction or adduction and an obviously enlarged horizontal rectus on CT scan. Enlarged extraocular muscles due to myositis may be differentiated from enlarged dysthyroid muscles by their CT scan appearance. Dysthyroid muscles are usually thickened at the orbital apex and the tendons appear normal. Myositic muscles have thickened tendons and appear normal at the orbital apex (see Chapter 13).

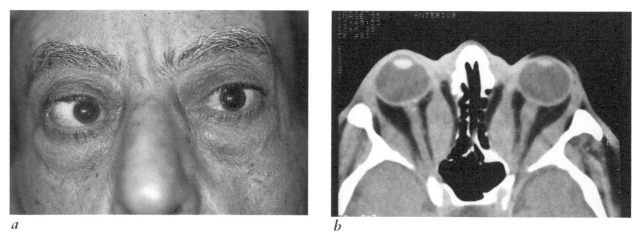

a   *b*

Figure 10.25 *Dysthyroid orbitopathy with markedly restricted ocular abduction (a). A CT scan demonstrates markedly enlarged medial recti (b).*

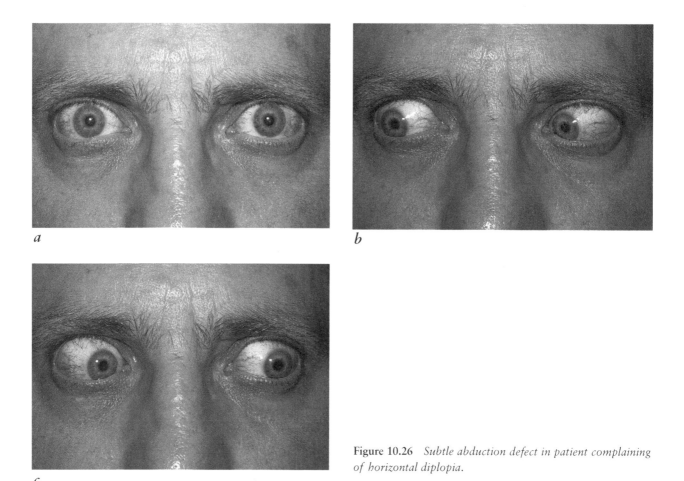

a   *b*

c

Figure 10.26 *Subtle abduction defect in patient complaining of horizontal diplopia.*

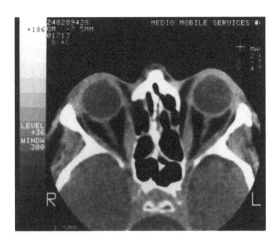

Figure 10.27 *A CT scan demonstrates mild enlargement of both medial recti.*

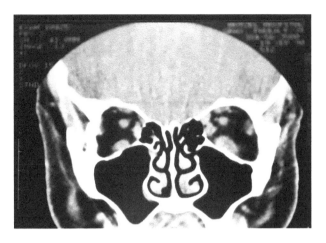

Figure 10.28 *Subtle enlargement of the inferior recti on a coronal CT scan. Note that the enlarged muscle bellies are convex and not concave like the normal muscle.*

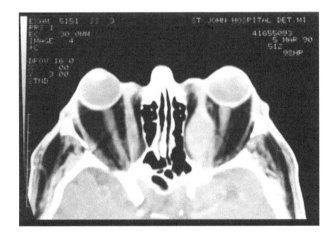

Figure 10.29 *Extreme enlargement of the medial rectus causing total restriction of abduction and a compressive optic neuropathy.*

MG

MG may mimic any extraocular motility defect. If an explanation is not apparent or the defect is atypical, perform a Tensilon test (Fig. 10.34). The Tensilon test is performed by injecting 10 mg of intravenous edrophonium (Tensilon) intravenously into the patient and observing the extraocular motility or eyelid response. Tensilon testing is basically safe and can easily be performed in an office setting. Several caveats make it safer. First, edrophonium may be premixed with 0.4 mg atropine/ml, obviating most potential side effects before they occur. If this combination is not available, keep 0.4 mg atropine

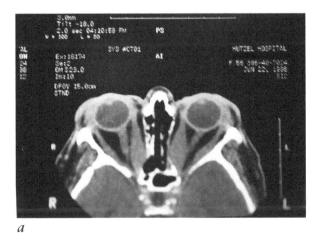

a

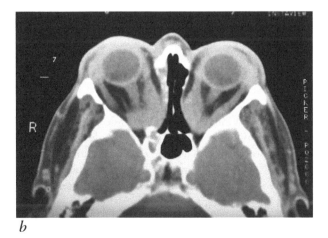

b

Figure 10.30 *A patient with dysthyroid orbitopathy, enlarged medial recti and normal visual function. A CT scan demonstrates enlarged medial recti without optic nerve compression at the orbital apex (a). After medial rectus recession, a CT scan demonstrates significant compression of the apical orbital optic nerve causing a compressive optic neuropathy (b).*

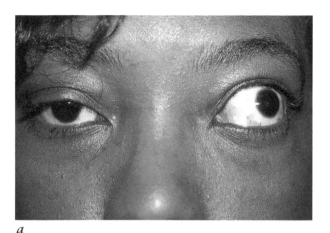
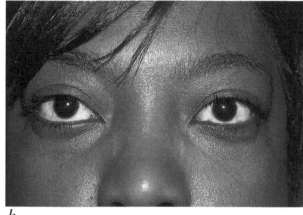

a   *b*

Figure 10.31 *A patient with known dysthyroid orbitopathy and an atypical extraocular motility pattern: an exotropia before (a) and after (b) administration of intravenous edrophonium.*

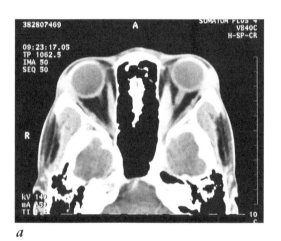
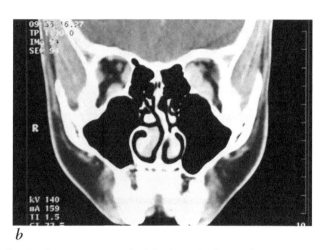

a   *b*

Figure 10.32 *A CT scan demonstrates enlargement of the medial and inferior recti, typical of dysthyroid orbitopathy.*

readily available as the edrophonium is injected and if excessive sweating, nausea or vomiting occur, inject the atropine: this will not affect the test result. Alternatively, a test dose of 2 mg edrophonium can be administered initially and if well tolerated the remainder can be injected. Most importantly, take an adequate history and make sure that the patient is not already being treated with Mestinon for MG. A Tensilon test administered to a patient taking cholinergic stimulants may result in excessive vagal stimulation, with resultant severe bradycardia for the patient and tachycardia for the examiner! A recent report describes excellent diagnostic results using much less edrophonium than the standard 10 mg. In this study only 3.3 mg edrophonium was needed to diagnose MG presenting as ptosis and 2.6 mg in MG presenting with extraocular motility dysfunction.[7]

A less definitive, but sometimes adequate alternative to the Tensilon test is the ice-cube test.[8,9] This is most effective in patients with isolated ptosis of the upper eyelid but may be helpful for screening patients with an extraocular motility defect.[10] A small plastic bag containing several ice cubes is placed upon each eye for 10–15 minutes. The patient is then examined to see if there is any change in either motility or eyelid function. A positive or equivocal ice-cube test then warrants a formal Tensilon test. Others believe that the ice-cube test is worthless and small doses of edrophonium are necessary to make the diagnosis.[8] Ice-cube testing may be helpful in patients with atypical ptosis but a Tensilon test is necessary to diagnose ocular myasthenia as the cause of extraocular motility dysfunction. Movaghar and Slavin[9] demonstrated that heat, cold and rest were

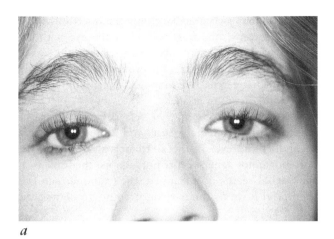

a

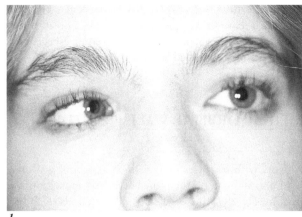

b

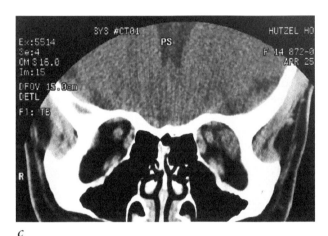

c

Figure 10.33 *A patient with restricted ocular abduction secondary to orbital myositis of the lateral rectus muscle (a and b). A CT scan demonstrates an enlarged lateral rectus muscle (c).*

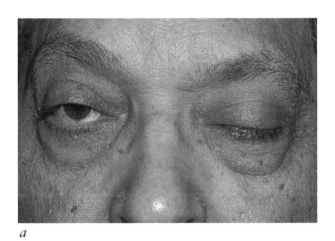

a

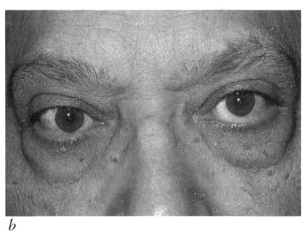

b

Figure 10.34 *A patient presenting with ptosis, diplopia and known dysthyroid orbitopathy (a). Ptosis markedly improved after 2 minutes of cooling with ice cubes (b), later confirmed by Tensilon test.*

equally effective (ineffective) in diagnosing ocular MG, and concluded that rest was the major factor in a positive test. The present author relies on Tensilon testing, especially at the lower doses described by Kupersmith et al.[8]

MEDIAL ORBITAL WALL FRACTURES

Patients with fractures of their medial orbital wall may have entrapment of their medial rectus muscle in the fracture site (Fig. 10.35—fighter). The eye fails to abduct and the patient complains of horizontal diplopia. CT imaging will demonstrate the fracture in the medial orbital wall and often the muscle entrapped in the fracture site (Fig. 10.36). If CT findings are equivocal, forced ductions and forced generations will differentiate medial rectus entrapment from a sixth-nerve paresis.

Forced ductions are performed by anesthetizing the eye over the insertion of the medial rectus with topical 4% xylocaine or cocaine. Grasping the insertion with a toothed forceps, one tries to abduct the eye with the forceps while the patient attempts to abduct the eye. If the lateral rectus is paretic, the eye can be moved easily, if the medial rectus is entrapped, it cannot be easily moved and often not at all.

Forced generations may be tested by grasping the insertion of the medial rectus and asking the patient to abduct the eye. If the sixth nerve is paretic, the patient cannot generate any pull against the forceps. If the medial rectus is entrapped, the examiner can feel the initial force as the patient attempts to abduct the eye.

SYNDROMES

To effectively diagnose and treat extraocular motility problems, one must be aware of certain syndromes.

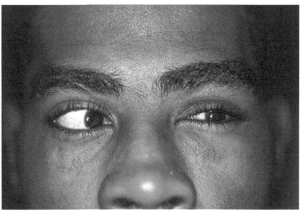

a

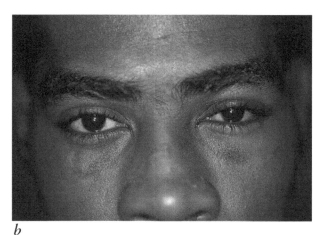

b

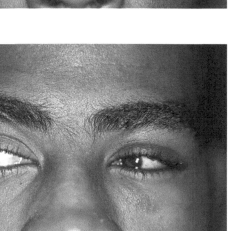

c

Figure 10.35 *A patient with restricted ocular abduction due to MR entrapment in a medial orbital wall fracture (a); eyes are straight in primary gaze (b); adduction is full (c).*

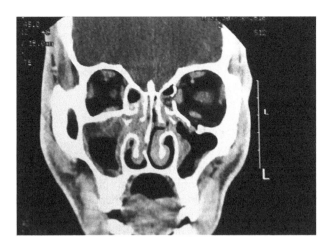

Figure 10.36 *Coronal CT scan demonstrates medial orbital wall fracture with entrapment of a portion of MR muscle.*

DUANE'S RETRACTION SYNDROME[11]

Patient's with Duane's type 1 (at least the two that have been autopsied) lack a sixth nerve nucleus and a sixth nerve:[12] the involved eye cannot be abducted (Fig. 10.37). Branches of the inferior division of the third nerve may innervate the lateral rectus; therefore, on attempted adduction of the involved eye, both the medial and the lateral recti contract (co-contraction syndrome) and the eye is tethered between the two contracting muscles. This causes the apparent retraction of the globe with attempted adduction (Figs 10.37c and 10.38), and slippage of the eye between the tethering muscles causes the typical upshooting and downshooting of the eye in adduction (Fig. 10.38). This diagnosis is often obvious (Figs 10.37 and 10.38); but it may be much more subtle (Fig. 10.39).

This is congenital. Patients rarely if ever have symptomatic diplopia. A compensatory head turn may be cosmetically or functionally disabling. Recessing the offending medial rectus muscle may treat this. Although

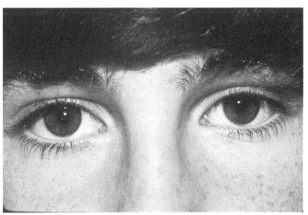

a

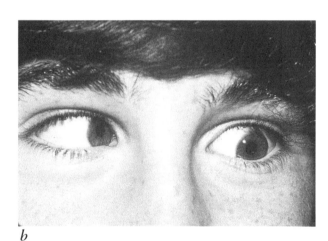

b

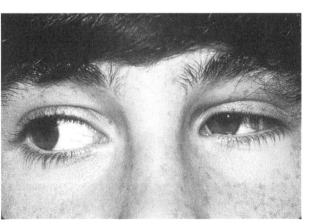

c

Figure 10.37 *Defective ocular abduction in patient with a left Duane's retraction syndrome. The patient's eyes are straight in primary gaze (a); abduction of the left eye is limited (b); retraction of the globe with adduction of the left eye (c).*

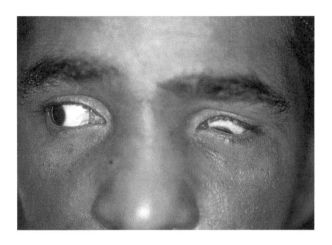

Figure 10.38 *The left eye overshoots in adduction due to slippage of the globe, tethered by the co-contracting horizontal recti.*

the upshooting of the eye in adduction may resemble an overacting inferior oblique muscle, avoid the temptation to recess it. It won't work since the upshooting is due to a tethering effect of the eye between the horizontal recti as they co-contract.

MÖBIUS SYNDROME[14]

Möbius syndrome is due to bilateral aplasia of the sixth-nerve nuclei and unilateral or bilateral aplasia of the facial nerve nuclei (Fig. 10.40).[13] These patients have bilateral abduction defects and unilateral or bilateral facial weakness. Associated ophthalmologic findings may include total external ophthalmoplegia, third-nerve paresis and bilateral ptosis. Lower cranial nerve involvement may result in dysphagia, arrhythmias and aspiration.

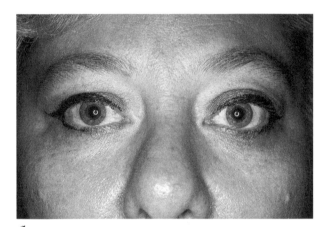

a

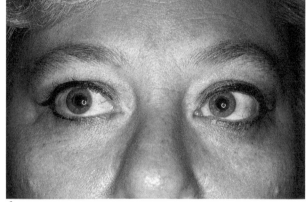

b

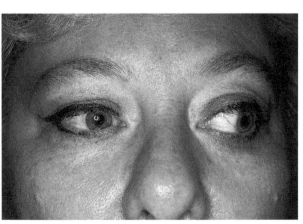

c

Figure 10.39 *A patient with a subtle right Duane's retraction syndrome. Eyes are straight in primary position (a); subtle abduction defect in right gaze (b); subtle retraction of the globe with adduction (c).*

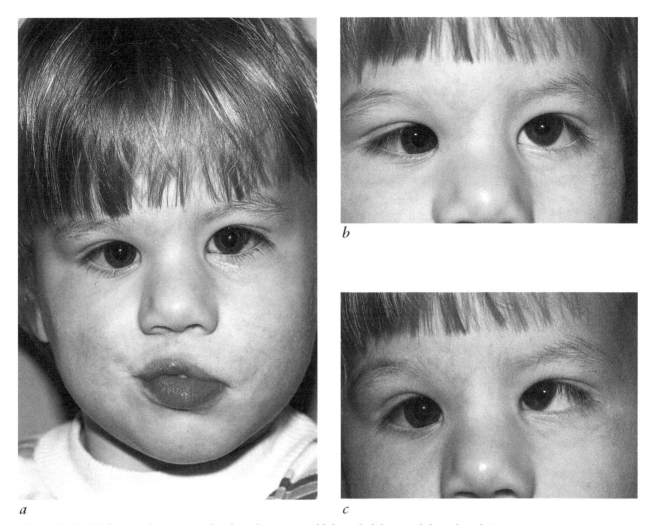

Figure 10.40 *Möbius syndrome: note facial weakness (a) and bilateral abduction defects (b and c).*

THIRD-NERVE PALSIES

The third nerve is the most complicated of the oculo-motor nerves, innervating four extraocular muscles—the superior rectus (SR), inferior rectus (IR), medial rectus (MR) and inferior oblique (IO)—the levator palpebrae superioris and the pupil. The third nerve originates in the midbrain with multiple subnuclei (Fig. 10.41). Warwicke first elucidated these in monkeys many years ago. The concept of nuclear third-nerve paresis has been of intellectual interest to neuro-ophthalmologists since Warwicke but of little practical importance. The subnuclei for the MR, IR and IO are paired and ipsilateral to the muscles innervated (Fig. 10.41).

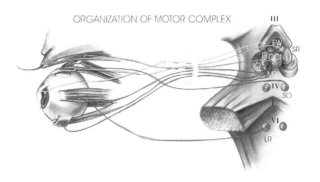

Figure 10.41 *Innervation of the extraocular muscles and pupil by the third-nerve subnuclei.*

The SR subnucleus is contralateral to the innervated muscle and there is one central caudal nuclei serving both upper eyelids (levator muscles). The Edinger-Westphal nucleus, serving the pupils, lies superior/rostral to the extraocular muscle subnuclei. Examples of a nuclear third-nerve paresis include an isolated lesion in the central caudal nuclei causing bilateral total ptosis (Fig. 10.42). This may resolve spontaneously if due to a lacunar infarction or demyelination. An ipsilateral third-nerve paresis (sparing levator) with a contralateral SR paresis is also nuclear in origin (Fig. 10.43), since the SR subnucleus is contralateral to the innervated muscle. These lesions are unusual and of little practical importance to most clinicians.[14]

Fascicles from the third-nerve subnuclei join in the brainstem to become the third-nerve fascicle (Fig. 10.44). The third nerve fascicle passes from dorsal to ventral midbrain, near the red nucleus dorsally and the corticospinal tract ventrally (Fig. 10.44). Involvement of the third-nerve fascicle in the dorsal midbrain may also involve the red nucleus, resulting in an ipsilateral third-nerve paresis and a contralateral tremor and ataxia

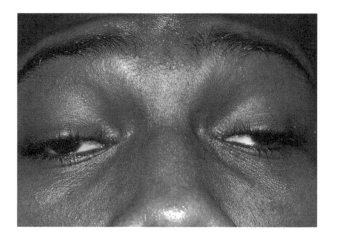

Figure 10.42 *Bilateral ptosis due to a lacunar infarct of the central caudal nucleus.*

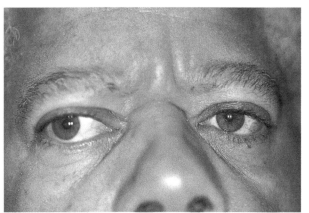

a

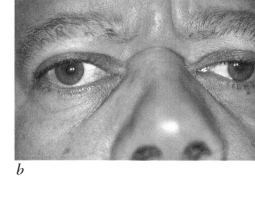

b

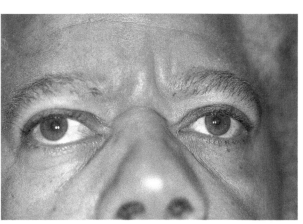

c

Figure 10.43 *Partial right nuclear third-nerve paresis. Right exotropia in primary gaze (a); mild pupillary dilatation and defective adduction of the right eye (b); bilateral upgaze paresis (c).*

CRANIAL NERVE III

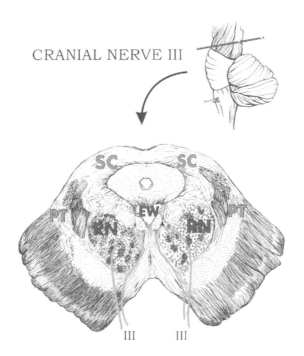

Figure 10.44 *Relationships of the third-nerve fascicle to midbrain structures: the red nucleus and cortico-spinal tract.*

(Benedict's syndrome) (Fig. 10.45). Involvement of the third-nerve fascicle in the ventral brainstem results in an ipsilateral third-nerve paresis and contralateral hemiparesis (Weber's syndrome) (Fig. 10.46). Awareness of these syndromes is important for they connote intrinsic and untreatable brainstem involvement as the cause of the third-nerve palsy. Although the majority of Weber's syndromes are due to intrinsic brainstem infarction or

Figure 10.45 *Benedict's syndrome—ipsilateral third-nerve paresis and contralateral ataxia and tremor due to infarction of the third-nerve fascicle and the adjacent red nucleus (see Fig. 10.44).*

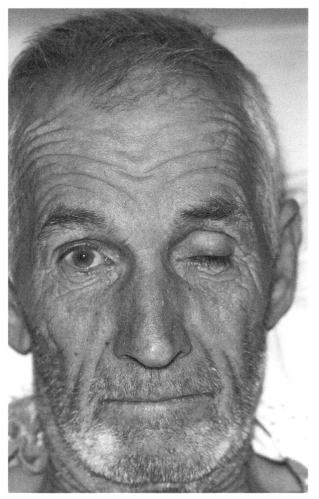

a

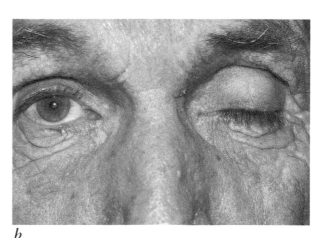

b

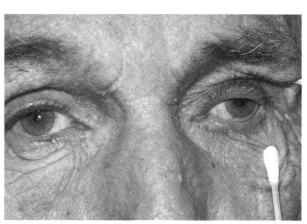

c

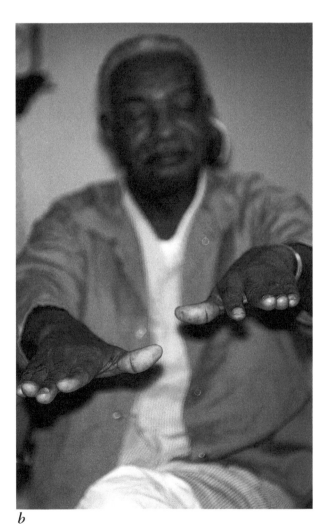

a

demyelination, both the third nerve and the cortico-spinal tract may be compressed by an extrinsic lesion or an aneurysm of the posterior cerebellar artery as it passes over the third nerve as it exits the midbrain or by an extrinsic tumor (Figs 10.47 and 10.48). These may be treatable lesions. Patients with Weber's syndrome require more vigorous imaging studies to rule out treatable lesions than patients with Benedict's syndrome, which is always intrinsic to the brainstem, untreatable and quite uncommon.[15]

As the third nerve exits the brainstem, the posterior cerebral and posterior cerebellar arteries encircle it (Fig. 10.47). Aneurysms of these arteries may cause an isolated third-nerve palsy or an extrinsic Weber's syndrome. As the third nerve passes from the brainstem to the cavernous sinus it is the site of isolated third-nerve palsies (Fig. 10.49). These may be practically divided into those involving or sparing the pupil. The classic third-nerve palsy with pupillary involvement is caused by an aneurysm at the juncture of the internal carotid and posterior communicating arteries (Fig. 10.50). These patients classically present with a headache and a total third-nerve palsy

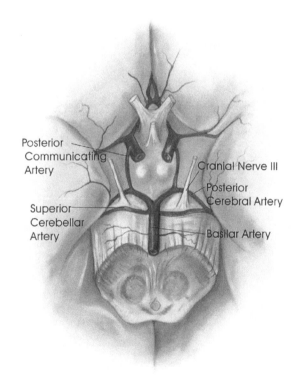

b

Figure 10.46 *Ventral brainstem infarction causing Weber's syndrome, ipsilateral third-nerve paresis and contralateral hemiparesis.*

Figure 10.47 *Anatomy diagram: third nerve exiting brainstem surrounded by the posterior cerebral and posterior cerebellar arteries.*

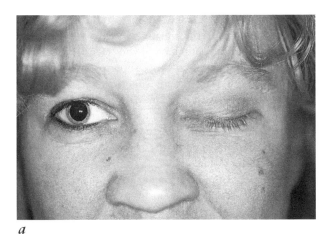

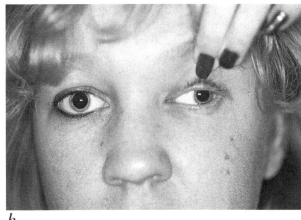

a

b

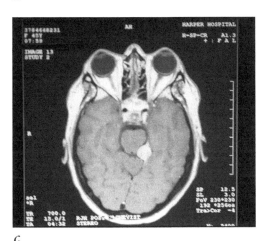

c

Figure 10.48 *Third-nerve palsy (a and b) due to compression of the third nerve as it exits the brainstem by a meningioma. A MRI scan demonstrates meningioma (c).*

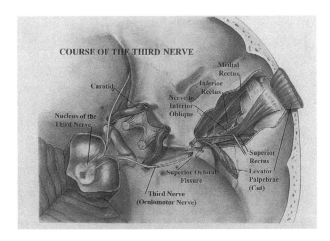

Figure 10.49 *Course of intrapeduncular third nerve from the brainstem to the orbit.*

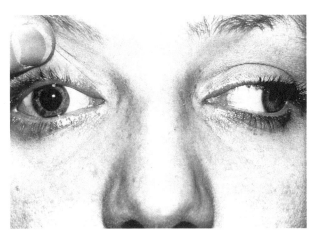

Figure 10.50 *Right third-nerve palsy with pupillary involvement. Note ptosis of the upper eyelid, a fixed dilated pupil and absent adduction of the right eye.*

with obvious pupillary involvement (Fig. 10.50). The eye is closed (ptosis). When opened the eye is exotropic and the pupil widely dilated (Fig. 10.50). Diagnosis and treatment of the offending aneurysm (Fig. 10.51) is often lifesaving. Unfortunately, the diagnosis is not always so obvious: the girl in Fig. 10.52 presented with diplopia, no headache, very subtle extraocular motility dysfunction and pupillary sign—all due to a posterior communicating/internal carotid artery aneurysm.

Pupil-sparing, third-nerve palsies result from microvascular disease due to diabetes or atherosclerosis. These vasculopathic third-nerve palsies may have total extraocular motility involvement, but the pupil is normal (Figs 10.53 and 10.54). Pain, severe at times, around the involved eye may be present. This will also resolve and may be treated with analgesics as necessary. Vasculopathic oculomotor palsies resolve spontaneously in 60–90 days, leaving no sequelae (Fig. 10.53f). There is never aberrant regeneration after a vasculopathic third-nerve palsy.

Seen early in its course, a vasculopathic third-nerve palsy may present as a partial paresis. The man in Fig. 10.55 complained of pain and diplopia. His right eye was exotropic and failed to adduct fully (Fig. 10.55). The present author was not familiar with painful internuclear ophthalmoplegia, so re-evaluated the patient several days later. By this time the diagnosis of vasculopathic third-nerve paresis (Fig. 10.56) in a diabetic was obvious. If, on the other hand, the partial third-nerve paresis does not progress rapidly (Fig. 10.57), or is accompanied by another oculomotor paresis (Fig. 10.15), suspect an infiltrative or compressive lesion in the cavernous sinus (Figs 10.57 and 10.58), even though the pupil is totally spared. Cavernous sinus lesions (carotid aneurysms, meningiomas and metastatic carcinomas) may present as a partial third-nerve paresis, often with or without minimal pupillary involvement (Fig. 10.57). Compressive lesions often cause superior division third-nerve palsies (levator and superior rectus). These patients should have a CT or MRI of both brain and orbits.[16,17] Remember, known diabetics are not immune to other causes of third-nerve paresis. If the pupil is involved, even minimally, be suspicious of a more ominous etiology (Fig. 10.59).

Diagnostic conundrums may arise when evaluating patients with total extraocular motility involvement and minimal but real pupillary involvement. The present author was taught during his fellowship that pupillary involvement should mirror motility involvement. If the pupil was only minimally involved in a patient with significant motility involvement (Fig. 10.59), the pupillary involvement was not significant, especially in known diabetics. This view fell from favor as clinicians realized that diabetes did not protect patients from aneurysms and tumors. For a number of years it was taught that any pupillary involvement was significant, and arteriograms of many patients with vasculopathic third-nerve palsies that were misfortunate enough to have just a little pupillary involvement were performed. A study has demonstrated that patients with minimal pupillary involvement rarely have aneurysms as the etiology.[18]

So what does the clinician do when confronted with a patient with a third-nerve palsy? If the pupil is obviously involved, immediate referral to a neurosurgeon for neuroimaging and arteriography is necessary. The patient in Fig. 10.50 has an internal carotid/posterior communicating junction aneurysm until proven otherwise. If there is

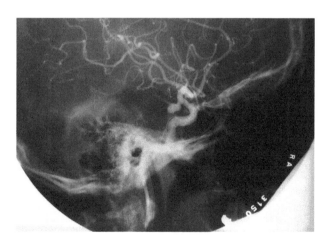

Figure 10.51 *Cerebral angiogram demonstrates aneurysm at the junction of the internal carotid and posterior communicating arteries.*

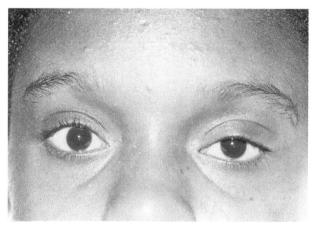

Figure 10.52 *Partial left third-nerve palsy with partial pupillary involvement also due to an aneurysm. Note the partial ptosis and pupillary involvement.*

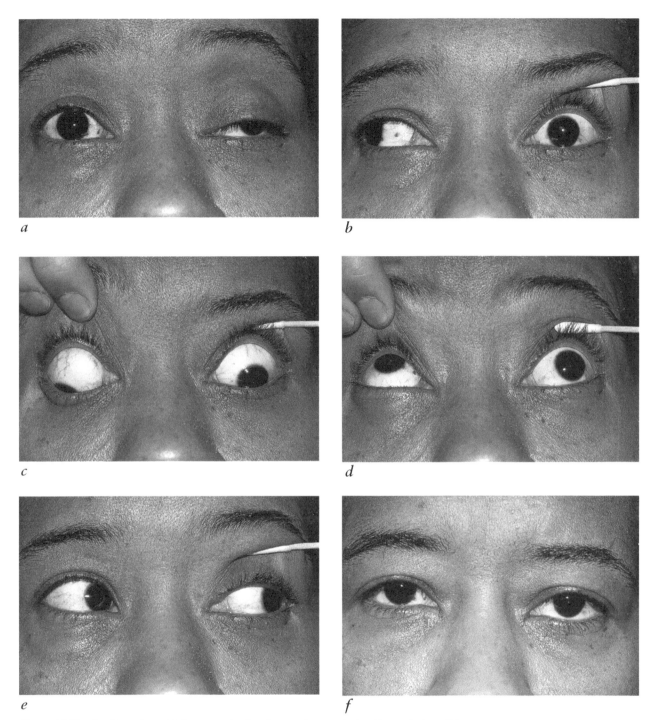

Figure 10.53 *Pupil-sparing, third-nerve palsy (a–e); complete resolution 2 months later (f).*

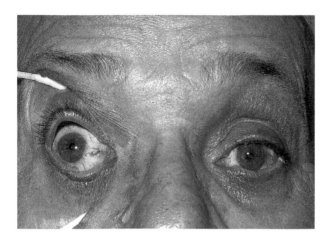

Figure 10.54   *Pupil-sparing, third-nerve palsy. Note that the pupils are equal and normal in spite of a total right third-nerve palsy.*

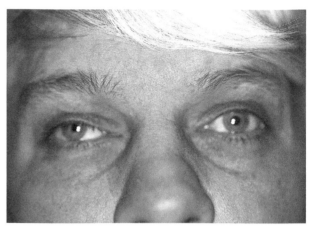

Figure 10.55   *Initial presentation of a vasculopathic third-nerve palsy mimicking an internuclear ophthalmoplegia.*

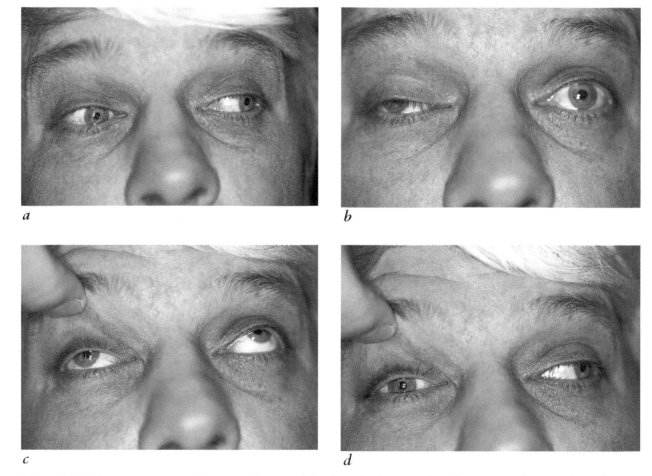

a   *b*

c   *d*

Figure 10.56   *The same patient as in Fig. 10.55 when several days later the diagnosis of pupil-sparing, third-nerve palsy is obvious.*

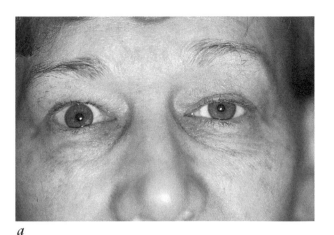

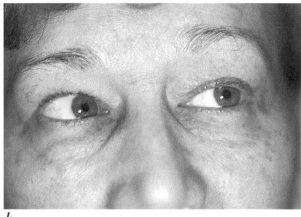

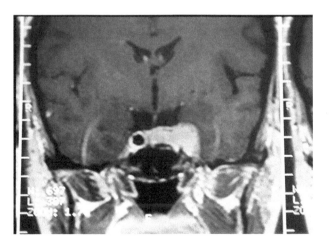

Figure 10.57   *A patient with a slowly progressive, partial third-nerve paresis is likely to have a compressive or infiltrative lesion in the cavernous sinus.*

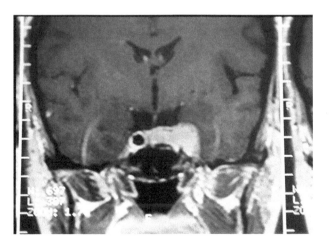

Figure 10.58   *MRI scan demonstrating an enhancing mass in the cavernous sinus.*

even a hint of contralateral hemiparesis, make sure that the posterior cerebral circulation is studied to rule out an aneurysm of the posterior superior cerebellar or posterior cerebral arteries compressing the third nerve as it exits the brainstem (external Weber's syndrome; Figs 10.47 and 10.48). A patient with a third-nerve palsy and a normal pupil (Figs 10.53 and 10.54) may be safely observed and followed, expecting spontaneous resolution in 60–90 days. This is especially true if the patient is a known diabetic. If not a known diabetic, the patient may be evaluated for possible diabetes or for other vasculopathic risk factors. The patient with partial pupil involvement may be challenging (Fig. 10.59). If the pupil involvement is minimal and does not correlate with the degree of motility involvement (Fig. 10.59), re-examine the patient several days later. If the pupil is unchanged, re-examine 1 week later. This is an especially safe approach

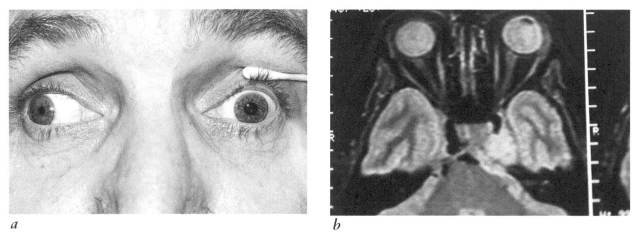

a *b*

Figure 10.59 *Known diabetic presenting with a complete third-nerve palsy with minimal but obvious pupillary involvement (a). An MRI scan demonstrates cavernous sinus metastasis (b).*

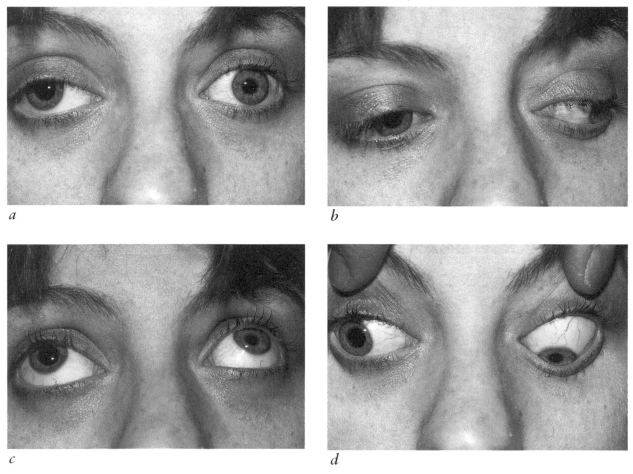

a *b*

c *d*

Figure 10.60 *A patient with traumatic third-nerve palsy. Note ptosis, pupillary dilatation (a), decreased adduction (b), elevation (c) and depression (d).*

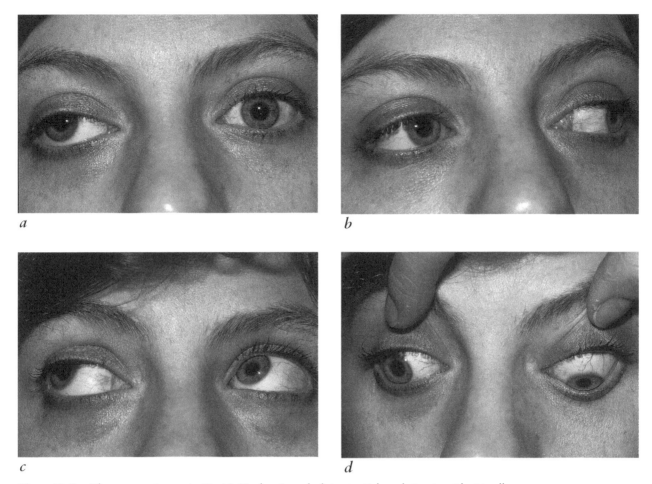

Figure 10.61 *The same patient as in Fig. 10.60 when 3 weeks later, partial resolution is evident in all gazes.*

in known diabetics. If the pupil changes (worsens) during the follow-up examinations, a full evaluation is necessary. This may include a contrast-enhanced MRI, MR angiography and four-vessel arteriography.[19] A simpler approach would be referral to a neuro-ophthalmologist to let him/her manage the patient in an appropriate fashion. Patients with previous intraocular surgery and damage to their iris sphincters may be particularly challenging to differentiate iatrogenic from neurologic pupillary dysfunction.

ABERRANT REGENERATION OF THE OCULOMOTOR NERVE[20]

Aberrant regeneration of the third nerve never occurs after a vasculopathic third-nerve palsy. It may occur after partial or complete resolution of a traumatic third-nerve palsy and may occur in the presence of a compressive lesion. The third nerve tries to regenerate its damaged fibers and miswires itself. The results are predictable, but may be confusing if not considered and recognized.

The patient in Fig. 10.60 has a traumatic third-nerve paresis that is partially resolving. Note the dilatation of the right pupil, ptosis of the upper eyelid, decreased adduction, depression and elevation of the right eye (Fig. 10.60a–d). Three weeks later the motility defects have partially resolved (Fig. 10.61a–d). Three months later there is apparent total resolution of the motility defects (Fig. 10.62), but subtle, aberrant regeneration is present (Figs 10.63 and 10.64). The right upper eyelid elevates with ocular depression due to miswiring between the superior division nerve fibers to the levator and the inferior division fibers to the inferior rectus (Fig. 10.63). There is pseudo-light-near dissociation of the pupils, with increased pupillary constriction with adduction of

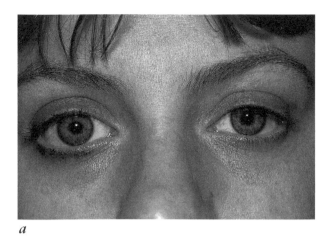

a

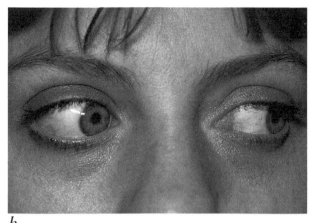

b

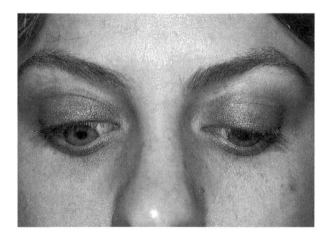

c

Figure 10.62 *The same patient as in Figs 10.60 and 10.61 when 3 months later third-nerve palsy appears to be totally resolved.*

the eye due to aberrant connections between nerve fibers directed to the medial rectus and the pupillary constrictor (Fig. 10.64). These motility findings may be subtle or very obvious. As with so many extraocular motility problems, considering the appropriate diagnosis greatly facilitates making the correct diagnosis!

Figure 10.63 *Upper eyelid retraction with attempted downgaze due to aberrant regeneration.*

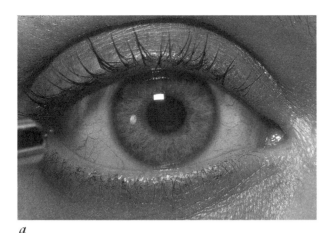
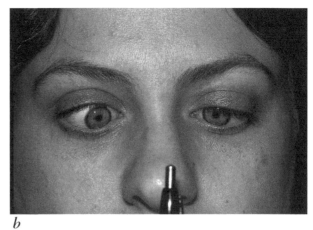

a *b*

Figure 10.64 *Pseudo-light-near dissociation of the pupils due to aberrant regeneration of the third nerve.*

REFERENCES

1. Silverman IE, Liu GT, Volpe NJ et al. The crossed paralyses: the original brainstem syndromes of Millard-Gubler, Foville, Weber and Raymond-Cestan. *Arch Neurol* 1995; **52**:635–8.

2. Moster ML, Savino PJ, Sergott RC et al. Isolated sixth nerve palsies in younger adults. *Arch Ophthalmol* 1984; **102**:1328–30.

3. Lee MS, Galetta SL, Volpe NJ et al. Sixth nerve palsies in children. *Pediatr Neurol* 1999; **20**:49–52.

4. Mutyala S, Holmes JM, Hodge DO et al. Spontaneous recovery rate in traumatic sixth nerve palsy. *Am J Ophthalmol* 1996; **122**:898–9.

5. Metz HS, Dickey CF. Treatment of unilateral sixth nerve palsy with botulinum toxin. *Am J Ophthalmol* 1991; **112**:381–4.

6. Galetta SL, Smith JL. Chronic isolated sixth nerve palsies. *Arch Neurol* 1989; **46**:79–82.

7. Holmes JM, Beck RW, Kip KE et al. Botulinum-A toxin vs conservative management in acute traumatic sixth nerve paresis. *JAAPOS* 2000; **3**:145–9.

8. Kupersmith MJ, Latkany R, Homel P. Development of generalized disease at 2 years in patients with ocular myasthenia gravis. *Arch Neurol* 2003; **60**:243–8.

9. Movaghar M, Slavin ML. Effect of local heat versus ice on blepharoptosis resulting from ocular myasthenia gravis. *Ophthalmology* 2001; **108**:1363–4.

10. Czoplinski A, Steck AJ, Fuhr P. Ice pack test for myasthenia gravis: a simple non-invasive safe diagnostic method. *J Neurol* 2003; **250**:883–4.

11. DeRespinis PA, Caputo AR, Wagner RS et al. Duane's retraction syndrome. *Surv Ophthalmol* 1993; **38**:257–88.

12. Ellis FD, Hoyt CS, Ellis EJ et al. Extraocular motility responses to orbital cooling for ocular myasthenia gravis. *JAAPOS* 2000; **4**:271–81.

13. Miller NR, Kiel SM, Green WR et al. Unilateral Duane's retraction syndrome (type 1). *Arch Ophthalmol* 1982; **100**:1468–72.

14. Ghabrial R, Versace P, Kourt G et al. Möbius' syndrome: features and etiology. *J Pediatr Ophthalmol Strabismus* 1998; **35**:304–11.

15. Pratt DV, Oreng-Nania S, Horowitz BL et al. MRI findings in a patient with nuclear oculomotor palsy. *Arch Ophthalmol* 1995; **113**:141–2.

16. Liu GT, Crenner CW, Logigian EL et al. Midbrain syndromes of Benedikt, Claude and Nothnagel: setting the record straight. *Neurology* 1992; **42**:1820–2.

17. Guy JR, Savino PJ, Schatz NJ et al. Superior division paresis of the oculomotor nerve. *Ophthalmology* 1985; **92**:777–84.

18. Guy JR, Day AL. Intracranial aneurysms with superior division paresis of the oculomotor nerve. *Ophthalmology* 1989; **96**:1071–6.

19. Capo H, Warren F, Kupersmith MJ. Evolution of oculomotor nerve palsies. *J Clin Neuro-Ophthalmol* 1992; **12**: 21–5.

20. Jacobson DM, Trobe JD. The emerging role of magnetic resonance angiography in the management of patients with third cranial nerve palsy. *Am J Ophthalmol* 1999; **128**:94–6.

21. Sibony PA, Lessell S, Gittinger JW Jr. Acquired oculomotor synkinesis. *Surv Ophthalmol* 1984; **28**:382–90.

Chapter 11 Vertical motility dysfunction

Patients with vertical motility dysfunction complain of vertical or torsional diplopia. It helps to quickly differentiate the motility disorders by simply asking the patient whether he or she sees double side by side or up and down, or 'Show me with your hands', 'Does it get worse (or better) when you look to the left or right?', 'Does it get worse (or better) when you tilt your head right or left)?', 'Does the double vision go away when you cover one eye?' If the latter is the case then this indicates a bona fide neuro-ophthalmologic/orbital problem. If it is not, the patient has uniocular diplopia (ghosting) and the etiology is almost always refractive—opacities in the cornea or lens—necessitating a careful dilated ocular examination to make the diagnosis (see Chapter 2).

Vertical motility dysfunction may result from neuro-ophthalmic or orbital disorders. Neuro-ophthalmic disorders include vertical gaze palsies, partial third- and fourth-nerve palsies, myasthenia gravis (MG) and skew deviation. Orbital etiologies include dysthyroid orbitopathy, orbital tumors, inflammation and muscle entrapment due to antecedent trauma. These are often easy to diagnose if they are considered, and if the appropriate imaging studies are ordered and reviewed.

The etiology of vertical diplopia is as variable as the individual practice environment. Keane,[1] a hospital-based neuro-ophthalmologist, has summarized his experience with vertical diplopia. The vast majority of patients had third (579 cases), fourth (133 cases), skew deviation (434 cases) or MG (94 cases) as the etiology of their diplopia. Orbital fractures and Graves's ophthalmopathy were present to a much lesser extent. These numbers are very different to the present author's experience in an ambulatory, referral neuro-ophthalmologic/orbital practice where the majority of patients have dysthyroid orbitopathy, fourth-nerve palsies, orbital trauma and progressing or resolving third-nerve paresis.

ORBITAL DISORDERS

Primary encapsulated orbital tumors (Figs 11.1 and 11.2), diffuse orbital infiltration (Fig. 11.3) or invasion from the adjacent sinuses (Fig. 11.4) may vertically displace the eye. Metastatic disease to the orbit may mimic vertical motility dysfunction (Fig. 11.5). Orbital neoplasms are usually obvious but may be overlooked if not considered and the appropriate imaging studies obtained (see Chapter 13).

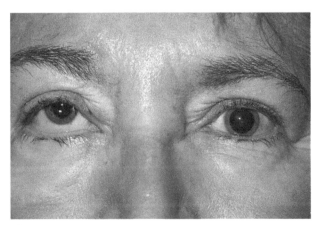

a

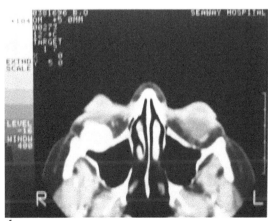

b

Figure 11.1 *Superior displacement of the right eye (a). A CT scan demonstrating a well-encapsulated inferior orbital tumor (b).*

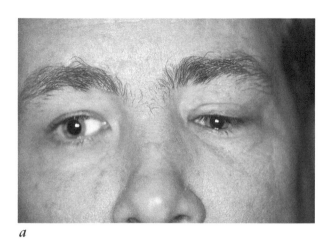

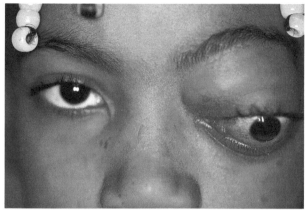

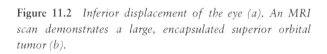

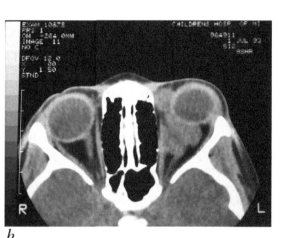

Figure 11.2 *Inferior displacement of the eye (a). An MRI scan demonstrates a large, encapsulated superior orbital tumor (b).*

Figure 11.3 *Inferior displacement of the eye (a) by a diffuse, infiltrating lymphangioma (b).*

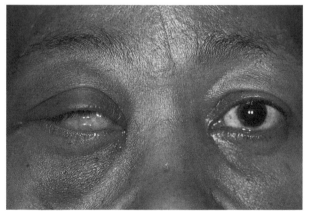

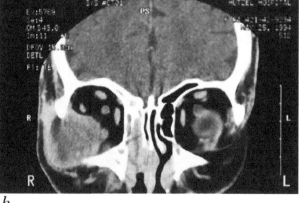

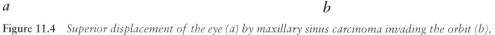

Figure 11.4 *Superior displacement of the eye (a) by maxillary sinus carcinoma invading the orbit (b).*

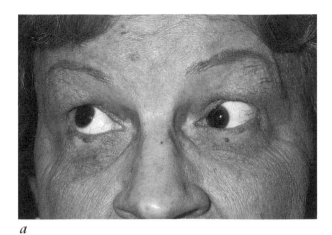
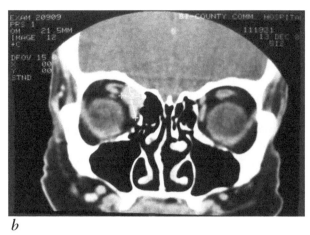

a

b

Figure 11.5 *Pseudo-Brown's syndrome with restriction of upgaze (a) by infiltration of the trochlea and superior oblique by metastatic breast carcinoma (b).*

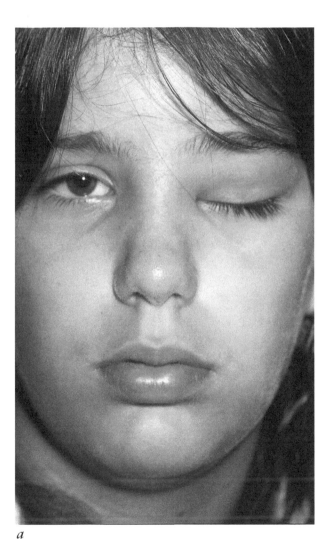

IDIOPATHIC ORBITAL INFLAMMATION

Patients with idiopathic orbital inflammation (orbital pseudo-tumor), may present with a variety of vertical motility dysfunctions. The girl in Fig. 11.6 presented with ptosis and upgaze paresis accompanied by erythema and swelling of the upper eyelid. After a comedy of diagnostic and therapeutic blunders (four-vessel cerebral angiogram, 10 days of intravenous antibiotics and suggested plastic surgery on her eyelid), her parents sought another opinion. The coronal computerized

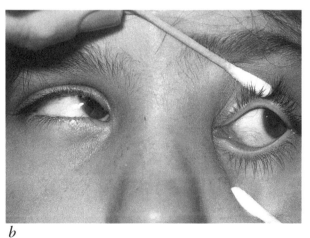

a

b

Figure 11.6 *A girl with orbital inflammation presenting with painful ptosis (a) and upgaze paresis (b).*

tomography (CT) scan demonstrated enlargement of the superior rectus/levator complex (Fig. 11.7). Symptoms and signs resolved promptly with oral corticosteroids. Orbital myositis may also involve the superior oblique and present as a pseudo-Brown's syndrome (Fig. 11.8). Awareness of the diagnosis and imaging the appropriate areas facilitate correct diagnosis.

Patients with recent or remote orbital trauma with a resultant orbital floor fracture may have vertical diplopia. The eye may have limited elevation, depression (Figs 11.9 and 11.10) or both secondary to entrapment of the inferior rectus or orbital septa in the fracture site (Fig. 11.11). CT scans are usually diagnostic but can be misleading. Forced ductions will differentiate restriction from paresis due to neural damage or loss of muscle.

In addition to orbital floor fracture with entrapment, the differential diagnosis of elevator paresis includes congenital double elevator palsy (Fig. 11.12) and congenital fibrosis (Fig. 11.13). Forced ductions differentiate the two, being positive in congenital fibrosis and negative in patients with double elevator paresis. An apparent double elevator paresis may be present in patients with dysthyroid orbitopathy (Fig. 11.14) but here the diagnosis should be obvious after CT scanning. Patients with acquired monocular elevator palsy present with acute onset of vertical diplopia. Unlike orbital etiologies, forced ductions and orbital imaging are negative.

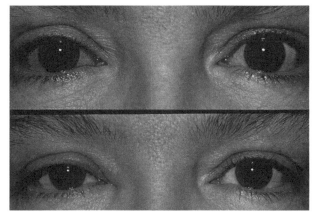

a

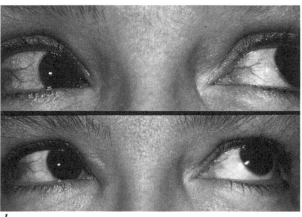

b

Figure 11.8 *Pseudo-Brown's syndrome caused by inflammation of the trochlea. Patient's eyes are straight in primary gaze (a), but note the decreased elevation in the field of the inferior oblique (b). Upper photos before treatment, lower photos demonstrate resolution after treatment with corticosteroids.*

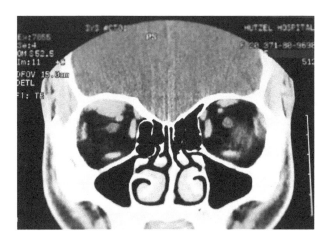

Figure 11.7 *Coronal CT scan demonstrates an enlarged superior rectus levator complex.*

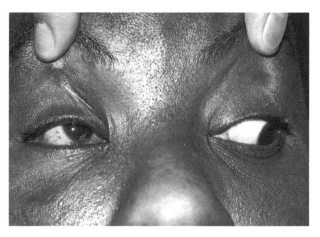

Figure 11.9 *Orbital floor fracture with hypertropia and restricted depression of the right eye.*

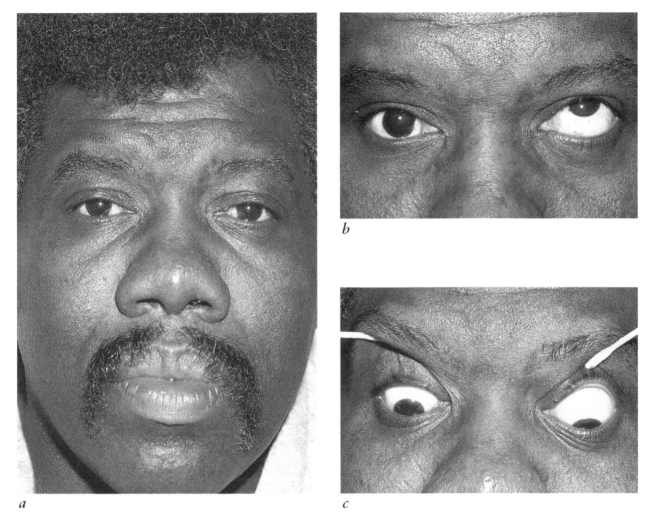

Figure 11.10 *A patient with remote orbital floor fracture. Eyes are straight in primary gaze (a); elevation is absent (b), depression is mildly limited (c).*

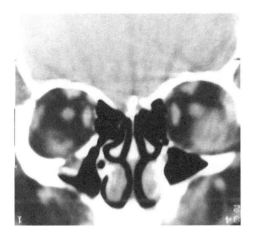

Figure 11.11 *Coronal CT scan demonstrates entrapment of the inferior rectus muscle and its septae.*

Dysthyroid orbitopathy is a common orbital etiology for vertical diplopia. Dysthyroid disease is often obvious (Fig. 11.15). Restrictive strabismus is usually accompanied by eyelid retraction, especially evident on attempted upward gaze (Fig. 11.16), and an enlarged inferior rectus is evident on a CT scan (Fig. 11.16b). The diagnosis may be obscured by normal or ptotic eyelids but is usually evident after testing the patient's versions and ductions and is confirmed by imaging studies (Fig. 11.17). Vertical motility defects caused by dysthyroid orbitopathy must be differentiated from an underacting superior rectus due to an ipsilateral partial third-nerve paresis and a contralateral fourth-nerve paresis. Testing both versions and ductions is important for underaction in upgaze due to inferior rectus

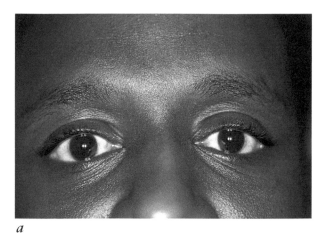

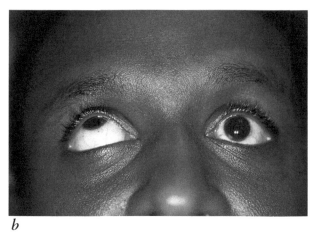

Figure 11.12 *Congenital fibrosis of the orbit (a) with restricted elevation of the left eye (b). Forced ductions are markedly positive.*

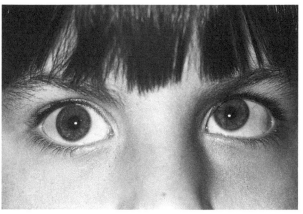

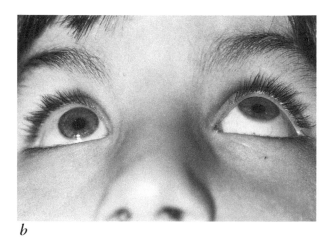

Figure 11.13 *Double elevator palsy. Right eye does not elevate in either abduction (a) or adduction (b). Forced ductions are negative.*

restriction may cause marked overaction of the contralateral inferior oblique mimicking a superior oblique palsy (Fig. 11.18). The restricted eye will not elevate when tested uniocularly (ductions) and forced duction testing will be positive. If the apparent restriction is due to inhibitional palsy of the contralateral antagonist, ductions and forced ductions would be normal (Fig. 11.19). Inhibitional palsy of the contralateral antagonist occurs because of Hering's law of equal innervation. A patient with dysthyroid infiltration of the left inferior rectus (Fig. 11.18) will require excessive innervation of the ipsilateral superior rectus as he/she tries to elevate that eye against the inertia of the enlarged dysfunctional muscle (Fig. 11.18). Since yoke muscles receive similar degrees of innervation, the contralateral inferior oblique muscle will appear to markedly overact (Fig. 11.18). This apparent overaction of the inferior oblique mimics a contralateral superior oblique paresis with an overacting right inferior oblique during version testing. If ductions are tested, the apparent overaction of the inferior oblique is no longer evident. The underaction of the left superior rectus working against the infiltrated left inferior rectus is obvious and restriction can be verified by forced duction testing. This apparent overaction of the inferior oblique may also occur in patients with a partially

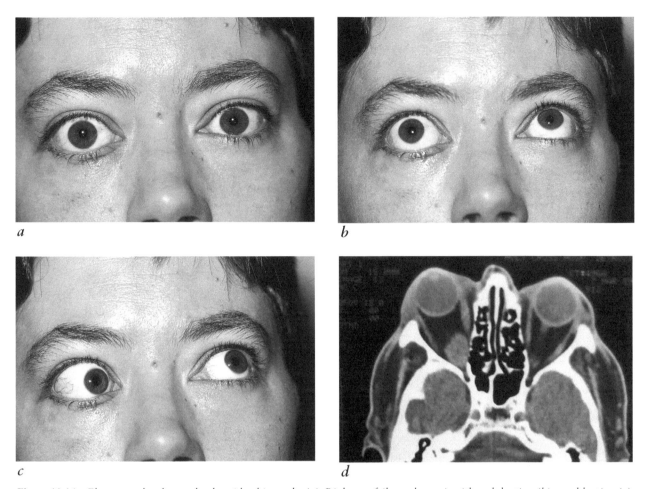

Figure 11.14 *Elevator palsy due to dysthyroid orbitopathy (a). Right eye fails to elevate in either abduction (b) or adduction (c). A CT scan is diagnostic, demonstrating marked enlargement of the right inferior rectus (d).*

resolved third-nerve paresis with underaction of the superior rectus. In these patients, forced ductions are negative (Fig. 11.19).

FORCED DUCTIONS

Forced ductions differentiate paretic from restrictive strabismus. The eye is anesthetized with a few drops of topical anesthetic. Pledgets from cotton-tipped applicators are soaked in 4% topical xylocaine or 4% cocaine. These small pledgets are then placed in the eye over the insertion of the rectus muscle you wish to grasp. If they are left in place for several minutes prior to testing, testing is painless. The insertion is grasped with a toothed forceps and the patient asked to look in the direction in which the eye is to be moved (Fig. 11.19b). The eye is gen-

tly moved in that direction with the forceps and restriction, if present, is evident. Forced ductions are most helpful in differentiating restrictive strabismus from paralytic strabismus (sixth-nerve palsy from medial rectus entrapment in a medial wall fracture, or restriction due to dysthyroid muscle enlargement from a contralateral superior oblique paresis or ipsilateral superior rectus paresis).

In summary, a patient with a partially resolved third-nerve paresis and deficient elevation of the left eye in adduction (Fig. 11.18) appears to have a 4+ overacting inferior oblique. Ductions differentiate the overacting inferior oblique from the underacting contralateral superior rectus. The marked secondary overaction of the inferior oblique is due to hypertrophy secondary to excessive innervation as the patient tries to fixate with the dominant left eye with its paretic

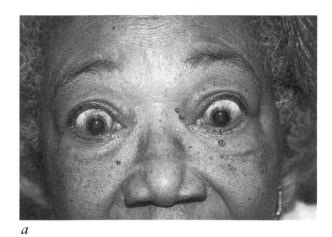

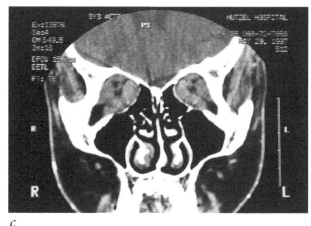

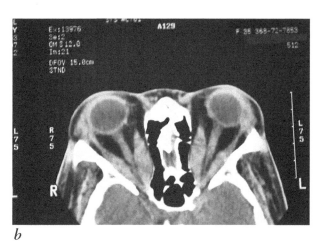

Figure 11.15 *A patient with obvious dysthyroid orbitopathy. Note retraction of the upper eyelids with attempted upgaze (a). CT scans demonstrate marked enlargement of all the extraocular muscles (b and c).*

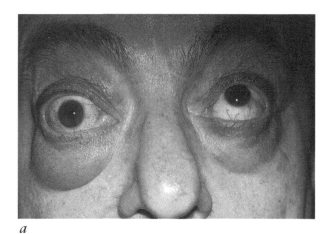

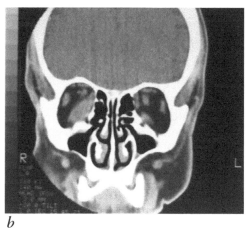

Figure 11.16 *Upgaze palsy due to dysthyroid orbitopathy (a). A CT scan demonstrates a markedly enlarged right inferior rectus (b).*

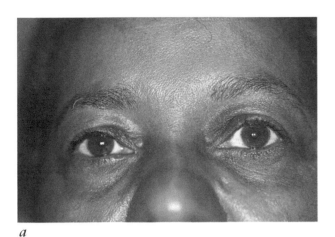

a

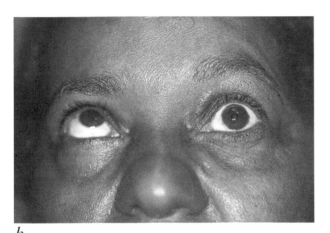

b

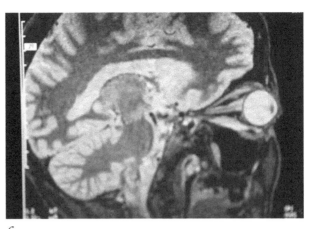

c

Figure 11.17 *A patient with subtle dysthyroid orbitopathy and partial upgaze paresis. Note absence of upper eyelid retraction (a and b); MRI scan demonstrates an enlarged left inferior rectus on sagittal view (c).*

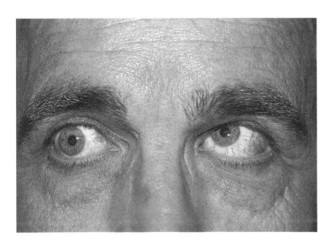

Figure 11.18 *A patient with right inferior rectus restriction demonstrates an overaction of the left inferior oblique with attempted upgaze.*

superior rectus muscle (Hering's law). Forced ductions (Fig. 11.19) differentiate the paretic superior rectus from the restricted inferior rectus (Fig. 11.18).

Finally, patients with primary overacting inferior oblique muscles (Fig. 11.20) are straight in primary gaze, i.e. there is no manifest vertical or cyclotorsional deviation. The deviation is only evident when they look in the field of action of the overacting muscle (Fig. 11.20). Patients with overacting inferior oblique muscles secondary to a paretic ipsilateral superior oblique or a paretic contralateral superior rectus often have a significant vertical deviation in primary gaze.

To the casual observer, a dissociated vertical deviation may mimic an overacting inferior oblique muscle (Fig. 11.21). As the eye adducts and elevates, the nose dissociates it and it shoots upward, mimicking an overacting inferior oblique. A patient with Duane's

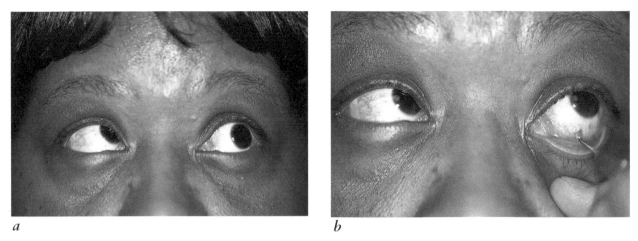

Figure 11.19   *Apparent overaction of the right inferior oblique in a patient with restricted upgaze due to a left superior rectus paresis residual from a partial third nerve paresis (a). Uniocular ductions and forced ductions are normal (b).*

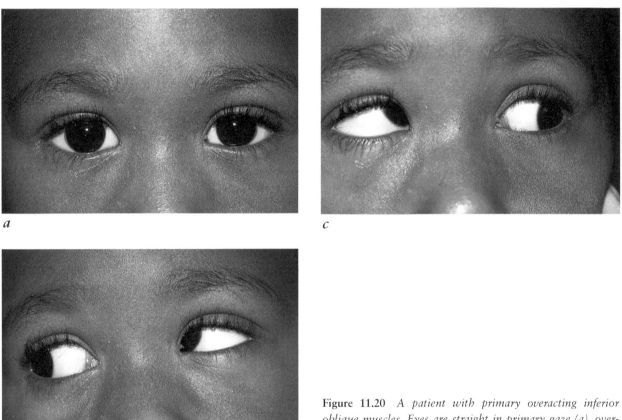

Figure 11.20   *A patient with primary overacting inferior oblique muscles. Eyes are straight in primary gaze (a), overacting inferior obliques are evident in both right (b) and left (c) gaze.*

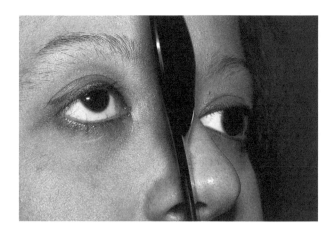

Figure 11.21 *Dissociated vertical deviation may mimic an overacting inferior oblique when the eye is dissociated by the patient's nose. Diagnosis is obvious when occluded.*

retraction syndrome (Duane's 1) may manifest marked apparent overaction of the inferior oblique muscle due to tethering of the globe by the co-contracting medial and lateral recti (Fig. 11.22). Other manifestations of Duane's—limited abduction and enophthalmos with adduction (Fig. 11.22) —should make the diagnosis obvious.

Patients with bilateral inferior rectus restriction often adopt a chin-elevated head position and have marked upper eyelid retraction (Fig. 11.23). Since the superior recti are constantly trying to elevate the eyes, levator overaction exacerbates the upper eyelid retraction. Recession of the inferior recti may completely or partially obviate the eyelid retraction.

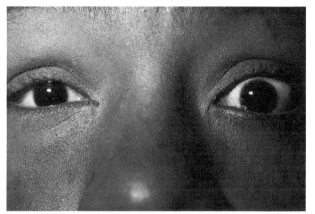

a

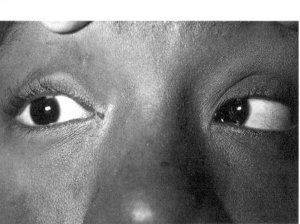

b

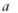

c

Figure 11.22 *Right Duane's retraction syndrome. Eyes are straight in primary gaze (a); abduction is limited in right gaze (b); pseudo-overaction of the inferior oblique muscle in left gaze due to tethering effect caused by co-contraction of the horizontal recti (c).*

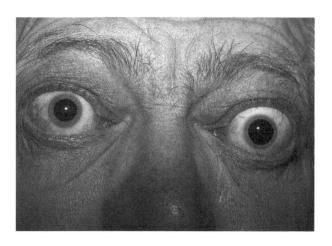

Figure 11.23 *Marked upper eyelid retraction with attempted upgaze in patient with bilateral inferior rectus restriction.*

Patients with dysthyroid involvement of the superior recti may manifest large hypertropias with restricted downgaze (Fig. 11.24). Normal or ptotic upper eyelids may obscure the diagnosis (Fig. 11.24) but imaging studies will demonstrate involvement of the appropriate muscles (Fig. 11.24c). The diagnosis of dysthyroid orbitopathy should be made with caution in the presence of normal or ptotic upper eyelids. Most patients with dysthyroid orbitopathy have upper eyelid retraction. If they do not, be careful. The patient in Fig. 11.25 was referred with the diagnosis of vertical diplopia secondary to dysthyroid orbitopathy. The normal-appearing upper eyelids prompted repeat imaging studies that revealed an intracranial aneurysm (Fig. 11.25b).

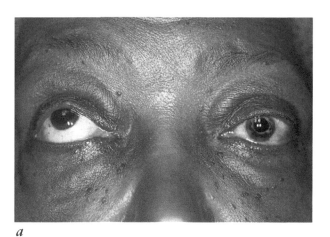

a

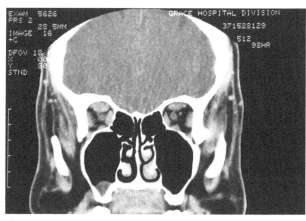

c

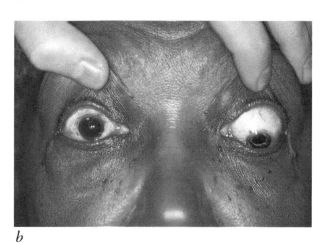

b

Figure 11.24 *A patient with dysthyroid orbitopathy presenting with a large right hypertropia (a) and limited depression of the right eye (b). A CT scan demonstrates enlargement of the right superior rectus (c).*

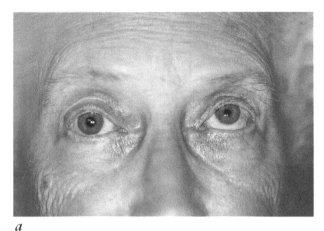

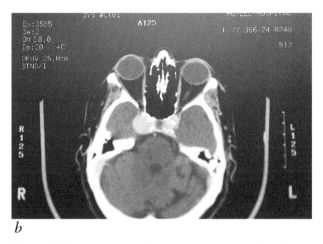

Figure 11.25 *A patient with decreased upgaze in the right eye and normal eyelids (a). A CT scan demonstrates a large intra-cavernous sinus carotid aneurysm (b).*

Figure 11.26 *Anatomy of vertical gaze.*

ANATOMY OF VERTICAL GAZE

The superior (trochlear nerve), inferior oblique muscles, and the superior and inferior recti (oculomotor nerve) accomplish vertical gaze. Vertical gaze is controlled in the upper midbrain in the vicinity of the peri-aqueductal region. Subsequently, vertical gaze dysfunction may result from peri-aqueductal or third or fourth cranial nerve dysfunction.

Unlike horizontal gaze, which is controlled in the pons, vertical gaze is generated in the midbrain. The rostral interstitial nucleus of the medial longitudinal fasciculus (riMLF nucleus) in the midbrain controls vertical gaze like the parapontine reticular formation (PPRF)

controls horizontal gaze in the pons. The riMLF nucleus is located at the junction of the diencephalon and the midbrain, just rostral to the oculomotor nucleus, dorsal to the red nucleus and ventral to the peri-aqueductal gray (Fig. 11.26). Upward gaze is controlled by neurons in the medial portion of the nucleus, downgaze by neurons in the lateral portion of the nucleus.[2] Downgaze fibers course medially through the upgaze neurons, so a medial lesion produces paralysis for both up- and downgaze, while a lateral lesion preferentially affects downgaze (Fig. 11.26).

The riMLF nuclei project to the oculomotor and trochlear nuclei. Upgaze palsies may result from lesions in the posterior commissure, bilateral pretectal region, unilateral thalamus or midbrain tegmentum and the peri-aqueductal gray (Fig. 11.26). An appropriately placed midbrain infarction or demyelinating plaque can produce paresis of upward and downward gaze.

SUN SETTING SIGN

Downwardly deviating eyes and retracted upper eyelids in an infant (Fig. 11.27) are a sign of hydrocephalus. This results from increased intracranial pressure (ICP) causing reversible dysfunction of the diencephalon or upper midbrain. Transient downward deviation of the eyes may be present in neonates and not a harbinger of hydrocephalus. Downwardly deviating eyes and upper eyelid retraction in an adult is much more likely caused by dysthyroid orbitopathy (Fig. 11.28). The enlarged dysfunctional inferior recti restrict upgaze. Attempts at upgaze cause excessive stimulation of the superior rectus/levator complex and resultant upper eyelid retraction. Forced duction testing easily differentiates these two causes of upgaze paresis if not obvious after clinical examination and imaging.

DOWNGAZE PALSY

Isolated downgaze palsy is rare and usually results from bilateral infarctions in the medial portion of the riMLF. If the lesions are incomplete, total or partial recovery may occur.

DORSAL MIDBRAIN SYNDROME (PARINAUD)

Lesions in the rostral portion of the dorsal midbrain may cause distinctive neuro-ophthalmologic signs involving supranuclear control of vertical gaze, light-near dissociation of the pupils, upper eyelid retraction and lag, upward gaze palsy and convergence retraction nystagmus elicited on attempted upward gaze. A bilateral upgaze palsy with doll's-head reflex or Bell's phenomenon intact indicates its supranuclear nature (Fig. 11.29). Accommodation and convergence may also be involved (Fig. 11.30). The most common causes of dorsal midbrain syndrome are pinealoma and midbrain infarctions. Patients with pinealomas may present with a dorsal midbrain syndrome accompanied by obstructive hydrocephalus and papilledema (Fig. 11.31). Other less common etiologies include multiple sclerosis, aqueductal stenosis, syphilis, midbrain hemorrhage, arteriovenous malformations, midbrain tumors and encephalitis.[3]

SKEW DEVIATION

Skew deviation is a vertical deviation resulting from a supranuclear or vestibulo-ocular disruption. It may be

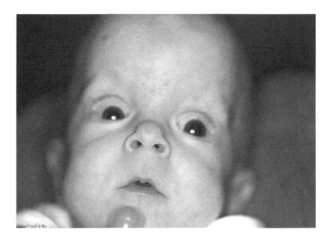

Figure 11.27   *Sunset sign infant with downward deviation of eyes and retracted upper eyelids due to congenital hydrocephalus.*

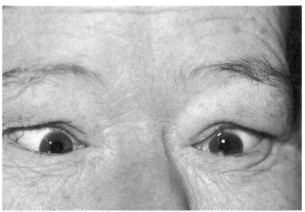

a

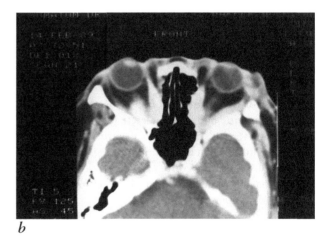

b

Figure 11.28   *Pseudo-sunset sign in an adult with dysthyroid orbitopathy (a). A CT scan demonstrates marked enlargement of extraocular muscles (b).*

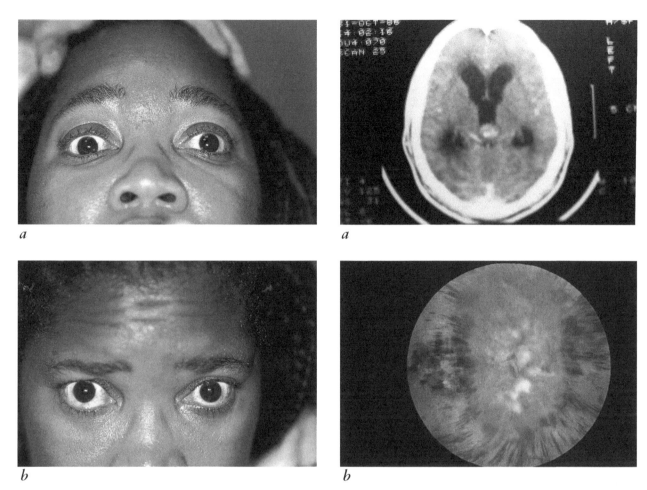

a

b

Figure 11.29 *Dorsal midbrain syndrome—upgaze palsy (a) with intact doll's-head maneuver (b).*

Figure 11.31 *A CT scan demonstrating a pinealoma and obstructive hydrocephalus (a) in a patient with severe papilledema (b).*

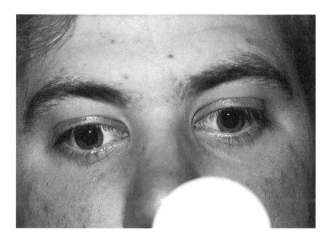

Figure 11.30 *Dorsal midbrain syndrome with severe accommodative convergence insufficiency and mydriatic pupils.*

comitant, incomitant or mimic an isolated vertical muscle paresis (Fig. 11.32). It is indicative of brainstem or cerebellar dysfunction, but has no other localizing value.[4]

It was found that the hypotropic eye in skew deviation was ipsilateral to the brainstem lesion in two-thirds of the patients studied. The brainstem lesion may be in the midbrain, pons or medulla; hence, there is no localizing value. Skew deviation may be mistaken for an isolated superior oblique paresis, but since cyclodeviation rarely occurs in skew deviation and almost always occurs in an isolated fourth-nerve palsy, the two should be readily differentiated.[5] It has also been reported in patients with elevated ICP and was reversible as the pressure was normalized.[6]

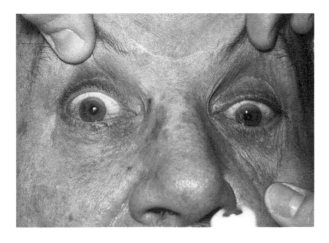

Figure 11.32   *Skew deviation due to brainstem infarction.*

ACQUIRED MONOCULAR ELEVATOR PALSY (AMPE)

Acquired monocular elevator palsy is a type of skew deviation resulting from a midbrain lesion immediately rostral to the oculomotor nuclei.[7] Patients experience sudden onset vertical diplopia. The lesion may be pretectal and supranuclear, leaving the doll's-head reflex and Bell's phenomenon intact (Fig. 11.29). It may also result from an infranuclear lesion of the fascicle with an absent doll's-head reflex and Bell's phenomenon.

BELL'S PHENOMENON

Upward and outward deviation of the eyes with forced eyelid closure results from unknown pathways between the seventh-nerve nucleus in the pons and the third-nerve nucleus in the rostral midbrain. In patients who cannot elevate their eyes (Fig. 11.29), the presence of eye elevation with forced eyelid closure indicates that the brainstem pathways, riMLF, motor neurons and extraocular muscles are functional. The upward gaze palsy must be due to a supranuclear lesion.

DOLL'S-HEAD REFLEX

As with Bell's phenomenon, an intact doll's-head reflex indicated that the vertical (or horizontal) gaze centers, motor neurons and extraocular muscles are functioning, and the lesion must be supranuclear. The patient with the vertical gaze palsy is asked to fixate an object and the chin is depressed (Fig. 11.29). If the eyes elevate, the doll's-

head reflex is present and the lesion is supranuclear. The same information can be obtained on comatose patients with bilateral warm- or cold-caloric testing. Cold water instilled into both ears causes a slow, tonic downward movement of both eyes. Warm water causes a slow, tonic upward movement of both eyes if the midbrain is intact.

FOURTH-NERVE PARESIS

The fourth (trochlear) nerve arises from the dorsal midbrain at the level of the inferior colliculi (Fig. 11.33). They cross in the anterior medullary velum in the roof of the fourth ventricle and sweep laterally around the midbrain to course rostrally toward the cavernous sinus. They enter it behind the posterior clinoid process, lying inferior to the third nerve and entering the orbit through the superior orbital fissure to innervate the superior oblique muscle.

Patients with acute fourth-nerve paresis present with vertical diplopia, often worse at near and in downgaze. They often complain of difficulty reading and walking downstairs, and adopt a compensatory head tilt (Fig. 11.34). Fourth-nerve pareses are the most common cause of acquired vertical strabismus in an ambulatory practice. Isolated fourth-nerve palsies are rarely of neuro-ophthalmologic significance. Most common etiologies are vasculopathic, traumatic and decompensated congenital pareses. Only rarely does an intracranial mass lesion present as a fourth-nerve paresis and even more rarely as an isolated palsy. Patients with isolated fourth-nerve palsies rarely require neuro-imaging. Orbital disorders that may mimic a fourth-nerve palsy include dysthyroid orbitopathy (Fig. 11.18),

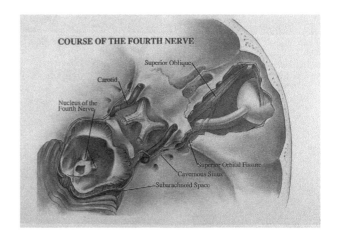

Figure 11.33   *Course of the fourth nerve from the brainstem to the superior oblique.*

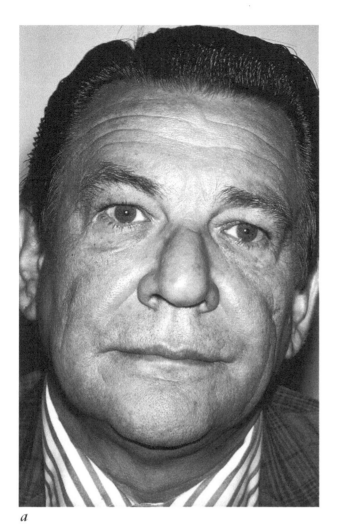

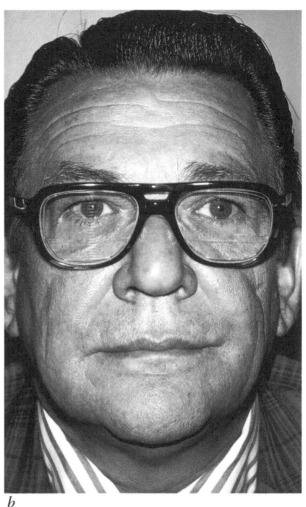

a   *b*

Figure 11.34   *A patient with right fourth-nerve palsy and a compensatory left head tilt (a). Head tilt resolved after treating hypertropia with a press-on prism (b).*

orbital tumors (Fig. 11.35) and orbital myositis of the superior oblique. These should be evident on clinical examination, imaged and treated appropriately. Brainstem lesions are an uncommon cause of isolated superior oblique palsies.[8]

Diagnosis of a recent-onset, isolated fourth-nerve paresis is clinical and should be obvious in most cases. Patients complain of vertical diplopia. The involved superior oblique may be detected utilizing the Parks' three-step test. A hypertropia is most always present in primary gaze (Fig. 11.36a). Make sure that the patient's head is in primary gaze before seeking the hypertropia. If a patient has adopted a compensatory head position, one may miss a subtle hypertropia if the head is not straightened during the examination. This is easily accomplished by placing your thumb in the patient's ear and fourth and fifth

fingers under the chin, thus straightening the head. The hypertropia increases in adduction of the involved eye (into the field of action of the underacting superior oblique and overacting inferior oblique) (Fig. 11.36b) and decreases in abduction of the involved eye (away from the field of action of the involved muscles) (Fig. 11.36c). The hypertropia increases when the head is tilted to the side of the involved muscle (Fig. 11.36d) and decreases when the head is tilted to the opposite side (Fig. 11.36e). If the three-step test localizes a paretic superior oblique, it is useful. The present author has not been impressed with its use to localize other cyclovertical deviations and has often been misled when using it to interpret anything but a superior oblique paresis.

The diagnosis of a superior oblique paresis may be obfuscated by spread of comitance with time. A careful

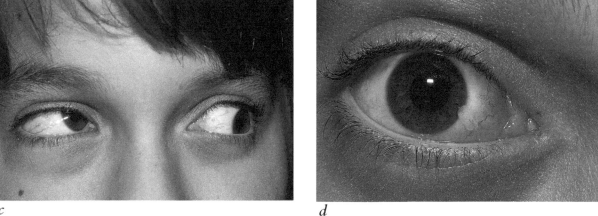

a

b

c

d

Figure 11.35 *A patient with a right hypertropia (a), underaction of the right superior oblique muscle (b) and overaction of the right inferior oblique (c) due to an anterior orbital lymphangioma (d).*

three-step test, with particular attention to the head tilt and measurement of the hypertropia in cardinal fields of gaze, will usually lead to the correct diagnosis.

Bilateral fourth-nerve palsies may present a diagnostic challenge. They should be suspected in any patient with significant antecedent head trauma. They almost exclusively occur after head trauma, although a small brain-stem infarction may involve both fourth-nerve nuclei. Patients with bilateral fourth-nerve paresis present differently to those with unilateral paresis. The vertical deviation is usually smaller and patients tend to adopt compensatory head positions permitting fusion in upgaze (Fig. 11.37). Excyclotorsion > 10° is present when measured with red and white Maddox prisms, and the head-tilt test is positive in both directions (Fig. 11.36). A right hypertropia increases with right head tilt and a left hypertropia is present on left head tilt.[9]

Head trauma, sometimes rather insignificant, is a common cause of fourth-nerve paresis (see Chapter 7).

The fourth nerve is susceptible to trauma in the midbrain at the anterior medullary velum and along its intracranial course to the cavernous sinus (Fig. 11.33). It is very susceptible to trauma in the region of the anterior cavernous sinus and orbital apex during cranio-orbital surgical procedures.

Patients with decompensated congenital or remotely acquired fourth-nerve palsies may present with complaints of acute onset vertical diplopia. A fourth-nerve paresis is diagnosed after performing the three-step test. The patient is asked to produce old, unposed photographs. These often reveal a longstanding head tilt, confirming the diagnosis of decompensated fourth-nerve paresis. Large amplitudes of vertical fusion are also indicative of a longstanding fourth-nerve paresis. No other evaluation is necessary. Treatment with prism or surgery can then be offered.

Vasculopathic fourth-nerve paresis may present in diabetics and other patients with vasculopathic risk factors.

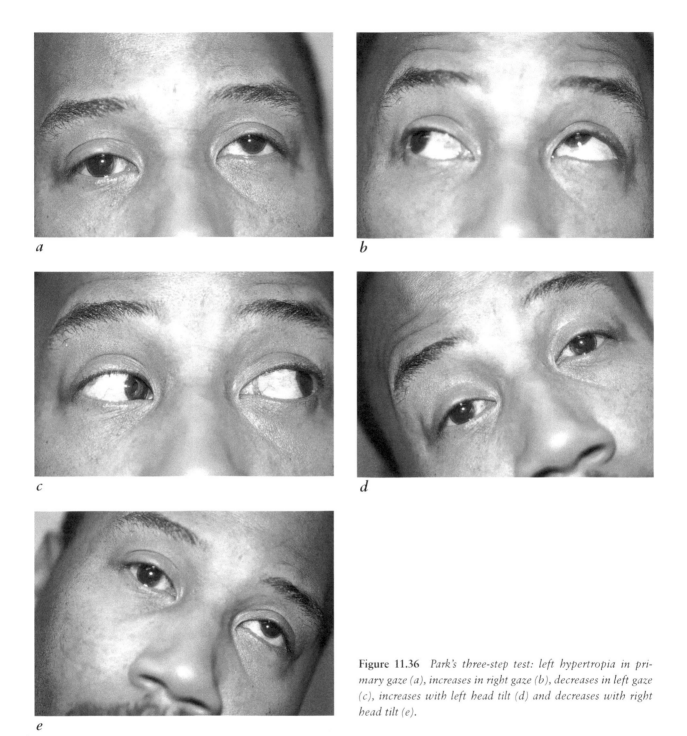

Figure 11.36 *Park's three-step test: left hypertropia in primary gaze (a), increases in right gaze (b), decreases in left gaze (c), increases with left head tilt (d) and decreases with right head tilt (e).*

Diabetic fourth-nerve palsies invariably get better in 60–90 days. Vasculopathic neuropathies in non-diabetics often improve spontaneously in 3–6 months. If stable, these may be treated with Fresnel press-on prisms (Fig.

11.34b). If they fail to resolve spontaneously, appropriate surgery is often successful. Patients with vasculopathic or traumatic fourth-nerve paresis will have normal amplitudes of vertical fusion, and an antecedent head tilt

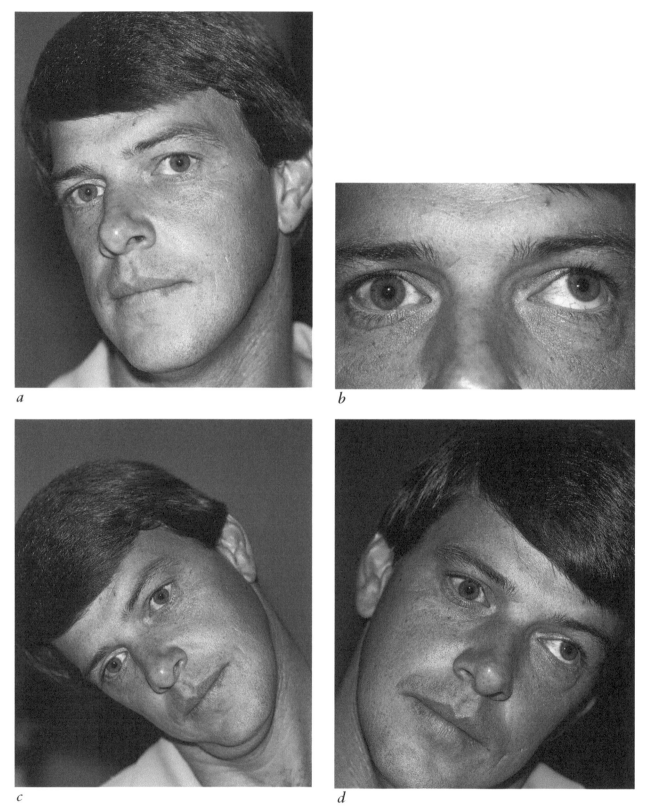

Figure 11.37   *Left superior oblique paresis superimposed upon a Duane's retraction syndrome type 2. The patient had adopted an unsightly head position (a). A large-angle left hypertropia was evident in primary gaze (b), and head tilt localized the left superior oblique paresis (c and d).*

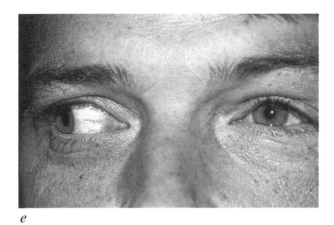
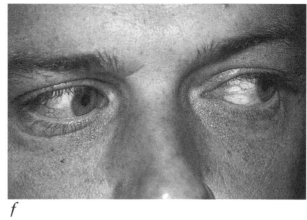

e   *f*

Figure 11.37 (cont.) *There was marked limitation of adduction and retraction of the globe (e). Ocular abduction was normal (f).*

will not be evident on review of old photographs. As with so many other disorders, the etiologies vary with the clinical environment.[10,11]

Fourth-nerve palsies may also be superimposed upon or coexist with other strabismus syndromes. Recognition will spare the patient the expense and anguish of an extensive neuroradiologic evaluation. A patient presented with an unsightly head position (Fig. 11.37a); straightening his head revealed a large left hypertropia (Fig. 11.37b), which on head-tilt testing localized to a left superior oblique palsy (Fig. 11.37c and d). Versions revealed marked limitation of adduction with retraction of the globe (Fig. 11.37e): ocular abduction was normal (Fig. 11.37f). This fourth-nerve palsy was superimposed upon a pre-existent Duane's retraction syndrome type 2.

OCULOMOTOR NERVE PALSIES

In Keane's series of patients with vertical diplopia, oculomotor nerve paresis was the most common etiology. Most third-nerve pareses are obvious (see Chapter 10); but a patient with an evolving or resolving third-nerve paresis may present complaining of vertical diplopia, and the etiology may not be obvious. Patients with isolated superior division third nerve palsies of either orbital or intracranial etiologies may also complain of vertical diplopia. This should be accompanied by ptosis of the upper eyelid (Fig. 11.38), since the third nerve divides into a superior and inferior branch as it enters the orbit. The superior division innervates the superior rectus and levator muscles. The inferior division innervates the medial rectus, inferior oblique, medial rectus, pupil and ciliary body. Isolated inferior (Fig. 11.39) or

superior division paresis (Fig. 11.38) often have an orbital etiology, but there have been well-documented reports of intracranial lesions presenting as isolated superior division third-nerve pareses.

EVOLVING OCULOMOTOR PARESIS

The patient in Fig. 11.40 complained of a recent-onset of vertical diplopia. He had adopted a mild chin-elevated head position. A small left hypertropia and exotropia was present in primary gaze (Fig. 11.40a). The extraocular motility deficit that increased in upgaze (Fig. 11.40b) did not localize. An orbital lesion was suspected and the patient sent for a CT scan. He returned 1 week later with a negative CT scan and an obvious pupil-sparing, right third-nerve paresis (Fig. 11.41). The small hypodeviation and limited elevation of the right eye (Fig. 11.40) was the initial manifestation of his vasculopathic third-nerve paresis.

A 60-year-old lady was referred with vertical diplopia. A small left hypertropia was present in primary gaze (Fig. 11.42a). Neuroimaging studies demonstrated a mass lesion in the left cavernous sinus (Fig. 11.42b) which proved to be undifferentiated carcinoma. An isolated vertical deviation may be the initial manifestation of a third-nerve paresis secondary to a mass lesion or even a vasculopathic process. If imaging studies of the appropriate areas are negative, edrophonium (Tensilon) testing should be done to rule out myasthenia gravis.

RESOLVING OCULOMOTOR PARESIS

A third-nerve paresis may resolve totally or partially. Partial resolution may result in a residual vertical or

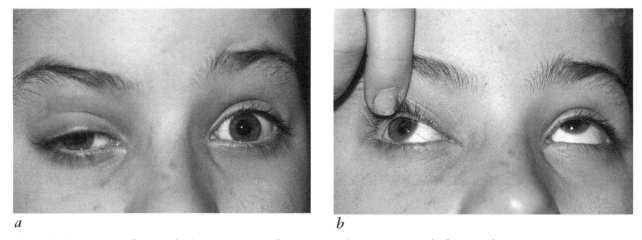

a

b

Figure 11.38 *Superior division third-nerve paresis with ptosis (a) and superior rectus dysfunction (b).*

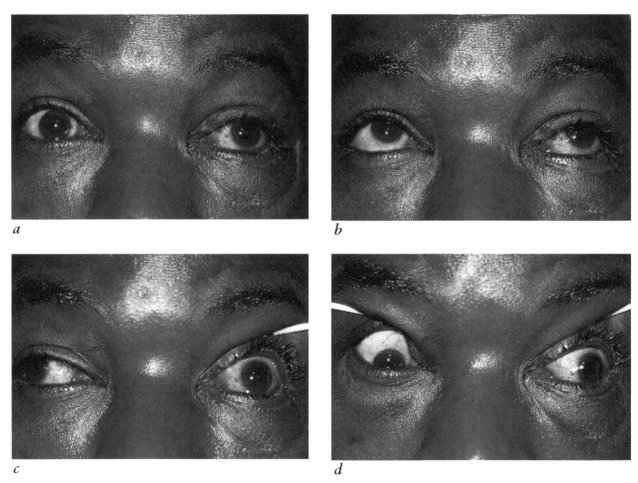

a

b

c

d

Figure 11.39 *Inferior division third-nerve paresis with an exotropia in primary gaze (a), normal elevation and upper eyelid function of the left eye (b), decreased adduction (c) and depression (d) of the left eye.*

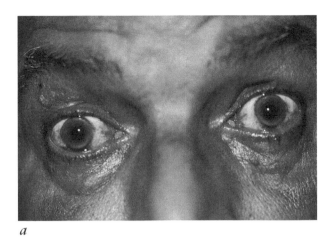
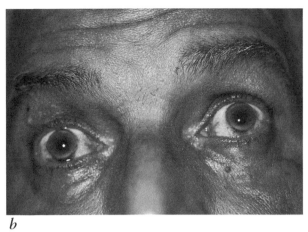

a   *b*

Figure 11.40   *Patient presenting with vertical diplopia, a right hypotropia (a) and decreased elevation of the right eye (b).*

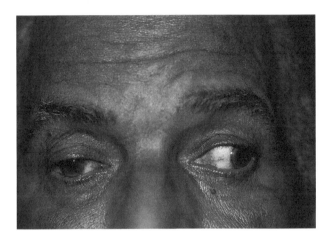

Figure 11.41   *The patient in Fig. 11.40 1 week later, with a vasculopathic third-nerve paresis evident.*

horizontal deviation. The pupil may remain dilated or normalize. If a previous third-nerve paresis was documented (Fig. 11.43), the diagnosis of a partially resolved third-nerve paresis is not difficult (Fig. 11.44). If an accurate history is not available, the diagnosis may be very difficult. Third-nerve palsies may also resolve with normal horizontal eye movements and partially or totally defective vertical motility (Fig. 11.45). After the motility defect has stabilized, appropriate eye muscle surgery may help restore some degree of binocular vision.

MYASTHENIA GRAVIS (MG)

MG may mimic any and all extraocular motility dysfunction and should be considered in any patient with

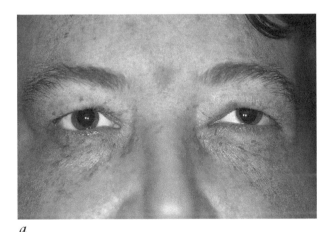
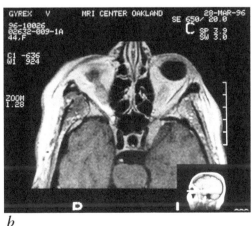

a   *b*

Figure 11.42   *A patient with vertical diplopia, a left hypertropia (a). An MRI scan demonstrates a cavernous sinus mass (b).*

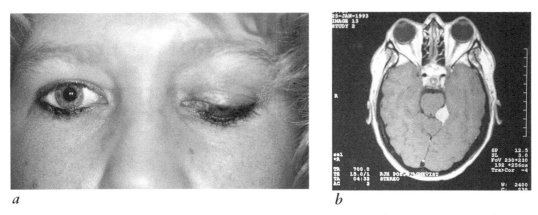

Figure 11.43 *Right third-nerve palsy (a) due to a meningioma compressing the nerve as it exits the brainstem (b).*

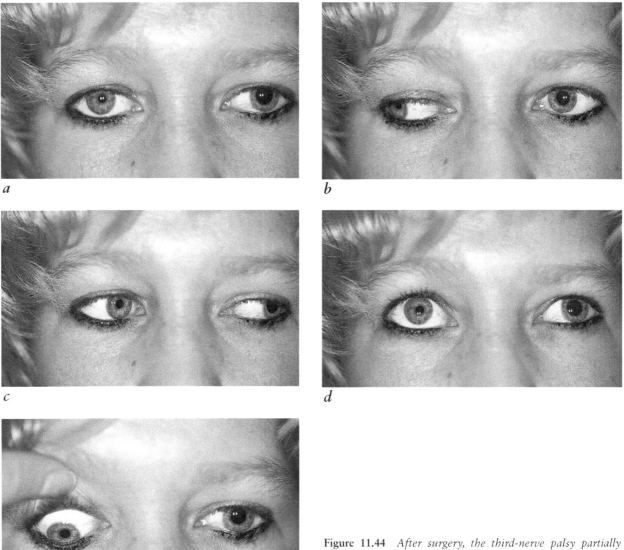

Figure 11.44 *After surgery, the third-nerve palsy partially resolved with normal levator function (a), improved adduction (b and c), decreased elevation (d) and absent depression (e). Note that the pupil remained fixed and dilated.*

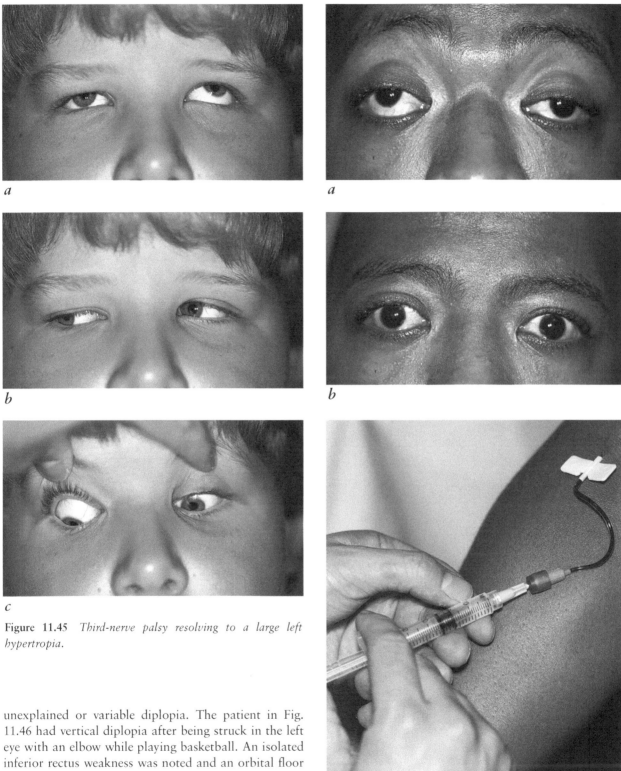

Figure 11.45 *Third-nerve palsy resolving to a large left hypertropia.*

unexplained or variable diplopia. The patient in Fig. 11.46 had vertical diplopia after being struck in the left eye with an elbow while playing basketball. An isolated inferior rectus weakness was noted and an orbital floor fracture suspected. A CT scan was normal and the vertical diplopia did not improve. On follow-up examination, he had obvious ptosis and a large exotropia (Fig. 11.46). A Tensilon test was markedly positive (Fig. 11.46b). When in doubt, consider MG.

Figure 11.46 *A patient with a right hypertropia and bilateral ptosis (a); ptosis and hypertropia completely resolved (b), after administration of intravenous Tensilon (c).*

REFERENCES

1. Keane JR. Vertical diplopia. *Semin Neurol* 1986; **6**:147–62.
2. Buttner-Ennever JA, Buttner U, Cohen B et al. Vertical gaze paralysis and the rostral interstitial nucleus of the medial longitudinal fasciculus. *Brain* 1982; **105**:125–35.
3. Keane JR. The pretectal syndrome: 206 patients. *Neurology* 1990; **40**:684–90.
4. Keane JR. Ocular skew deviation. *Arch Neurol* 1975; **32**:185.
5. Trobe JD. Cyclodeviation in acquired vertical strabismus. *Arch Ophthalmol* 1984; **102**:717.
6. Frohman LP, Kupersmith MJ. Reversible vertical ocular deviations associated with raised intracranial pressure. *J Clin Neuro-ophthalmol* 1985; **5**:158.
7. Ford CS, Schwartze GM Weaver RG et al. Monocular elevation paresis caused by an ipsilateral lesion. *Neurology* 1984; **34**:1264.
8. Thomke F, Ringel K. Isolated superior oblique palsies with brainstem lesions. *Neurology* 1999; **53**:682–5.
9. Kushner BJ. The diagnosis and treatment of bilateral masked superior oblique palsy. *Am J Ophthalmol* 1988; **105**:186–94.
10. Keane JR. Fourth nerve palsy: historical review and study of 215 inpatients. *Neurology* 1993; **43**:2439–43.
11. Von Noorden GK, Murray E, Wong SY. Superior oblique paresis: a review of 270 cases. *Arch Ophthalmol* 1986; **104**:1771–6.

Chapter 12 **Parasellar syndromes**

PARASELLAR SYNDROME (MULTIPLE OCULOMOTOR PARESES)[1]

The third, fourth and sixth branches of the fifth cranial nerves merge into the cavernous sinus (Fig. 12.1a and b). Patients with a combination of oculomotor nerve pareses have a cavernous sinus lesion until proven otherwise (Fig. 12.2).

A 43-year-old man was referred for evaluation of ptosis (Fig. 12.2). Examination demonstrated ptosis, an enlarged pupil, and adduction and abduction deficits (Fig. 12.2a and b). There was an obvious third- and sixth-nerve paresis. Imaging was directed at the cavernous sinus, which demonstrated a diffuse mass extending laterally (Fig. 12.3). At biopsy, it proved to be an undifferentiated carcinoma.

Patients with cavernous sinus lesions may also present with isolated cranial nerve paresis but these are often

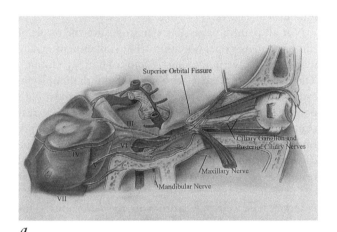

a

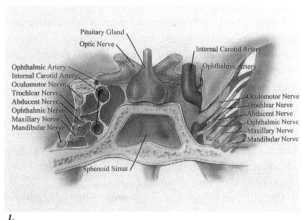

b

Figure 12.1 *Confluence of the oculomotor nerves in the cavernous sinus: lateral view (a); coronal view (b).*

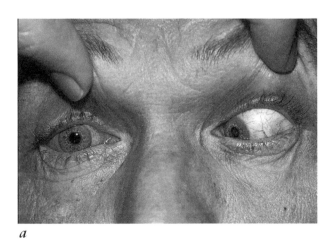

a

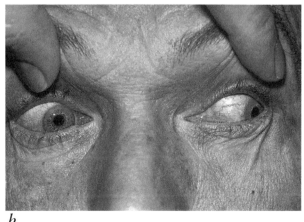

b

Figure 12.2 *Multiple oculomotor nerve palsies (third and sixth) are hallmarks of cavernous sinus lesions.*

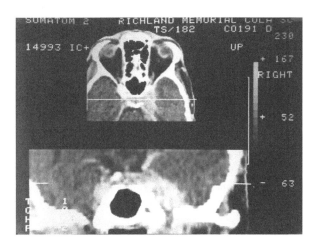

Figure 12.3 *A CT scan demonstrates a diffuse, enhancing mass in the right cavernous sinus.*

atypical, i.e. a partial third-nerve paresis that neither evolves nor improves (Fig. 12.4).

A 48-year-old lady presented with a left sixth-nerve paresis for several years prior to evaluation. Neuro-radiologic evaluation, albeit limited, was normal. She underwent eye muscle surgery for treatment of a large-angle esotropia. This obviated her diplopia. Several years later, diplopia recurred and she was referred for evaluation. A partial, pupil-sparing third-nerve paresis was evident (Fig. 12.5), as was a hint of left sixth-nerve paresis. A better computerized tomography (CT) scan visualizing the cavernous sinus demonstrated a mass (Fig. 12.6), which proved to be a carotid aneurysm.

The most common cavernous sinus lesions are carotid aneurysms, carotid–cavernous fistulae, meningiomas and metastatic carcinomas. Pituitary tumors can extend laterally and involve the cavernous sinus. Sphenoid sinus neoplasms can extend superiorly and involve the cavernous sinus, as can nasopharyngeal carcinomas.

Primary tumors in the lung, breast and prostate may metastasize to involve the cavernous sinus. These patients may present with periorbital pain along the distribution of the trigeminal nerve. Careful imaging of the cavernous sinus demonstrates an enhancing mass bulging the wall of the cavernous sinus laterally, appearing convex on coronal sections (Fig. 12.4b).

Squamous cell carcinomas from the facial skin, tongue or tonsil may extend perineurally and involve the cavernous sinus even years after 'complete' surgical excision ('cancer along a nerve'). These patients present with periorbital pain and cranial nerve findings. Initial imaging studies are often negative, or initially interpreted as negative. Eventually, symptoms and signs progress, the appropriate areas are imaged with contrast-enhanced magnetic resonance imaging (MRI), and the diagnosis established (Fig. 12.7).

Not all painful parasellar symptoms are the result of tumor or aneurysm. Idiopathic orbital inflammation may involve the cavernous sinus (Tolosa-Hunt syndrome). These patients present with painful ophthalmoplegia, exquisitely responsive to systemic corticosteroids, with pain being relieved almost immediately. The extra-ocular motility defects are a bit slower to respond. Imaging studies demonstrate enhancement of the cavernous sinus (Fig. 12.8). Failure to respond or partial response to corticosteroids should prompt further evaluation.

Other less welcome visitors to the cavernous sinus include infections due to syphilis, Lyme disease, fungi

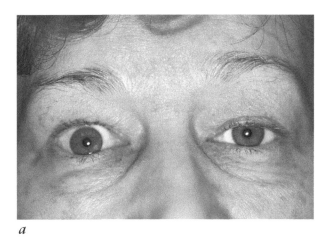

a

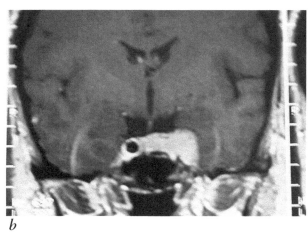

b

Figure 12.4 *Longstanding, pupil-sparing partial third-nerve paresis (a) in patient with a cavernous sinus meningioma evident on MRI (b).*

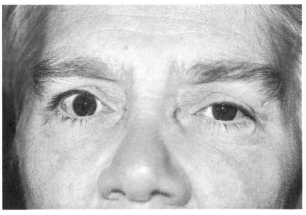

a

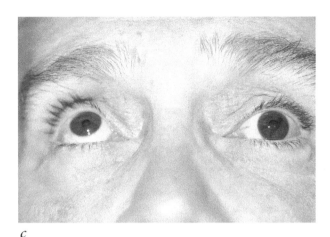

c

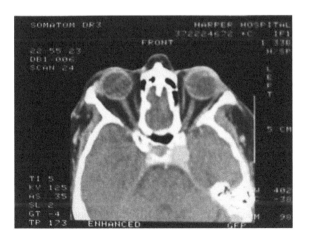

b

Figure 12.5   *Partial pupil-sparing, third-nerve paresis.*

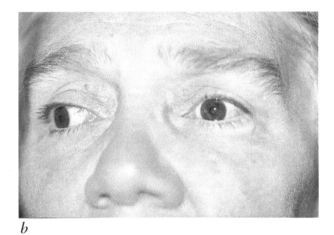

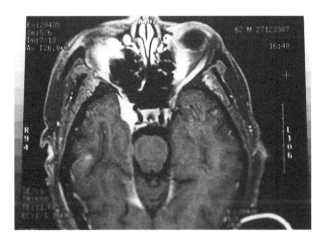

Figure 12.6   *A CT scan demonstrates an enhancing mass that proved to be an intracavernous carotid aneurysm.*

Figure 12.7   *An MRI scan demonstrating enhancement of the right cavernous sinus.*

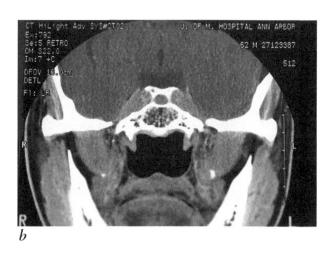

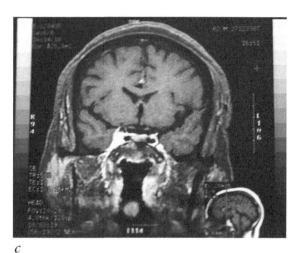

Figure 12.8 *A patient presenting with painful diplopia and a right sixth-nerve palsy (a). A CT scan demonstrates bilateral enlargement of the cavernous sinus (b); an enhanced MRI localizes inflammation to the right cavernous sinus (c).*

(aspergillosis, cryptococcosis), sarcoidosis, meningeal carcinomatosis and toxoplasmosis. The infectious elements should be especially suspected in patients with altered immunity.

CASE STUDY

A 36-year-old physician was referred with a painful sixth-nerve paresis (Fig. 12.9) after failing a trial of steroids. MRI demonstrated multiple intracranial lesions compatible with toxoplasmosis (Fig. 12.10). Further evaluation revealed HIV disease, which was known but

not volunteered. The patient refused further treatment and died of his disease.

CAROTID–CAVERNOUS FISTULAE[2–4]

Carotid artery–cavernous sinus fistulae may be a subtle (Fig. 12.11) or very obvious clinical diagnosis (Fig. 12.12). Subtle carotid–cavernous fistulae usually result from communication between a small dural arteriole (from the external carotid circulation) and the cavernous

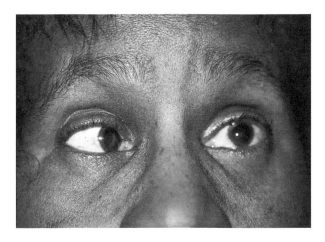

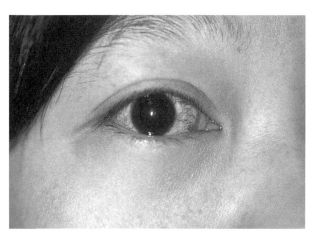

Figure 12.9 *Painful right sixth-nerve palsy as the presenting sign of diffuse cerebral toxoplasmosis.*

Figure 12.11 *A patient with a low-flow dural cavernous sinus fistula presenting as chronic conjunctivitis.*

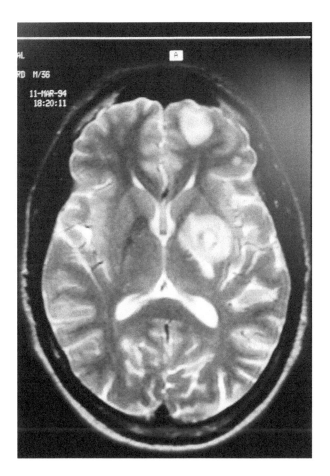

Figure 12.10 *An MRI scan demonstrates multiple toxoplasmosis lesions.*

sinus. This is a low-flow fistula, which is often misdiagnosed as a chronic red eye (Fig. 12.11), and should be considered in the differential diagnosis of a patient with chronic non-responsive 'conjunctivitis'. The most common findings are arterialized conjunctival vessels, proptosis and elevated intraocular pressure (IOP); but diplopia, ptosis, visual changes, venous stasis retinopathy and eyelid swelling may also occur.

If considered, the diagnosis is usually obvious and can be verified by carotid angiography. Angiography is usually diagnostic but the fistulae may be difficult to visualize, especially if the external carotid circulation is not imaged. Subtraction techniques may be very helpful in visualizing elusive fistulae. Twenty to 50% of the dural cavernous fistulae close spontaneously or after angiography.[2] Others may be closed by embolization techniques that are highly successful in skilled hands. These patients may also manifest enlargement of their superior ophthalmic veins on CT scan (Fig. 12.13) on ultrasonography. Although not diagnostic, this finding is highly suggestive in the appropriate clinical setting.

Obvious carotid–cavernous fistulae result from direct communication between the intracavernous carotid artery and the cavernous sinus. Symptoms are usually abrupt and progressive and include headache, ocular or orbital pain, blurred vision, diplopia and a subjective bruit. These patients have obvious arteriolization of their conjunctival vessels (Figs 12.12 and 12.14), an audible bruit and often multiple oculomotor nerve palsies or a frozen globe. Initial presentation may be

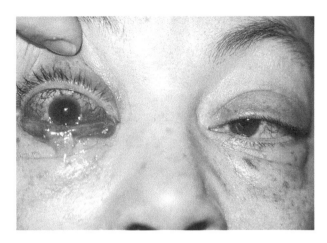

Figure 12.12 *Obvious carotid cavernous fistula with arteriolization of the conjunctival vessels.*

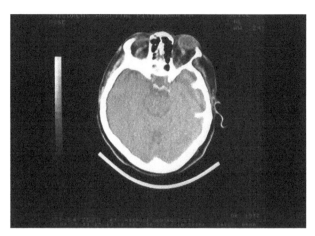

Figure 12.13 *A CT scan demonstrates enlargement of the superior ophthalmic vein, a soft but valid sign of a dural cavernous fistula.*

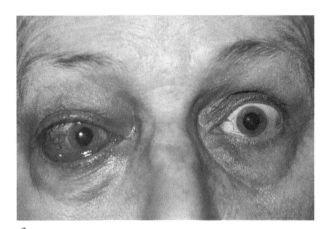

a   *b*

Figure 12.14 *A patient with a carotid–cavernous fistula presenting with proptosis (a) and a sixth-nerve paresis (b).*

much subtler, as in the lady in Fig. 12.15, who presented with a partial third-nerve palsy that developed into total ophthalmoplegia and partial visual loss over the course of 1 month.

In the cavernous sinus (Fig. 12.1b), sympathetic nerves innervating the pupil surround the carotid artery. The sixth nerve and the third nerve lie adjacent to the carotid artery. Subsequently, enlargement of fistulae from the carotid artery may initially present as an isolated third- or sixth-nerve paresis or a combination of the two (Figs 12.14 and 12.15).

CAROTID ANEURYSMS

Intracavernous carotid artery aneurysms rarely rupture, occur in older individuals and do not require the same degree of urgency as other intracranial aneurysms.[2,5] Patients may present with diplopia in extremes of gaze (sixth-nerve paresis), coupled with a partial third-nerve paresis (Fig. 12.5). Extreme periocular pain or dysesthesia (fifth nerve) may also accompany these signs. Pupillary findings are variable:

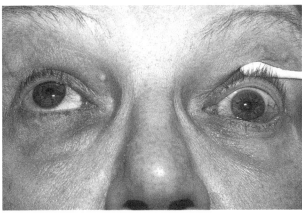

a

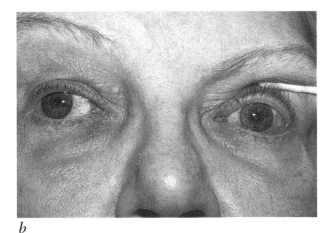

b

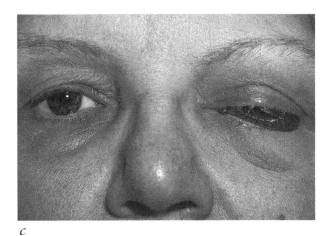

c

Figure 12.15 *A patient with a carotid–cavernous fistula presenting initially as a partial, pupil-sparing third-nerve paresis (a and b); 1 month later, extensive proptosis and conjunctival chemosis are evident (c).*

pupils may be partially dilated (third nerve) or constricted (sympathetic nerves along the carotid artery). Aberrant regeneration of the third nerve may be evident and, in the absence of an antecedent traumatic third-nerve paresis, primary aberrant regeneration should alert the clinician to a cavernous sinus tumor or aneurysm, especially in middle-aged to elderly women.

REFERENCES

1. Keane JR. Cavernous sinus syndrome. An analysis of 151 cases. *Arch Neurol* 1996; 53:967–71.
2. Kupersmith MJ. Neuro-vascular Neuro-ophthalmology. (Springer-Verlag; Berlin, 1993.)
3. Lewis AI, Tomsick TA, Tew JM Jr. Management of 100 direct carotid–cavernous sinus fistulas: results of treatment with detachable balloons. *Neurosurgery* 1995; 36:239–45.
4. Guo WY, Pan DH, Wu HM et al. Radiosurgery as a treatment alternative for dural arteriovenous fistulas of the cavernous sinus. *Am J Neuroradiol* 1998; 19:1081–7.
5. Linsky ME, Sekhar LN, Hirssch WL Jr et al. Aneurysms of the intracavernous carotid artery: natural history and indications for treatment. *Neurosurgery* 1990; 26:933–7.

Chapter 13 Orbital disorders

The orbit is a region of confluence for many surgical specialties. This is both an advantage and disadvantage to the unsuspecting patient. Surgeons may have a tendency to exceed the limits of their expertise as they delve from their area of expertise, i.e. sinus, mouth, brain or eyelid, into the orbit. These transgressions may cause anxiety for the surgeon and significant loss of visual function for the unsuspecting patient. Experienced orbital surgeons have developed great respect for potential complications and techniques to minimize potential loss of visual function. The occasional orbital surgeon often represents trouble waiting to happen.

Structures intrinsic or extrinsic to the orbit may result in proptosis and visual dysfunction. Understanding orbital disorders is facilitated by understanding its relationship to adjacent extrinsic structures (Figs 13.1 and 13.2), as well as intrinsic orbital anatomy. Superior to the orbit lies the anterior cranial fossa and frontal lobe of

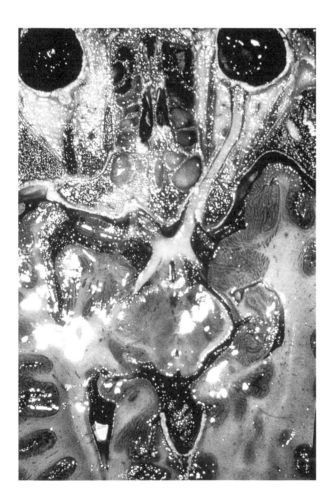

Figure 13.1 *Axial cadaver section demonstrates the relationship of the orbit to the ethmoid sinus medially, lateral orbital wall, optic canal, cavernous sinus and middle cranial fossa.*

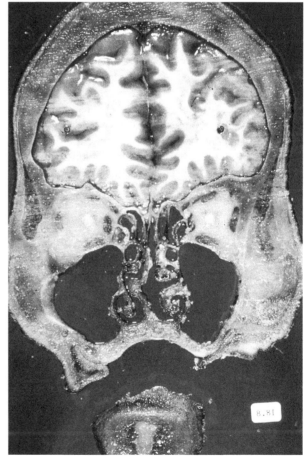

Figure 13.2 *Coronal cadaver section demonstrates the relationship between the orbit and the anterior cranial fossa, ethmoid sinus and the maxillary sinus.*

the brain. The maxillary sinus is inferior to the orbit. Medial to the orbit, separated by the thin lamina papyraciae, is the ethmoid sinus. Deep to the orbit is the middle cranial fossa, cavernous sinus, optic nerve and chiasm. Thinking of these adjacent structures and their relationship to the orbit is very helpful in delineating the cause and results of orbital dysfunction.

Infection, inflammation or tumor in the ethmoid, frontal or maxillary sinus, often initially presents as orbital dysfunction. Patients with a sinus mucocele often present with proptosis and deviation of the eye away from the involved sinus (Fig. 13.3). Computerized tomography (CT) scans demonstrate the contiguous sinus pathology (Fig. 13.4).

Tumors originating in the anterior or middle cranial fossae may involve the optic nerve or the orbit (Figs 13.5 and 13.6). Carotid–cavernous fistulae may have a dramatic orbital presentation (Fig. 13.7), while dural–cavernous fistulae present in a much more subtle fashion (Fig. 13.8). Periorbital trauma may involve the anterior or middle cranial fossae, transforming a seemingly trivial orbital injury into significant neurosurgical trauma (Fig. 13.9). Intrinsic orbital structures may also result in proptosis and visual dysfunction. Patients with disorders of the extraocular muscle, lacrimal gland, optic nerve and ciliary nerves will present with proptosis and visual dysfunction.

Once orbital dysfunction has been recognized and imaged, the clinician must decide if and how to treat the patient. Is it medical or surgical disease? If surgical, is it resectable and curable or should it be biopsied as conservatively as feasible? The present author's guidelines after 20 years of treating orbital disease remain that common things are common, but expect the unexpected. Secondly, if a patient has a history of cancer, regardless

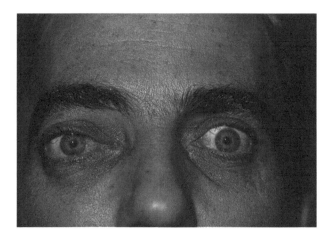

Figure 13.3 *Patient presenting with proptosis and exotropia.*

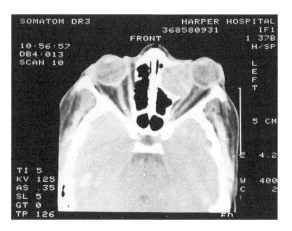

Figure 13.4 *A CT scan demonstrates a large ethmoid sinus mucocele.*

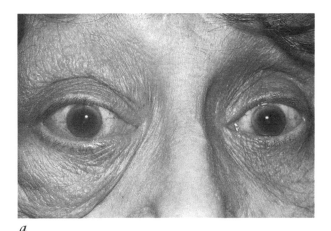

a

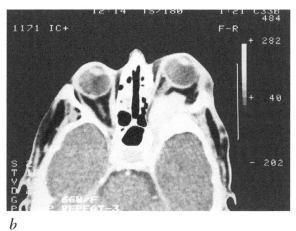

b

Figure 13.5 *A patient with proptosis and visual loss (a). A CT scan demonstrates a sphenoid ridge meningioma with intraorbital extension (b).*

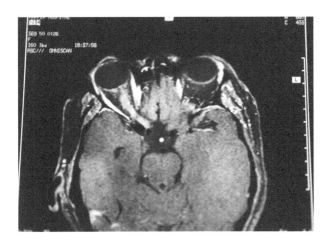

Figure 13.6 *MRI scan demonstrates enhancement of the intraorbital and intracranial optic nerve by a perioptic meningioma.*

of how remote, neuro-ophthalmologic and orbital manifestations are secondary to the malignancy until proven otherwise. Finally, a decision to totally resect or to only biopsy a lesion should be made prior to surgery based upon the imaging studies, and the selected surgical approach should keep the lesion between the surgeon's hands and the optic nerve.

In the past a great deal was made about evaluating the patient with orbital disease. Advances in neuro-imaging from CT to magnetic resonance imaging (MRI) and their widespread availability have made the prolonged examination of the proptotic patient all but obsolete. If a patient presents with proptosis, imaging is mandatory. It is equally important to personally review the imaging studies, especially when looking for subtle evidence for orbital disease. In a referral practice, patients present with two types of scans: great quality

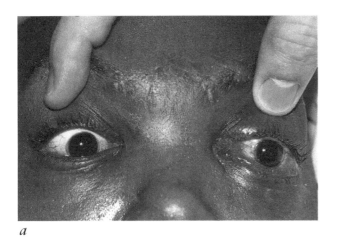

a

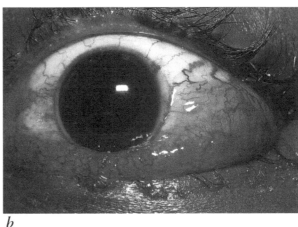

b

Figure 13.7 *A patient with traumatic carotid–cavernous fistula (a) and not so subtle (b) red eyes. Note the extensive arterialization of the conjunctival vessels.*

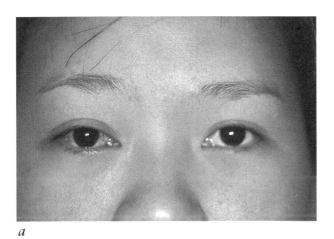

a

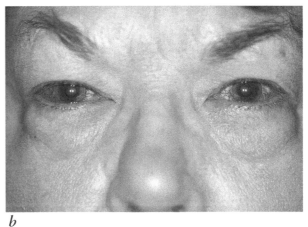

b

Figure 13.8 *A patient with a dural cavernous sinus fistula presenting with a more subtle, chronic red eye as opposed to the obvious arteriolized vessels (a). CT scans demonstrated enlarged superior ophthalmic veins in both patients.*

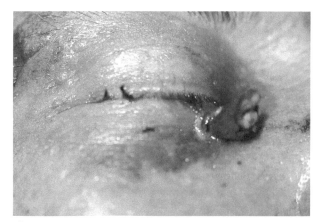

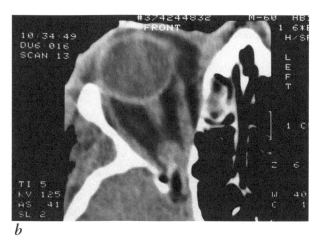

Figure 13.9 *A patient with a penetrating wound to the orbit (a). A CT scan demonstrates entry into the middle cranial fossa (b).*

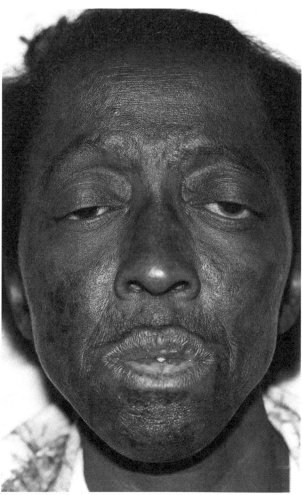

scans of the wrong area and poor quality scans of the appropriate region. This caveat has not changed from the CT to the MRI era.

A little common sense and clinical evaluation may spare the system the expense of an imaging study, or at least direct the clinician to order the appropriate imaging study. Which orbit is abnormal, the proptotic or the contralateral side? Pseudo-proptosis may result from an enlarged eye secondary to axial myopia (Fig. 13.10), ipsilateral eyelid retraction (Fig. 13.11) or contralateral ptosis (Fig. 13.12). Patients with contralateral enophthalmos due to orbital trauma, chronic maxillary sinusitis (Fig. 13.13) or metastatic scirrhous carcinoma (Fig. 13.14) may present or be referred with apparent proptosis of the normal eye. Scirrhous enophthalmos may result from metastatic breast or gastric carcinomas, or the scirrhous variety of idiopathic orbital inflammation.

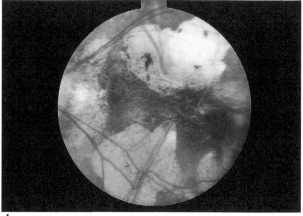

Figure 13.10 *Pseudoproptosis (a) secondary to unilateral high myopia (b).*

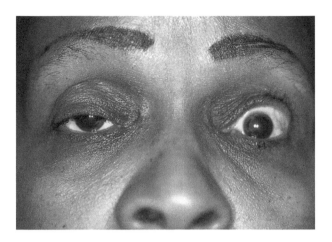

Figure 13.11 *Pseudoproptosis due to upper eyelid retraction.*

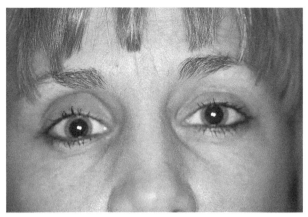

a

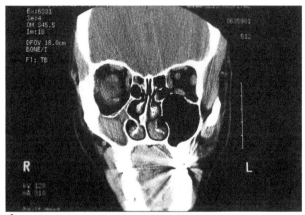

b

Figure 13.13 *Pseudoproptosis due to enophthalmus caused by contralateral chronic maxillary sinusitis.*

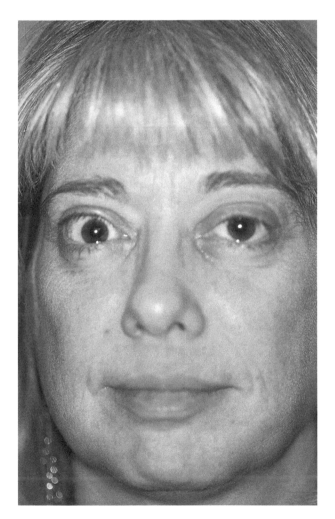

Figure 13.12 *Pseudoproptosis due to ptosis of the contralateral upper eyelid.*

CT scans should be obtained on any patient with real proptosis, a palpable orbital mass, orbital infection, inflammation or adjacent sinus disease involving the orbit. The present author prefers CT to MRI for the initial evaluation of orbital disorders. The CT scan allows one to discern the density, location and extent of the lesion, and any abnormalities of the orbital bones or adjacent sinuses. The MRI scan allows one to differentiate an encapsulated lesion from the adjacent optic nerve (Fig. 13.15). This can be invaluable in surgical decision-making. An encapsulated lesion that is separate from the optic nerve is resectable and should be completely removed.

Papers describing the incidence and frequency of any orbital disorder are marred by the referral bias of the practice or institution from where the data were obtained. An institution with a prominent ENT oncology program will have an overwhelming number of sinus tumors

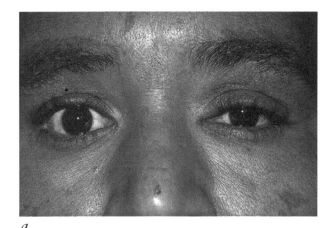
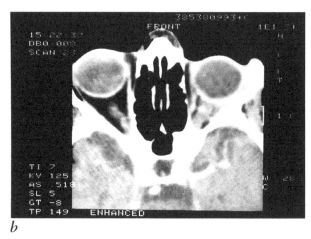

a *b*

Figure 13.14 *Pseudoproptosis (a) due to contralateral enophthalmos due to scirrhous breast carcinoma (b).*

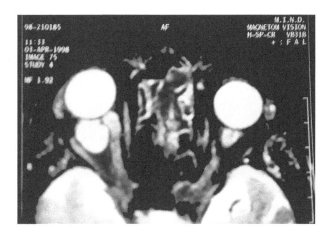

Figure 13.15 *An MRI scan differentiates encapsulated orbital mass from the adjacent optic nerve.*

involving the orbit, while an institution with a strong neurosurgical department will be biased towards intracranial meningiomas and gliomas with secondary orbital involvement. An ophthalmologic orbital practice will be biased towards primary orbital diseases and tumors: dysthyroid orbitopathy, orbital inflammation, cellulitis and encapsulated tumors.

SECONDARY ORBITAL TUMORS

Paranasal sinuses lie superior, inferior and medial to the orbit. Tumors, infections and inflammations of the paranasal sinuses may present with orbital manifesta-

tions of proptosis, pain, decreased vision or double vision. CT scans will delineate the pathology and direct appropriate treatment by the appropriate specialist.

ORBITAL CELLULITIS

Orbital cellulitis is usually the result of infection in the ethmoid sinus. Infection enters the orbit through the thin medial orbital wall (see Fig. 13.1) resulting in a diffuse orbital infection or a localized sub-periosteal abscess (Figs 13.16 and 13.17). Orbital infections anterior to the orbital septum are much more benign than infections posterior to the orbital septum. A patient with a preseptal cellulitis presents with pain, erythema and swelling of the anterior orbit (Fig. 13.18). The key issue is that there is no visual dysfunction. Specifically, there is no evidence for optic nerve or extraocular motility dysfunction. Patients with postseptal cellulitis may have decreased vision, a relative afferent pupillary defect (RAPD), extraocular motility dysfunction and proptosis (Figs 13.16 and 13.17). This represents a relative ophthalmologic emergency and requires prompt aggressive treatment with appropriate doses of intravenous antibiotics and occasionally timely surgery, especially if a sub-periosteal abscess is present and visual function does not improve shortly after initiation of antibiotic therapy. There is controversy in the literature as to when and if surgery is necessary,[1] but certainly a patient with a sub-periosteal abscess whose visual function does not improve or has deteriorating visual function during medical treatment deserves drainage of their abscess. These

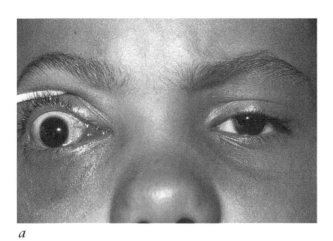

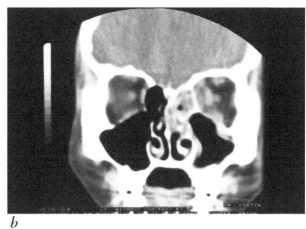

a   *b*

Figure 13.16 *Orbital cellulitis due to a subperiosteal abscess (a). A coronal CT scan demonstrates adjacent ethmoid sinusitis (b).*

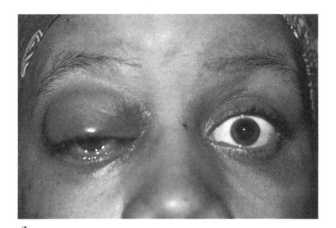

a

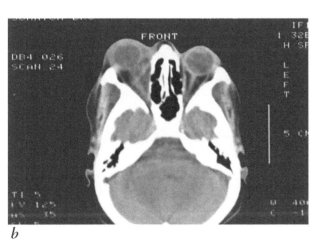

b

Figure 13.17 *A patient with orbital cellulitis (a). A CT scan demonstrates a subperiosteal abscess with no evidence of ethmoiditis (b).*

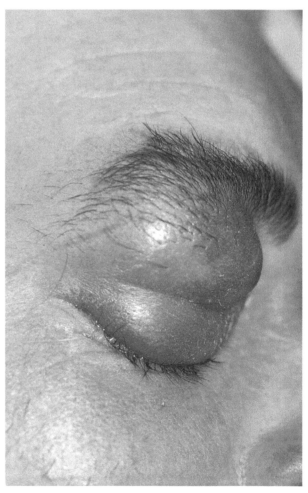

Figure 13.18 *Preseptal cellulitis.*

lesions are easily and safely accessible in the appropriate sub-periosteal space.

Orbital infections need to be differentiated from dacryocystitis—an infection of the lacrimal sac that is confined within the sac and its surrounding periosteum (Fig. 13.19). Patients with acute dacryocystitis should not undergo lacrimal probing and attempted irrigation, for such manipulation may violate the periosteum and spread the confined lacrimal sac infection into the orbit (Fig. 13.20). Appropriate treatment for dacryocystitis is parenteral antibiotics and external incision and drainage if necessary (Fig. 13.21).

MENINGIOMAS

Sphenoid ridge meningiomas may compress the adjacent orbit by enlargement of the sphenoid ridge, causing proptosis and diplopia due to extraocular motility dysfunction

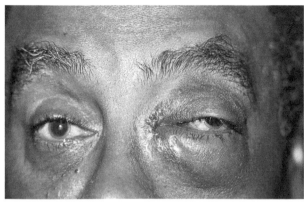

a

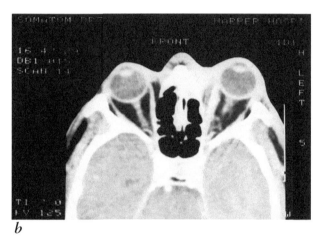

b

Figure 13.20 *Orbital cellulitis after misguided probing in patient with dacryocystitis (a). A CT scan demonstrates orbital abscess (b).*

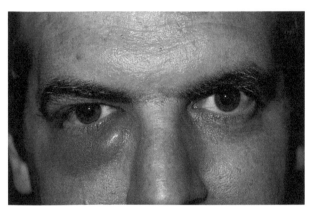

a

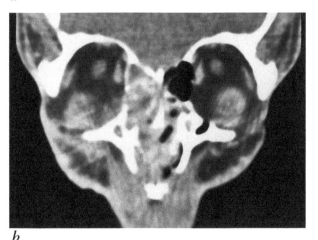

b

Figure 13.19 *Atypical dacryocystitis with extensive pansinusitis present on a CT scan.*

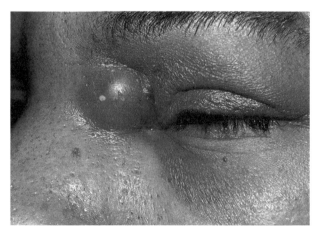

Figure 13.21 *Acute dacryocystitis. Appropriate treatment entails incision and drainage and parenteral antibiotics.*

(Fig. 13.22). This sphenoid ridge enlargement must be differentiated from fibrous dysplasia (Fig. 13.23) and an uncommon, osteoblastic form of metastatic prostate carcinoma (Fig. 13.24). Sphenoid ridge meningiomas may also invade the orbit as well as compress it. These patients present with proptosis, motility dysfunction and eyelid edema (Figs 13.5 and 13.22). Treatment is primarily neurosurgical extirpation of the tumor, with careful removal of the orbital component if present (Fig. 13.25).

Perioptic and planum sphenoidale meningiomas (Fig. 13.6) are discussed in the section on optic neuropathies since that is their primary mode of presentation.

ORBITAL INFLAMMATION

Orbital inflammatory disease may affect any portion of the orbit and often presents with pain and visual dys-

function. The entire orbit may be diffusely involved (Fig. 13.26) or just one orbital structure (Fig. 13.27). Orbital inflammation may have a specific etiology—sarcoidosis, vasculitis or Wegener's granulomatosis (Fig. 13.28)—but is most often idiopathic, occurring without an obvious cause.

Idiopathic orbital inflammation (IOI) may affect any and all orbital structures. Presenting signs and symptoms depend upon which orbital structures are inflamed. Patients with very anterior orbital inflammation present with the ultimate red eye. Patients with periscleritis present with an intensely painful inflamed eye (Fig. 13.26). Vision may or may not be affected; decreased vision usually results from macular edema, exudation and stria caused by posterior periscleral inflammation (Fig. 13.26c).

If the optic nerve is involved, patients may have profound, painful visual loss accompanied by a painful, red eye (Fig. 13.29a and b). The optic disc may appear swollen or normal (Fig. 13.29c). If only the optic nerve sheath is swollen (perineuritis), visual function may be

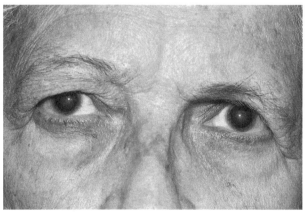

a

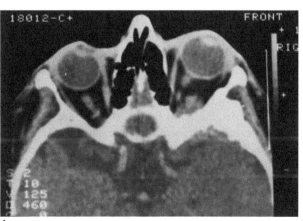

b

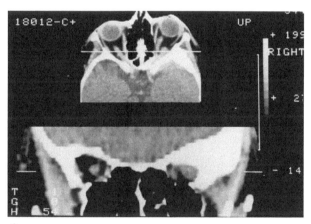

c

Figure 13.22 *A patient with a sphenoid ridge meningioma (a). CT scans demonstrate hyperostosis of the sphenoid ridge and orbital invasion (b and c).*

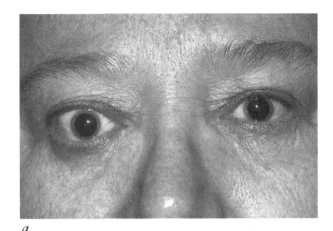

a

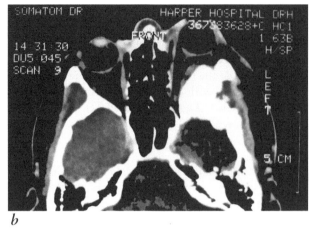

b

Figure 13.23 *A patient with isolated proptosis (a) as a presenting sign of fibrous dysplasia of the sphenoid ridge (b).*

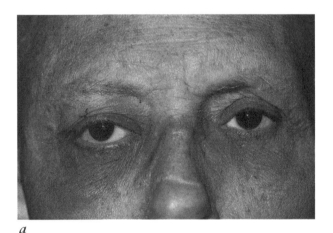

a

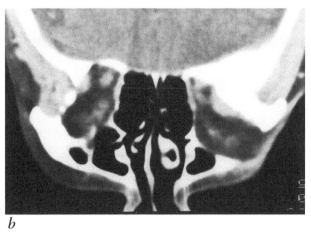

b

Figure 13.24 *A patient with metastatic prostatic carcinoma (a). A CT scan demonstrates osteoblastic metastasis with orbital involvement (b).*

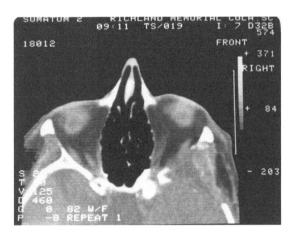

Figure 13.25 *A postoperative CT scan demonstrating total removal of the sphenoid ridge and orbital tumor in the patient shown in Fig. 13.22.*

quite normal. Patients with posterior orbital/cavernous sinus inflammation present with painful extraocular motility dysfunction with or without visual loss and a quiet eye (Figs 13.30 and 13.31).

Orbital myositis represents inflammation of one, several or all extraocular muscles. The presenting ocular motility dysfunction depends upon which extraocular muscles are inflamed. Patients with isolated medial rectus involvement will present with painful abduction or adduction defects (Fig. 13.32). CT scans demonstrate enlargement of the involved medial rectus muscle (Fig. 13.32c). Extraocular muscle enlargement secondary to IOI usually involves the tendon inserting upon the globe (Fig. 13.33a), whereas muscles enlarged by dysthyroid orbitopathy spare the tendon (Fig. 13.33b).

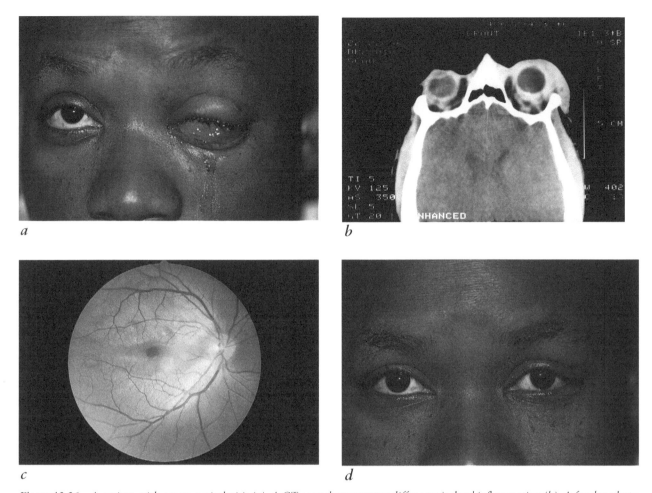

Figure 13.26 *A patient with severe periscleritis (a). A CT scan demonstrates diffuse periscleral inflammation (b). A fundus photo demonstrates macular edema and stria secondary to adjacent inflammation (c). Total resolution several days after parenteral corticosteroids (d).*

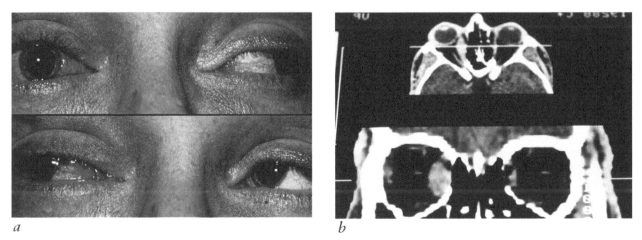

Figure 13.27 *Orbital myositis involving the medial rectus muscle causing painful restriction of ocular adduction (a). A CT scan demonstrates isolated enlargement of the medial rectus muscle (b).*

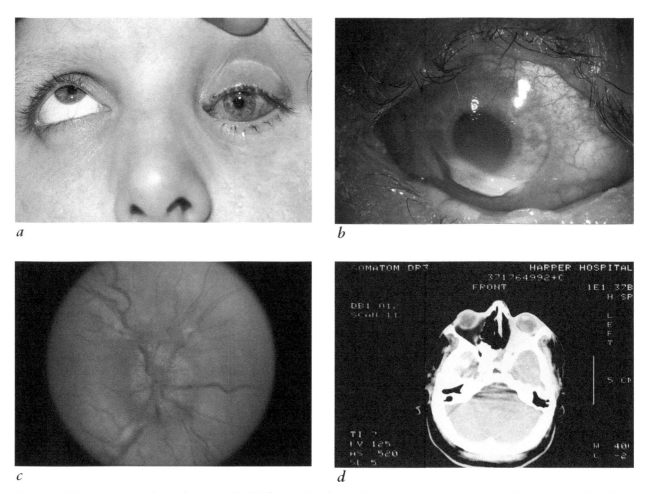

Figure 13.28 *A patient with unrelenting orbital inflammation due to Wegener's granulomatosis (a). Visual loss resulting from peripheral corneal melts (b) and optic disc edema (c). A CT scan demonstrates diffuse orbital inflammation with intracranial extension (d).*

Patients with isolated lacrimal gland involvement present with orbital pain and an 'S' ptosis (Fig. 13.34a). CT scans demonstrate enlargement of the orbital lobe of the lacrimal gland (Fig. 13.34b).

Idiopathic orbital inflammation—posterior or anterior, diffuse or localized—should respond quickly, dramatically and completely to appropriate corticosteroid therapy (Fig. 13.35). Patients who fail to respond, respond incompletely or whose imaging studies do not normalize should be biopsied. Lymphomas may partially respond to corticosteroid treatment (Fig. 13.36), as may metastatic tumors (Fig. 13.37). Incomplete response or recrudescence of symptoms while steroids are being tapered should prompt repeat imaging studies and biopsy of suspicious lesions (Fig. 13.38).

The most common error the present author has observed in the management of IOI is inappropriate steroid treatment, usually too little for too short a time. Prednisone 80 mg/day should be continued for 2 weeks then tapered by 20 mg every 2 weeks.[2] Patients who respond initially and then have a recurrence of symptoms should be re-imaged. Suspicious lesions should be biopsied. If the diagnosis remains IOI, the dose of prednisone may be increased. Doubling the present dose seems to be a reasonable and effective approach, i.e. if symptoms recur while the patient is taking 20 mg/day, increase the dose to 40 mg/day. Patients who fail to respond to corticosteroids may respond to low-dose (2000 G) orbital irradiation.[3]

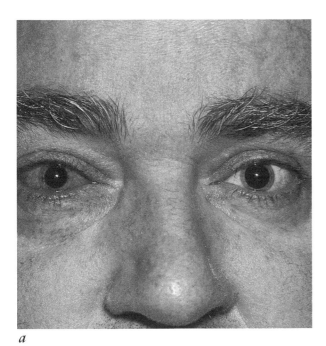

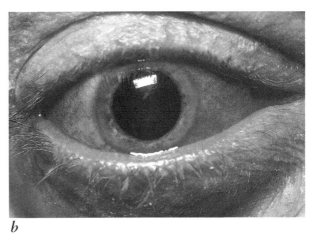

Figure 13.29 *A patient with periscleritis (a), the ultimate painful, red eye (b). Contiguous optic nerve sheath inflammation presents with optic disc swelling and normal visual function (perineuritis) (c).*

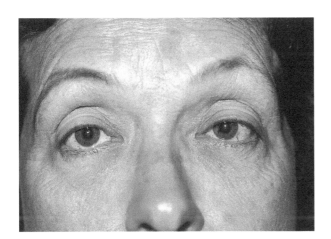

Figure 13.30 *A patient with acute-onset, painful left esotropia due to sixth-nerve paresis caused by cavernous sinus inflammation (Tolosa-Hunt syndrome).*

DYSTHYROID ORBITOPATHY

Thyroid eye disease is one of the great imitators in ophthalmology. If not considered, the diagnosis is often missed by a variety of subspecialists. Thyroid eye disease is a clinical diagnosis, sometimes confirmed by laboratory findings.

EYELIDS

Dysthyroid eyelid retraction of upper or lower lids or both is often the clinically obvious cause of a patient's complaints of irritated eyes (Fig. 13.39). Eyelid findings can be much more subtle and subtle eyelid retraction is often overlooked (Fig. 13.40). The diagnosis of dysthyroid eyelid retraction should be actively sought in

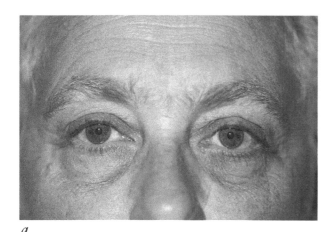
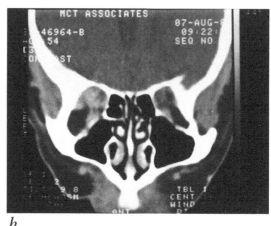

Figure 13.31 *A patient presenting with painful proptosis and a quiet eye (a) due to posterior orbital inflammation, evidenced on a CT scan (b).*

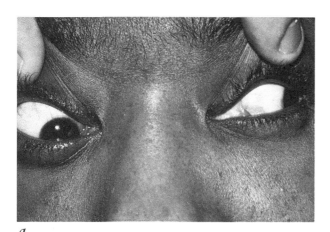
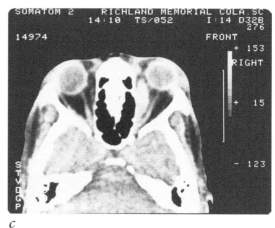

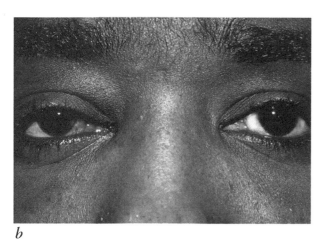

Figure 13.32 *A patient presenting with painful diplopia and defective ocular adduction (a). Note the sector inflammation over the medial rectus muscle insertion (b). A CT scan demonstrates marked enlargement of the medial rectus and its tendon (c).*

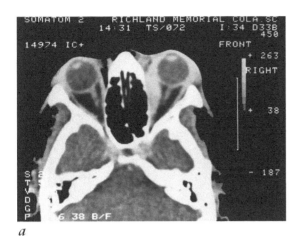
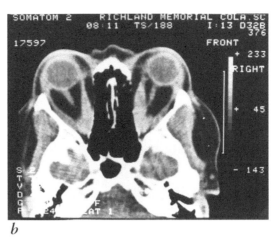

a   *b*

Figure 13.33   *A CT scan comparing orbital myositis (a) and dysthyroid orbitopathy (b). Note that the muscle tendon is involved anteriorly in myositis (a), while the muscle tendons are spared in dysthyroid orbitopathy (b). Also note that the muscle enlargement is primarily anterior in myositis and posterior in dysthyroid orbitopathy.*

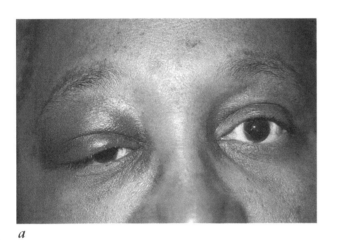
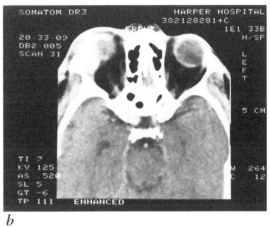

a   *b*

Figure 13.34   *Orbital inflammation with the distinctive S-ptosis in patient with dacryoadenitis (a). A CT scan demonstrates diffuse enlargement of the lacrimal gland (b).*

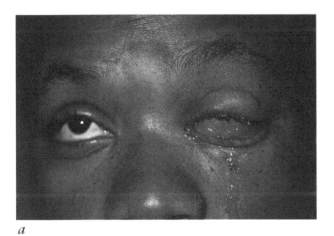
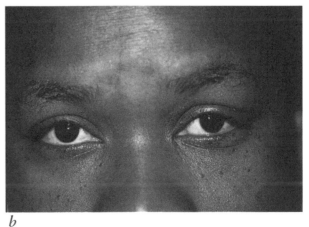

a   *b*

Figure 13.35   *Patients with idiopathic orbital inflammation (a) should have a rapid and total resolution after appropriate steroid therapy (b).*

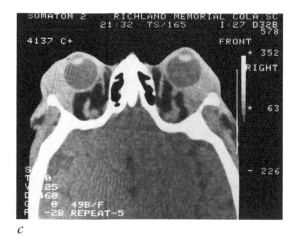

a

b

c

Figure 13.36 *A patient with presumed, bilateral dacryo-adenitis (a) only partially responded to 2 weeks of appropriate steroid therapy (b). A CT scan demonstrates well-demarcated lacrimal gland enlargement (c) that proved to be malignant lymphoma.*

any patient complaining of ocular irritation, photo-phobia, foreign-body sensation or other dry-eye symptoms.

KERATOPATHY

A 65-year-old lady was referred to a corneal specialist with the diagnosis of neurotropic keratitis. Her corneas were eroded and stained with fluorescein. She was referred to the neuro-ophthalmology service for evaluation of her extraocular motility dysfunction which was thought to be progressive external ophthalmoplegia. Horizontal and vertical gaze were both significantly restricted and corneal erosions were evident, as was marked eyelid retraction (Fig. 13.41). Eyelid retraction is not compatible with the diagnosis of chronic progressive external ophthalmoplegia. The patient also had a history of a recent 20-pound weight loss and was very tachycardic. Endocrinologic evaluation confirmed hyperthyroidism. A CT scan demonstrated marked enlargement of her extraocular muscles (Fig. 13.42), causing her motility dysfunction.

PROPTOSIS

Most patients with proptosis secondary to dysthyroid orbitopathy with eyelid retraction or eyelid signs probably have another cause for their proptosis and should be imaged by CT or MRI scans. This distinction is academic since the present author images the orbits of all patients with apparent proptosis. A patient with proptosis, eyelid retraction, equivocal clinical optic nerve compression and very significant enlargement of the apical orbital extraocular muscles (Fig. 13.43) would be treated initially for dysthyroid optic neuropathy by surgical decompression of the orbital apex (external ethmoidectomy and medial orbital wall decompression). If there were no significant extraocular muscle enlargement at the orbital apex, eye muscle or eyelid surgery would be performed as indicated rather than orbital decompression.

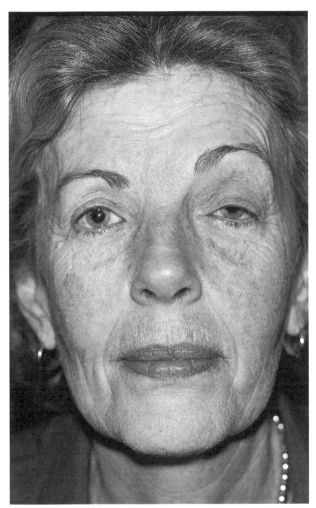

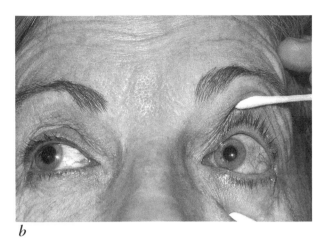

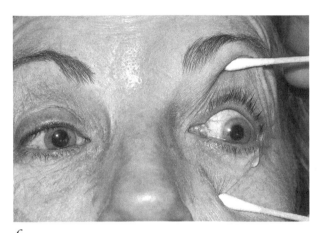

Figure 13.37 *A patient presented with painful ptosis (a), diplopia with restricted ductions (b and c). A CT scan demonstrates a ring-enhancing medial orbital mass (d).*

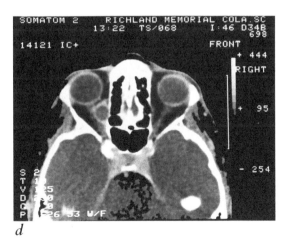

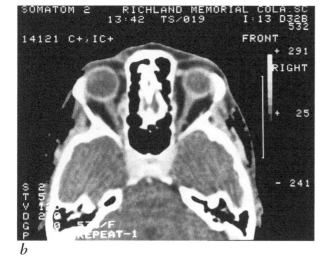

a

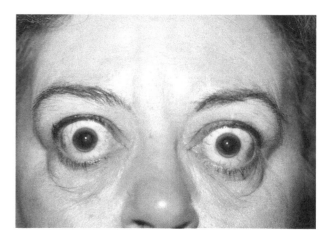

Figure 13.39 *Dysthyroid orbitopathy with obvious retraction of all four eyelids.*

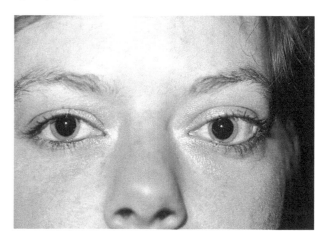

Figure 13.40 *Subtle dysthyroid orbitopathy with temporal retraction of the left upper eyelid.*

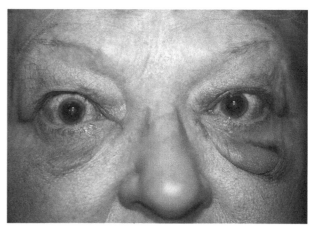

b

Figure 13.38 *Total resolution of signs and symptoms in the patient shown in Fig. 13.37 after an appropriate course of corticosteroids (a). A repeat CT scan demonstrates a residual orbital mass (b) that proved to be metastatic melanoma.*

Figure 13.41 *Patient with upper eyelid retraction, exposure keratopathy and restriction of extraocular motility due to dysthyroid orbitopathy.*

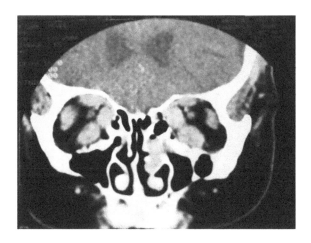

Figure 13.42 *A CT scan demonstrates marked enlargement of the extraocular muscles.*

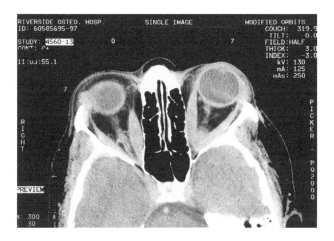

Figure 13.43 *A CT scan demonstrates enlargement of the posterior extraocular muscles compressing the optic nerves at the orbital apex, left side more than right.*

OCULAR HYPERTENSION

Ocular hypertension is common in patients with thyroid-associated orbitopathy (TAO), occurring in 24% of patients in a recent large series.[4,5] Although ocular hypertension is common, progression to glaucomatous damage is rare, occurring only in patients with persistent, active orbital involvement and chronically elevated intraocular pressure (IOP). The majority of patients with TAO and elevated IOP do not develop glaucomatous optic nerve or visual field changes. Elevated IOP in patients with TAO may occur due to tethering of the globe by fibrotic rectus muscles, orbital congestion causing elevated episcleral venous pressure decreasing aqueous outflow, mucopolysaccaride deposition in the trabecular meshwork or a direct thyrotoxic effect.[5]

Patients with ocular hypertension and TAO are often overtreated for their ocular hypertension, especially if the thyroid orbitopathy is unrecognized. Illustrative cases may be found in the section on pseudoglaucoma.

The diagnosis of TAO should be considered in patients with ocular hypertension, where it may be a presenting sign. The ocular hypertension is unlikely to cause glaucomatous visual field or optic nerve changes and so should not be treated aggressively. Visual field changes in a patient with TAO are much more likely due to optic nerve compression at the orbital apex and should be treated accordingly (see below).

DYSTHYROID OPTIC NEUROPATHY (DON)

Compression of the optic nerve at the orbital apex by enlarged extraocular muscles (Fig. 13.43) should be considered in any patient with TAO and may be the initial manifestation. Patients may have obvious TAO (Fig. 13.44) and visual loss. Visual dysfunction may be much more subtle and occur in the absence of other manifestations of TAO. The patient in Fig. 13.45 was referred with progressive visual loss of unknown etiology. There was minimal proptosis but a definite RAPD. The CT scan (Fig. 13.45b) demonstrated bilateral apical orbital compression by enlarged extraocular muscles. Her oriental lid creases and dermatochalasis masked eyelid retraction (Fig. 13.45a).

The patient in Fig. 13.46 was followed for many years with vague visual complaints treated with new refractions. He sought a second opinion. The presence of a left RAPD and mild proptosis prompted a visual field, which demonstrated a peripheral defect, and a CT scan (Fig. 13.46b and c), which demonstrated apical orbital optic nerve compression by a markedly enlarged left medial rectus muscle. Additional illustrative case histories may be found in the section on compressive optic neuropathies.

Patients with TAO may develop optic nerve compression at any time regardless of the status of their disease and thyroid function. Patients most commonly develop orbitopathy within 18 months of treatment of their thyroid dysfunction and the disease often runs its course within 36 months, but this is not universal.[6,7]

There is no consensus of opinion as to the appropriate treatment for patients with DON. There are vocative advocates of corticosteroids—oral and intravenous

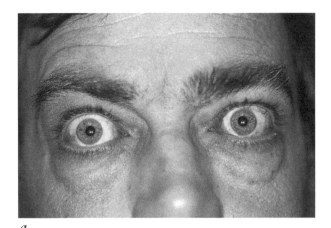
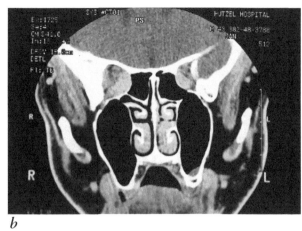

a   *b*

Figure 13.44   *A patient with severe dysthyroid orbitopathy (a). A CT scan demonstrates total compression of the optic nerve by enlarged extraocular muscles (b).*

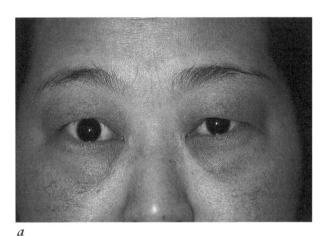
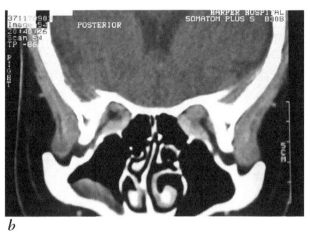

a   *b*

Figure 13.45   *A patient with dysthyroid orbitopathy and minimal eyelid signs masked by an oriental lid crease and dermatochalasis (a). A CT scan demonstrates apical orbital optic nerve compression (b).*

—orbital apical irradiation[8] and surgical decompression of the orbital apex.[9,10]

Many patients initially respond to corticosteroids, which actually shrink the inflamed extraocular muscles and decompress the orbital apex. As steroids are tapered, some patients maintain their improvement but others have a recrudescence of visual dysfunction. These patients may be treated with irradiation of the orbital apex (2000 rads). This is ostensibly a safe dose for the optic nerve and retina. However, radiation retinopathy is a well-described complication of this treatment, especially in myopic patients whose eyes are a bit longer and extend into the field of irradiation. Additionally, a recent prospective, randomized study from the Mayo clinic questions whether external beam irradiation has any benefit at all in patients with TAO.[11]

The present author prefers to take risks up front and decompress the orbital apex surgically in patients refractory to or intolerant of corticosteroids. This may be safely performed under direct visualization via an external ethmoidectomy and removal of the medial orbital wall back to the orbital apex. Orbital irradiation is reserved for those patients with DON refractory to an adequate orbital apical decompression documented by a postoperative CT scan. Extraocular muscles may enlarge so much that they are refractory to decompression (Fig. 13.47). The medial wall of the orbit must be removed and the periorbita incised to adequately decompress the orbital apex. This may be accomplished via external ethmoidectomy or a transantral–transethmoidal procedure. Removal of the orbital floor or lateral wall does not adequately decompress the orbital apex and does

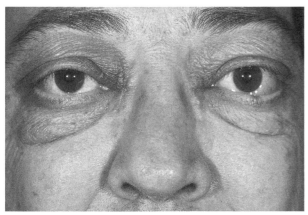

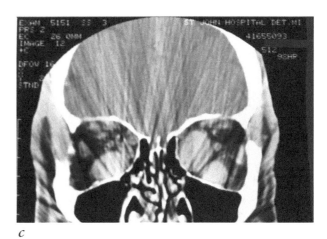

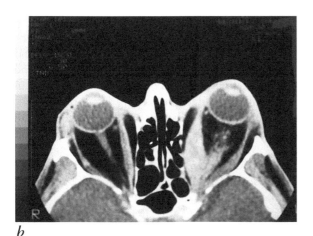

Figure 13.46 *Minimal proptosis and no evidence for eyelid retraction (a) in a patient with optic nerve compression by a markedly enlarged left medial rectus muscle evident on axial and coronal CT scans (b and c).*

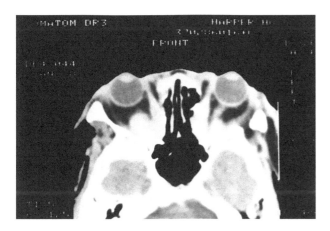

Figure 13.47 *A CT scan demonstrates optic nerve compression by massively enlarged extraocular muscles.*

not allow for incision of the medial periorbita, so they are inadequate procedures for patients with DON.

The back wall of the maxillary sinus usually lies 10 mm anterior to the orbital apex, hence removal of the orbital floor by itself cannot decompress the optic nerve. In-fracture and removal of the medial orbital wall may be accomplished with difficulty, but the medial periorbita cannot be easily or safely incised. Removal of the lateral orbital wall cannot decompress the orbital apex.

A 60-year-old lady with DON underwent orbital decompression for severe visual loss. Decompression was accomplished through a fornix incision. She failed to regain visual function after surgery and sought a second opinion. Visual acuity was 20/40 in the right eye and 20/200 in the left eye. Both pupils reacted sluggishly and there was a RAPD on the left. A CT scan (Fig. 13.48)

Figure 13.48 *A CT scan demonstrates an incomplete apical orbital decompression that failed to resolve the compressive optic neuropathy. Note the intact left medial orbital wall and the partially intact right medial orbital wall.*

demonstrated an intact medial orbital wall on the left and partial removal of the medial orbital wall on the right. She underwent an external ethmoidectomy and orbital apical decompression on the left side. Visual acuity promptly improved to 20/30 and the RAPD reversed. She then underwent an external ethmoidectomy and orbital apical decompression on the right side. Although it was evident that the previous surgeon had removed most of the medial orbital wall, the posterior medial wall was intact and the periorbita had not been incised. Vision improved to 20/20 in both eyes postoperatively and has been stable for 6 years. Patients with residual

visual dysfunction after orbital decompression should have a repeat CT scan to ensure that the decompression was indeed adequate before offering them any other form of therapy.

PRIMARY ORBITAL TUMORS

Primary orbital tumors may be well encapsulated and surgically resectable or diffusely infiltrative and not amenable to a surgical cure. Encapsulated orbital tumors include cavernous hemangiomas, schwannomas, hemangiopericytomas and benign mixed tumors of the lacrimal gland.

Cavernous hemangiomas are the most common primary orbital tumor. They are slow-growing tumors, and patients present with slowly progressive proptosis and visual dysfunction (Fig. 13.49). Imaging studies demonstrate a well-encapsulated mass (Fig. 13.50) that may be differentiated from the adjacent optic nerve by MRI scan (Fig. 13.51). Treatment is complete surgical removal, which is usually quite easy, as these tumors are rarely adherent to adjacent orbital structures.

Schwannomas are also well encapsulated tumors (Fig. 13.52) that may grow to a rather large size and be difficult to extract by the standard lateral orbitotomy. These tumors should be removed completely and should not be biopsied or partially removed as they may bleed profusely.

Hemangiopericytomas (Fig. 13.53) and benign mixed tumors of the lacrimal gland (Fig. 13.54) are also well-encapsulated tumors. If partially removed or if the capsule is violated, they have the potential for malignant

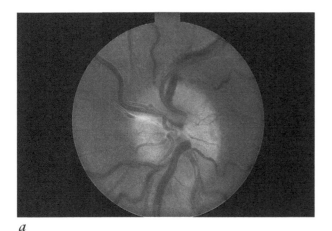

a

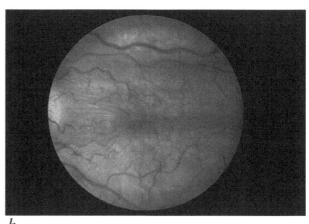

b

Figure 13.49 *Mild optic disc edema and macular pigment changes in a patient with chronic compression due to a cavernous hemangioma.*

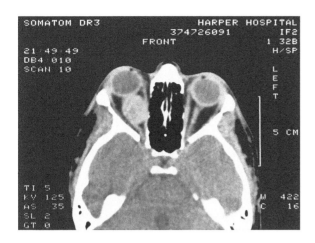

Figure 13.50 *A CT scan demonstrates a large encapsulated orbital mass.*

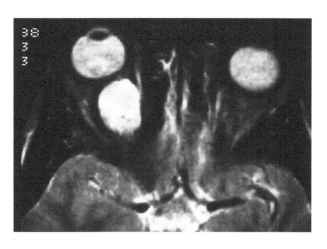

Figure 13.51 *An MRI scan—T2 weighted—easily differentiates the mass from the adjacent optic nerve.*

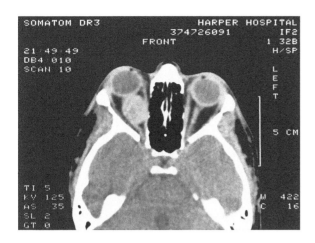

a

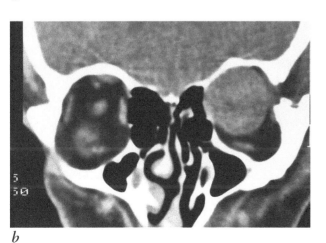

b

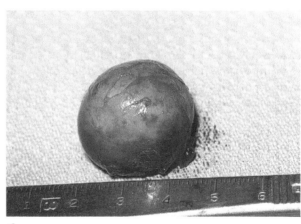

c

Figure 13.52 *Well-encapsulated orbital schwannoma on axial (a) and coronal (b) CT scans. A well-encapsulated orbital mass was removed via craniotomy (c).*

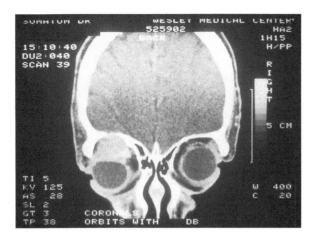

Figure 13.53 *A coronal CT scan demonstrates a well-encapsulated hemangiopericytoma.*

recurrence. If an orbital tumor appears encapsulated, every effort should be made to remove it completely. Occasionally the surgeon will be fooled by a pseudo-encapsulated tumor (Fig. 13.55), but this should not occur often and may often be avoided by careful review of the imaging studies.

Lymphangiomas (Fig. 13.56) and capillary hemangiomas (Fig. 13.57) are infiltrative orbital lesions that are rarely totally resectable. Both have a tendency to involute with age but are often difficult to manage while awaiting divine intervention. Fortunately, many capillary hemangiomas respond to intralesional corticosteroid injections (Fig. 13.57b and c). Patients with lymphangiomas may present with acute, painful proptosis secondary to hem-

orrhage within the tumor (Fig. 13.58). If visual function is threatened, surgical drainage may be indicated, but there is literature supporting observation alone. The present author prefers to drain the hemorrhage and remove as much of the tumor as feasible with a CO_2 laser.

Orbital varices (Fig. 13.59a) may be difficult to distinguish from lymphangiomas histopathologically but they may appear pseudoencapsulated on a CT scan (Fig. 13.59b). The presence of a phlebolith on a CT scan is diagnostic (Fig. 13.59c).

Lymphomas may be confined to the orbit (Fig. 13.60) or involve the orbit as part of widespread systemic disease (Fig. 13.61). Biopsy of the orbital lesion with fresh tissue examination by the alerted pathologist distinguishes between malignant lymphoma and benign lymphoid hyperplasia. Oncology evaluation determines whether there is any systemic involvement and what treatment should be offered. Isolated orbital lymphomas respond well to local irradiation. Systemic disease warrants the appropriate chemotherapy regimen.

LACRIMAL FOSSA TUMORS

A mass in the supero-temporal orbit involves the lacrimal gland until proven otherwise. It may be as benign as an orbital dermoid cyst (Figs 13.62 and 13.63) or a prolapsed lacrimal gland (Fig. 13.64). A normal lacrimal gland falls from the lacrimal fossa and presents as a palpable mass in the lateral upper eyelid. If recognized, it is easily repaired through an eyelid crease incision. If it appears abnormal at surgery then it can be

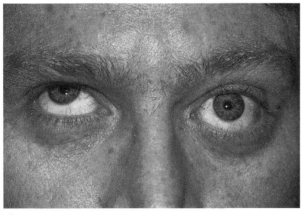

a

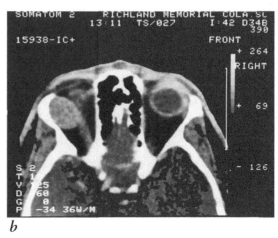

b

Figure 13.54 *Proptosis and limited upgaze (a) in a patient with CT scan evidence of a benign mixed tumor (b). Note that the mass is encapsulated and the orbital wall is fossified but not eroded by the long-standing mass.*

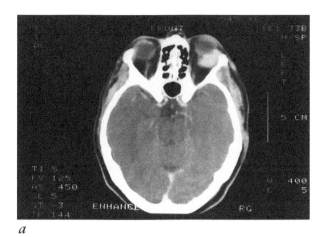

a

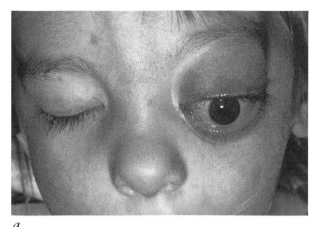

a

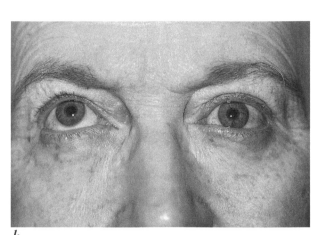

b

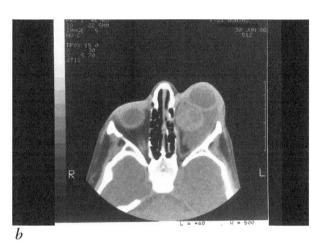

b

Figure 13.56 *Massive proptosis due to an orbital lymphangioma (a). A CT scan demonstrates a diffuse orbital mass with an encapsulated area of recent hemorrhage (chocolate cyst) (b).*

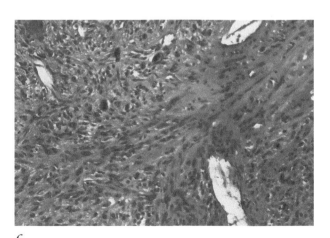

c

Figure 13.55 *A CT scan demonstrates a calcified, pseudo-encapsulated orbital mass (a) in a patient with metastatic leiomyosarcoma (b). Intrinsic calcification in the mass indicated that this was not the typical benign, encapsulated lacrimal fossa mass (compare with Fig. 13.54b). Histopathology of leiomyosarcoma (c).*

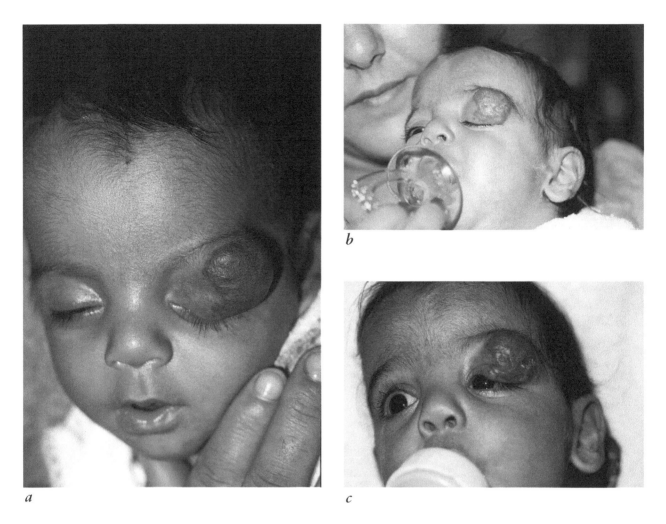

Figure 13.57 *Large capillary hemangioma causing amblyopia (a). Partial involution 3 weeks after treatment with intralesional steroids (b). Further involution 6 weeks after treatment. Note that the visual axis is no longer occluded (c).*

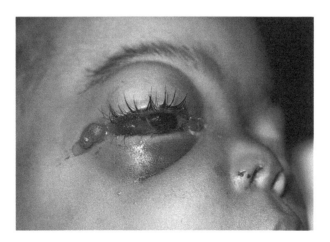

Figure 13.58 *Sudden onset of painful proptosis due to hemorrhage into a lymphangioma.*

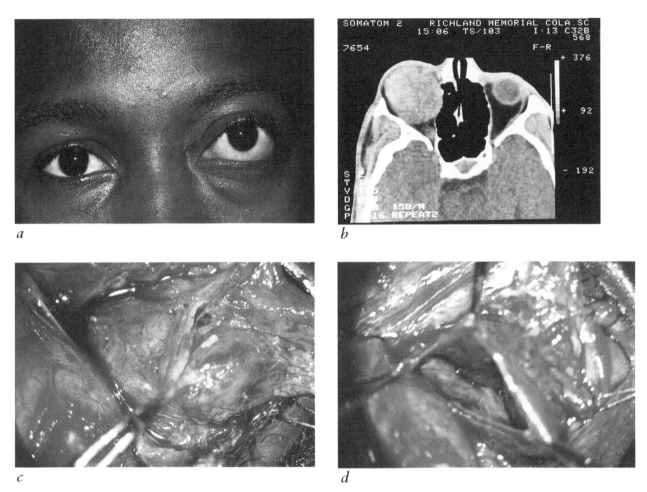

Figure 13.59 *A patient with slowly progressive visual loss secondary to a longstanding orbital varix (a). A CT scan demonstrates a large pseudo-encapsulated mass and phlebolith (b). Appearance of the mass after surgical exposure (c). Cystic nature is evident after incision and occlusion of feeder vessels (d).*

biopsied, as sarcoidosis, lymphoma or idiopathic orbital inflammation may also enlarge the prolapsed gland. Patients with dacryoadenitis (inflammation of the lacrimal gland) have pain and evidence for acute orbital inflammation (Fig. 13.65a). The lacrimal gland is diffusely enlarged on a CT scan and adjacent orbital structures may enhance due to the contiguous inflammation (Fig. 13.65b). Oral steroids are curative (Fig. 13.65c). Patients with lymphomas of the lacrimal gland may mimic dacryoadenitis but there is rarely an acute inflammatory reaction, and the response to steroid therapy is incomplete (Fig. 13.66). Lacrimal gland biopsy is often diagnostic. If lymphoma is even remotely suspected, furnish the pathologist with a fresh tissue specimen so appropriate immunocytology studies can be done to determine the type of lymphoma.

An encapsulated lacrimal fossa mass is most likely a benign mixed tumor of the lacrimal gland. Patients have a history of painless, slowly progressive proptosis. A CT scan demonstrates a well-encapsulated mass and fossification of the lacrimal fossa (Fig. 13.67): there is no erosion of the adjacent bone. Isolated involvement of the palpebral lobe of the lacrimal gland may also occur (Fig. 13.68). Treatment is complete surgical removal without violation of the capsule. Partial removal, biopsy or violation of the capsule may result in malignant transformation years later (Fig. 13.69).

Adenocarcinoma (Fig. 13.70a–c) or adenocystic carcinoma of the lacrimal gland (Fig. 13.71a–c) is a devastating malignancy. Patients present with rapid, painful proptosis. A CT scan demonstrates a diffuse, infiltrating lacrimal fossa mass eroding the adjacent bone

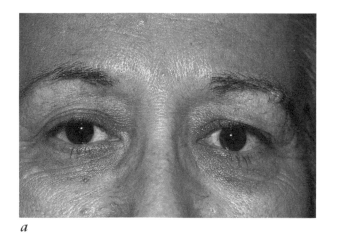

a

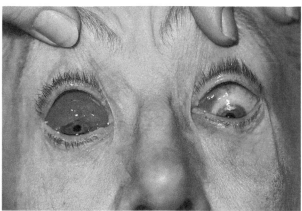

a

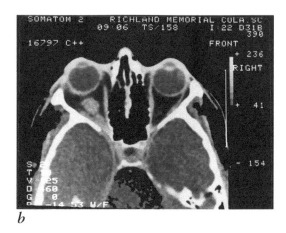

b

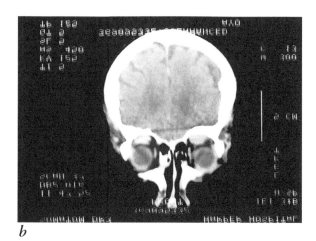

b

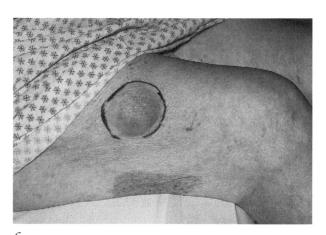

c

c

Figure 13.60 *A patient with mild proptosis due to an isolated orbital lymphoma (a). A CT scan demonstrates a diffuse mass in the inferior orbit (b and c).*

Figure 13.61 *A patient with bilateral orbital involvement (a), a CT scan (b) shows manifestation of disseminated systemic lymphoma with multiple cutaneous lesion (c).*

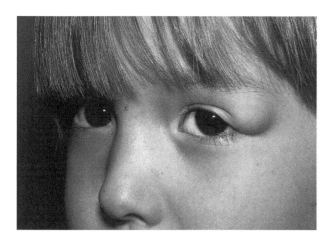

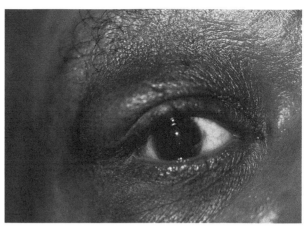

Figure 13.62 *Classic dermoid cyst presenting as a well-encapsulated, superficial orbital mass in a child.*

Figure 13.64 *Prolapsed lacrimal gland.*

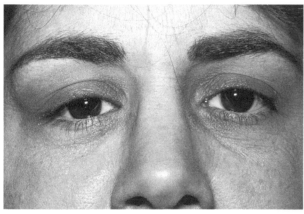

a

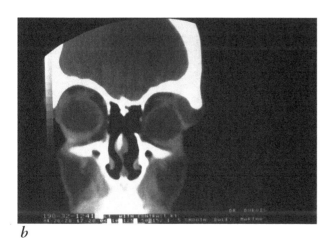

b

Figure 13.63 *An adult with a dermoid cyst presenting in the deeper orbit (a). A CT scan demonstrates a cystic anterior orbital mass (b).*

(Fig. 13.71b), and calcification may also be evident (Fig. 13.70b). There is no good treatment for these carcinomas. Treatments range from high-dose orbital irradiation (Fig. 13.72) and chemotherapy to radical orbitectomy (orbital exenteration with adjacent craniectomy) (Fig. 13.73) and all have their advocates and success stories. This is an often fatal and disfiguring disease (Figs 13.72 and 13.73).

METASTATIC ORBITAL TUMORS

A patient presenting with orbital dysfunction and a history of a primary malignancy has metastatic disease to the orbit until proven otherwise. Metastatic breast carcinoma is most common. It may present as proptosis (Fig. 13.74) or motility dysfunction (Fig. 13.75). Scirrhous breast or gastric carcinoma may present as enophthalmos (Fig. 13.76).

Prostate cancer is rapidly replacing lung cancer as the most common metastatic carcinoma to the orbit in males. Patients with metastatic prostate carcinoma may present with an acutely inflamed orbit (Fig. 13.77) or osteoblastic metastasis mimicking a sphenoid-ridge meningioma (Figs 13.24 and 13.78). Orbital soft tissue or the adjacent bone may be involved. These patients often present with an acutely inflamed orbit (Figs 13.77 and 13.78) and metastatic prostate carcinoma should be included in the differential diagnosis of the acute orbit. Patients with metastasis to the cavernous sinus or more posterior orbit, however, may present with an

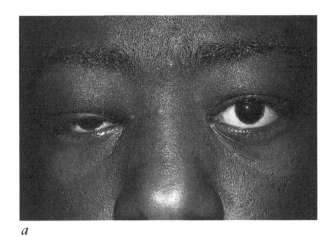
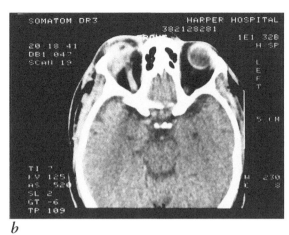

a

b

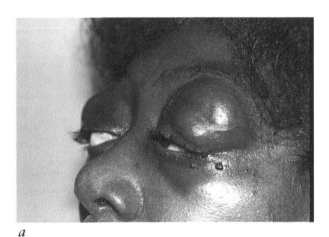

c

Figure 13.65 *A patient with acute dacryoadenitis (a). A CT scan demonstrates diffuse enlargement of the lacrimal gland (b). Total resolution after corticosteroid therapy (c).*

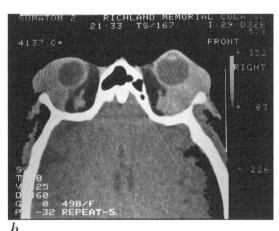

a

b

Figure 13.66 *A patient with lymphoma of the lacrimal gland (a). A CT scan demonstrates enlargement of the lacrimal glands well confined by the septated structures of the orbit (b).*

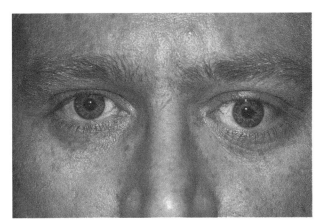

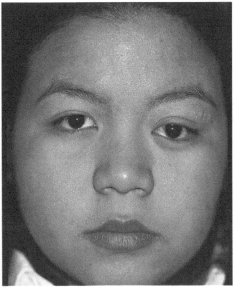

a

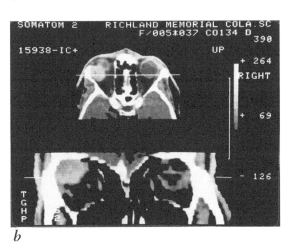

b

Figure 13.67 *Proptosis and downward displacement of the globe in a patient with a benign mixed tumor of the lacrimal gland (a). A CT scan demonstrates a well-encapsulated tumor in the lacrimal fossa (b).*

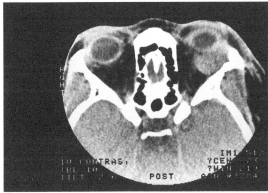

b

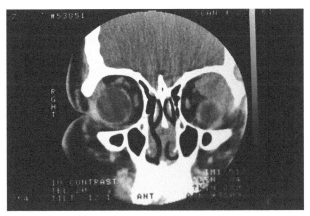

c

Figure 13.69 *A patient who had a partial excision of a benign mixed tumor years before (a). CT scans demonstrate a less than perfectly encapsulated mass with a hint of bony erosion (b and c) (compare with Figs 13.54b and 13.67b). Excisional biopsy revealed a benign mixed tumor with malignant transformation.*

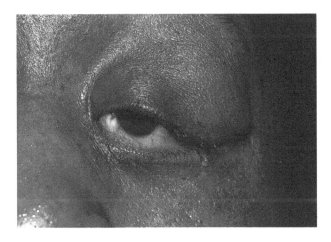

Figure 13.68 *Benign mixed tumor of the palpebral lobe of the lacrimal gland.*

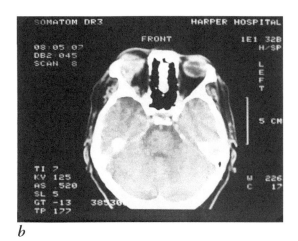

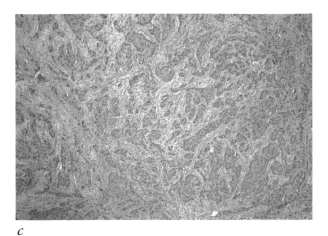

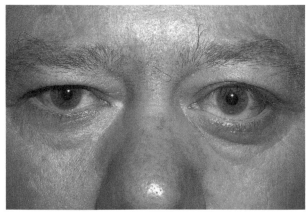

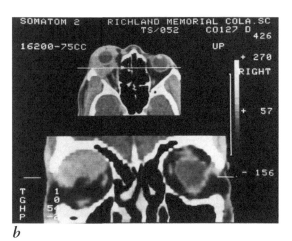

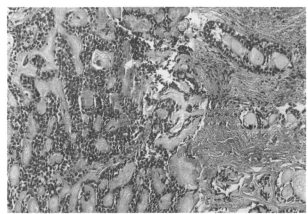

Figure 13.70   *A patient presenting with neurotropic keratitis and an upgaze palsy (a). A CT scan demonstrates a pseudo-encapsulated mass with areas of calcification (b). Histopathology demonstrated adenocarcinoma of the lacrimal gland (c).*

Figure 13.71   *A patient presenting with rapid-onset, painful proptosis due to adenocystic carcinoma of the lacrimal gland (a). A CT scan demonstrates a diffuse mass eroding the lateral orbital wall (b) (compare with Figs 13.54b and 13.66b). Histopathology demonstrates adenocystic carcinoma of the lacrimal gland (c).*

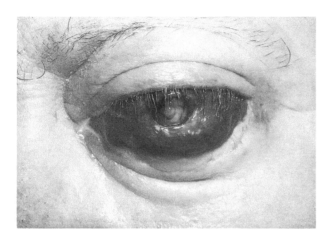

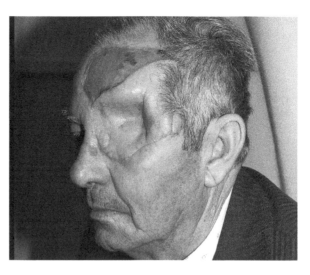

Figure 13.72 *The patient shown in Fig. 13.71a after biopsy and local irradiation therapy.*

Figure 13.73 *A patient after radical orbitectomy for adeno-cystic carcinoma of the lacrimal gland.*

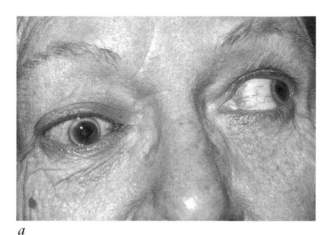

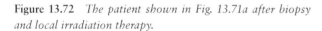

a

b

Figure 13.74 *A patient presenting with proptosis and diplopia 10 years after the diagnosis of breast carcinoma (a). A CT scan demonstrates diffuse orbital involvement (b).*

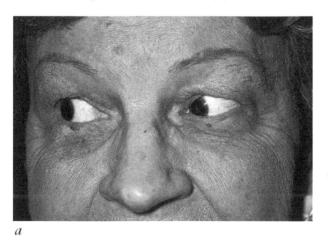

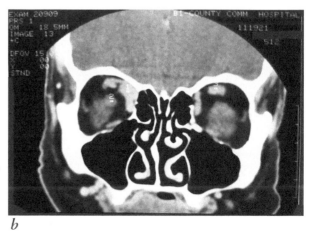

a

b

Figure 13.75 *A patient presenting with diplopia and a pseudo-Brown's syndrome (a) due to metastatic breast carcinoma to the superior oblique muscle (b).*

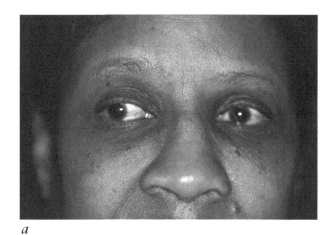

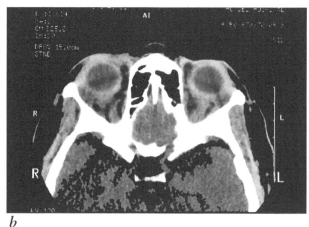

a   *b*

Figure 13.76 *Enophthalmos (a) due to bilateral orbital metastasis of scirrhous breast carcinoma (b).*

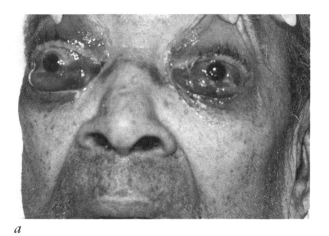

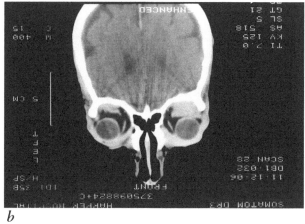

a   *b*

Figure 13.77 *Metastatic prostate carcinoma presenting as an acutely inflamed orbit (a). A CT scan demonstrates bilateral superior orbital masses (b).*

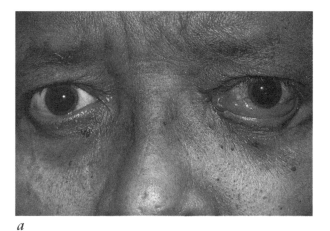

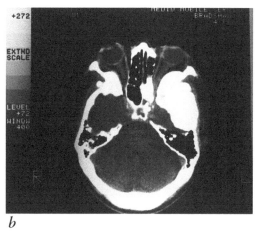

a   *b*

Figure 13.78 *A patient presenting with an inflamed orbit (a) due to massive osteoblastic prostatic carcinoma metastasis (b).*

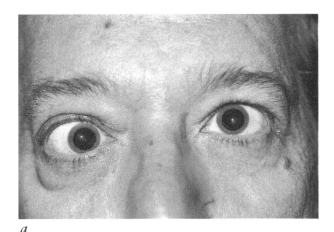
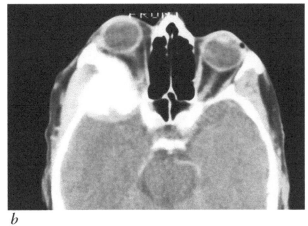

a   b

Figure 13.79   *Sixth-nerve palsy and proptosis (a) due to intracranial and intraorbital prostatic metastasis (b).*

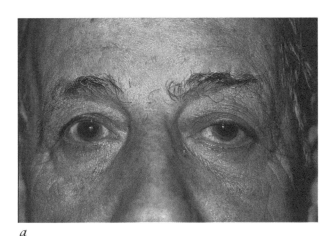
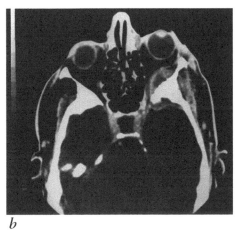

a   b

Figure 13.80   *Subtle proptosis (a) due to posterior orbital and intracranial metastasis of prostatic carcinoma (b).*

isolated cranial nerve paresis (Fig. 13.79) with or without proptosis (Fig. 13.80).

Less common but often perplexing metastasis to the orbit occurs from cutaneous melanoma (Figs 13.37 and 13.81), often years after the primary tumor was excised. Renal cell carcinoma may metastasize to the orbit. These lesions may bleed profusely when biopsied. Patients may present with an obvious orbital lesion and no history of a primary malignancy. The orbital pathology then leads to discovery of the primary tumor. Orbital destruction with bony metastasis and erosion may also result from systemic plasmacytoma (Fig. 13.83a). This tumor may initially have a favorable response to systemic steroid therapy but the appearance of the CT scans leaves little question as to the gravity of the diagnosis (Fig. 13.82b and c).

ORBITAL DISORDERS IN CHILDREN

RHABDOMYOSARCOMA

A rapidly expanding orbital mass in a child is a rhabdomyosarcoma until proven otherwise (Fig. 13.83). This tumor may be confined to the orbit or involve the adjacent sinuses and brain. Clinical findings may be obvious, with extensive brain and sinus involvement, or subtle. The present author has seen orbital rhabdomyosarcoma initially present as isolated ptosis with normal imaging until repeated and reviewed in detail with attention to the levator superior rectus complex (Fig. 13.84).

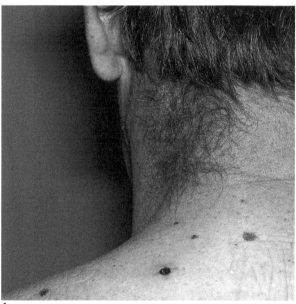

a

b

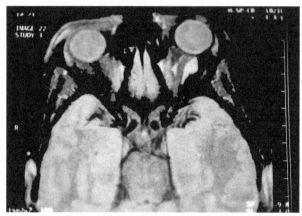

c

Figure 13.81 *Metastatic melanoma. A patient presented with painful diplopia (a), examination revealed melanotic cutaneous lesions (b). MRI demonstrates an enhancing mass inferior to the optic nerve (c).*

ORBITAL CELLULITIS

Orbital infections in children, as in adults, may mimic isolated eyelid infections (a hot chalazion) and acute dacryocystitis, neither of which are orbital infections and should be differentiated from pre- and postseptal orbital cellulitis. This differentiation may be especially difficult in young children who are squirming and screaming to avoid examination. If in doubt, treat as an orbital infection, obtain a CT scan and treat with appropriate intravenous antibiotics. Specific regimens will not be offered, for they will be obsolete by the time this chapter is published, but remember to cover Hemophilus in young children.[9,10]

IOI

Children with IOI may appear systemically ill with fever and an elevated white blood cell (WBC) count. They may be lethargic complaining of abdominal pain and vomiting. It may be very difficult to distinguish between orbital cellulitis and IOI. The child in Fig. 13.85 was referred for pain in the right orbit; she was afebrile and had a normal WBC count. Clinical diagnosis was IOI, but a CT scan demonstrated obvious sinusitis with minimal orbital involvement. Treatment with antibiotics was appropriate. The child in Fig. 13.86 also had painful proptosis, but was febrile with an elevated WBC count. Her diagnosis was orbital cellulitis until her CT scan demonstrated obvious enlargement and inflammation of the lateral rectus muscle. The diagnosis was promptly changed to the orbital myositis subgroup of IOI and treatment with corticosteroids was appropriate. Differentiating orbital infection from idiopathic inflammation may be quite difficult in children and is greatly facilitated by CT scanning. A CT scan is essential in the diagnosis of an inflamed orbit in adults as well as children, and rendering an opinion without the help of a scan is fraught with danger for both you and your patient.[11]

Evaluation and treatment of patients with orbital disorders is one of the most challenging areas of ophthalmology. The relative rarity of these cases and the relative plethora of 'specialists' in orbital disorders makes it difficult for any single practitioner to be comfortable diagnosing and treating these patients. General guidelines that the present author has taught his residents and fellows over the past 25 years will be briefly reviewed.

If you are at all suspicious of orbital dysfunction, image the orbit with CT or MRI. CT is still the best screen for orbital disorders as it not only visualizes the

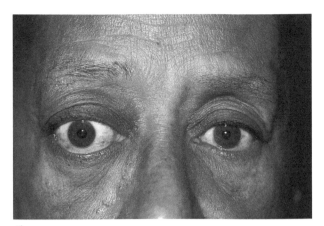

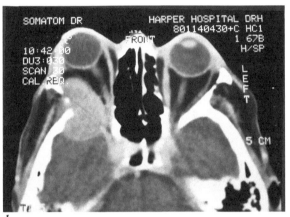

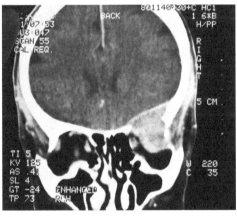

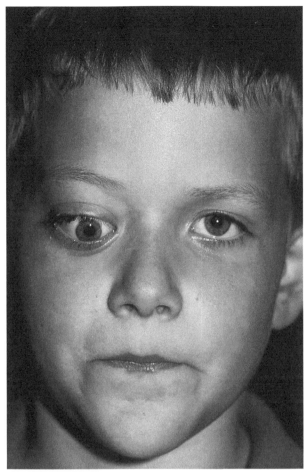

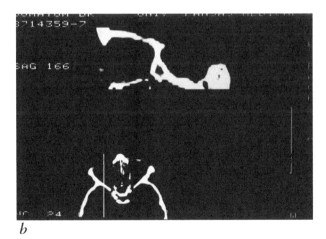

Figure 13.82 *Proptosis and visual dysfunction (a) due to plasmacytoma metastatic to the orbit. CT scans demonstrate intracranial and intraorbital metastasis with erosion of the sphenoid ridge, lateral orbital wall and orbital roof (b and c).*

Figure 13.83 *Rapidly progressive proptosis (a) after incidental trauma as the presenting manifestation of orbital rhabdomyosarcoma (b).*

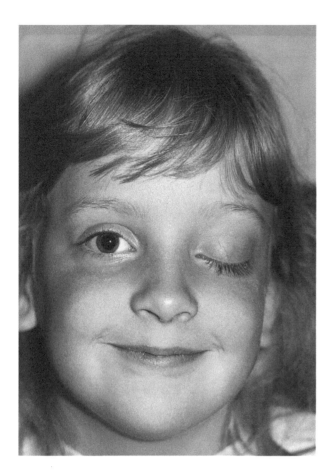

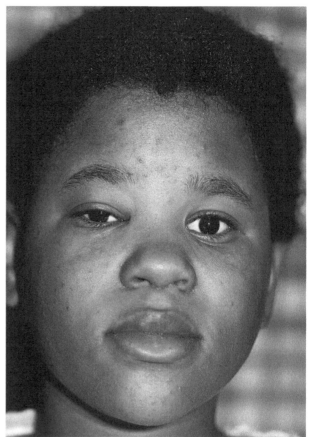

a

Figure 13.84 *Isolated ptosis with total loss of levator function as the initial manifestation of orbital rhabdomyosarcoma.*

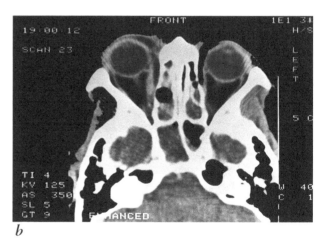

b

Figure 13.85 *Afebrile patient with normal WBC count (a). A CT scan demonstrates orbital cellulitis with adjacent ethmoiditis (b).*

orbital soft tissue but also the adjacent sinuses and bone. The present author reserves orbital MRI for differentiating orbital masses from the optic nerve. Prior to operating on an orbital lesion, review your imaging and decide whether the lesion is totally resectable or should only be biopsied and treated with chemotherapy or radiation therapy. An encapsulated lesion is surgical disease and should be removed in its entirety, choosing a surgical approach that keeps the lesion between the surgeon's instruments and the optic nerve. A diffuse lesion is either inflammatory, metastatic or lymphoma, and as such is not surgically curable. These should be biopsied to obtain the appropriate diagnosis then referred to the appropriate specialist for treatment. It sounds trite, but remember medical treatment for medical disease and reserve surgical treatment for surgical disease.

Finally, do not forget to take a history. Even a remote history of a primary malignancy may be very helpful in establishing the diagnosis of metastatic disease to the orbit.

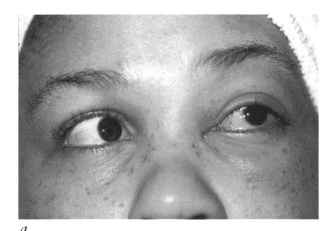
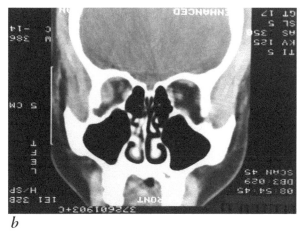

a   *b*

Figure 13.86 *Febrile patient with elevated WBC count due to orbital myositis (a). A CT scan demonstrates normal sinuses and an enlarged lateral rectus muscle (b).*

REFERENCES

1. Hornblass A, Herschorn ML, Stern K et al. Orbital abscess. *Surv Ophthalmol* 984; **29**:169–78.
2. Leone CR, Lloyd WC. Treatment protocol for orbital inflammatory disease. *Ophthalmology* 1985; **92**:1325–31.
3. Lanciano R, Fowble B, Sergott RC et al. Treatment of orbital pseudotumor by radiation therapy. *Int J Radiat Oncol Biol Phys* 1990; **18**:407–11.
4. Peele-Cockerham K, Pal C, Kennerdell JS. The prevalence and implications of ocular hypertension in thyroid associated orbitopathy. *Ophthalmology* 1997; **104**:914–17.
5. Kazim M, Kennerdell JS. Elevated intraocular pressure and dysthyroid orbitopathy. *Orbit* 1991; **10**:211–15.
6. Bartley GB, Fatourechi V, Kadrmas EF et al. The treatment of Graves' ophthalmopathy in an incidence cohort. *Am J Ophthalmol* 1996; **121**:200–6.
7. Perros P, Crombie AL, Kendall Taylor P. Natural history of thyroid associated ophthalmopathy. *Clin Endocri (Oxf)* 1995; **42**:45–50.
8. Kazim M, Trokel S, Moore S. Treatment of acute Graves' orbitopathy. *Ophthalmology* 1991; **98**:1443–8.
9. Garrity JA, Fatourechi V, Bergstralh EJ et al. Results of transantral orbital decompression in 428 patients with severe Graves' ophthalmopathy. *Am J Ophthalmol* 1993; **116**:533–47.
10. Soares-Welch CV, Fatourechi V, Bartley GB et al. Optic neuropathy of Graves' disease: results of transantral orbital decompression long term follow-up in 215 patients. *Am J Ophthalmol* 2003; **136**:433–41.
11. Gorum C, Garrity JA, Fatourechi V et al. A prospective, randomized, double blind placebo controlled study of orbital radiotherapy for Graves' orbitopathy. *Ophthalmology* 2001; **108**:525–34.
12. Chang CH, Lai YH, Wang HZ et al. Antibiotic treatment of orbital cellulitis: an analysis of pathogenic bacteria and susceptibility. *J Ocul Pharmacol Ther* 2000; **16**:75–9.
13. Starkey CR, Steele RW. Medical management of orbital cellulitis. *Pediatr Infect Dis J* 2001; **10**:1002–5.
14. Uehara F, Ohba N. Diagnostic imaging in patients with orbital cellulitis and inflammatory pseudotumor. *Int Ophthalmol Clin* 2002; **42**:133–42.

Index

T - #0038 - 311024 - C0 - 276/219/18 - PB - 9780367394349 - Gloss Lamination